Logotherapy and Existential Analysis: Proceedings of the Viktor Frankl Institute Vienna

Volume 2

Series Editor
Alexander Batthyány, Vienna, Austria

The Viktor Frankl Institute, established in Vienna in 1992 by an international group of colleagues and friends, is a scientific society dedicated to preserving and promoting the life's work of Viktor Frankl. Its mission includes providing authentic information about logotherapy and existential analysis. The Institute holds exclusive access to Viktor Frankl's private archives, which represent the world's largest collection of texts and research on logotherapy and existential analysis.

As a recognized member of the UNESCO Archives Portal in Paris, the Institute is committed to cataloging Viktor Frankl's private archives from the period of 1925 to 1997. This comprehensive task involves the digitization of historical audio and video recordings. In addition, the Institute meticulously compiles a comprehensive bibliography that includes dissertations, theses, journal articles, and media reports. An integral part of its work also involves chronicling the international development and impact of logotherapy and existential analysis.

http://www.viktorfrankl.org

Charles L. McLafferty, Jr. • Jay I. Levinson
Editors

Logotherapy and Existential Analysis

Springer

Editors
Charles L. McLafferty, Jr.
President, Purpose Research
Charlottesville, VA, USA

Faculty Member, Viktor Frankl Institute of Logotherapy
Stamford, TX, USA

Jay I. Levinson
Private Practice
Baltimore, MD, USA

ISSN 2366-7559 ISSN 2366-7567 (electronic)
Logotherapy and Existential Analysis: Proceedings of the Viktor Frankl Institute Vienna
ISBN 978-3-031-48921-1 ISBN 978-3-031-48922-8 (eBook)
https://doi.org/10.1007/978-3-031-48922-8

This Springer imprint is published by the registered company Springer Nature Switzerland AG
The registered company address is: Gewerbestrasse 11, 6330 Cham, Switzerland

Paper in this product is recyclable.

Preface

Each of us has a "beginning point" in the pursuit of meaning. For many, it was reading Viktor Frankl's book *Man's Search for Meaning*. For others, it was an encounter with a person who pointed us to meaning. It is conceivable that it could be found in reading this volume in which the reader can encounter Viktor Frankl (and his beginning point) as well as the experiences of others who knew him. The types of research presented in other chapters range from empirical and scientific to case studies and ethnographic reports. The authors not only seek to confirm the theoretical assumptions, but to expand them and connect them with other theories. The principles of logotherapy are applied to education, workplace and educational environments, the tragic triad of fear, suffering, and death—even to international relations. In still other chapters, the depth of Frankl's philosophical foundation is expanded.

Across this volume, several themes emerge. The first is *the legacy of Viktor Frankl*. Though this entire book is (by definition) Frankl's legacy, it opens with three chapters that provide perspectives of the development of (a) logotherapy itself, (b) a close working friendship with Frankl, and (c) the digital archives of Frankl's work.

The second theme is the application of *logotherapy in the prevention and amelioration of suffering*. Every person on this planet must face their own mortality and the ever-present potential for suffering. But the vast range of ways in which individuals suffer is echoed by the topics presented by the authors: the first-person perspective of the loss of an intimate partner; the death of a "battle buddy" in combat, accompanied with the life-altering experience of posttraumatic stress disorder; the loss of innocence in cases of childhood abuse; the pain of mental illness and involuntary confinement; the experience of life-threatening illness; the experience of moral injury in trying to treat that illness; the suffering of members of a third-world nation; even the suffering of entire nations that yearn for meaningful conflict resolution. Such is the range of suffering—and the applicability of the principles of logotherapy.

The third theme (which of necessity overlaps with the second) is *research on logotherapy*, which was important to Frankl (e.g., see Batthyány & Guttmann, 2005; Thir & Batthyány, 2016). There are two discrete branches of research in logotherapy: qualitative (ethnographic, phenomenological, case study) and empirical (statistical) research.

Qualitative research is of necessity in understanding logotherapy; 60 years ago, Frankl used case studies extensively in his lectures and books. These case studies are critical to the understanding of logotherapy because of its adaptable, flexible nature. Frankl (1969/2014) insisted that, because each person is unique, there could be no "one size fits all" approach to applying logotherapy:

> Not each and every method is applicable to each and every patient with the same success, nor is each and every therapist capable of handling each and every method with equal success. As to adjusting the method to the patient, the great psychiatrist Beard once said: "If you have treated 2 cases of neurasthenia in the same way, you have mistreated at least one of them. (p. 163)

Thus, case studies are helpful (imperative, even) in helping to convey the variety of unique ways in which logotherapy can be applied… not to demonstrate a method per se as much as demonstrating to the practitioner how creativity, adaptation, discernment, and intuition can be used to apply the principles of logotherapy.

This volume contains several chapters of qualitative research using a variety of modalities that incorporate logotherapy, from writing therapy to autoethnography to case studies; addressing a range of conditions, from suicidality to terminal illness and, as mentioned, from childhood abuse to posttraumatic stress disorder. These qualitative studies give context and perspective for the application of logotherapy—uniquely—to each unique encounter.

The scientific study of logotherapy was also important to Frankl, as was demonstrated by the extensive listing of research in the appendices of several of his books. This volume extends the empirical base of logotherapy in examining: altruism and service motivations in college students, translated adaptations of the Purpose in Life test on two continents, as well as qualities of meaning in highly intelligent and gifted individuals.

The third theme that emerged is *practical applications of logotherapy*. To be sure, many of the research topics above are the direct result of the process of applying logotherapy, and this theme overlaps considerably with research as well as the alleviation of suffering. The two main areas in which this theme is uniquely suited is in working with children/young adults and in the workplace.

In working with children and young adults, the use of superheroes is discussed as a gateway to helping the individual to understand the true self. The principles of logotherapy are also applied to helping at-risk students find meaning in the educational process.

The modern workplace is rapidly changing, and workers are increasingly seeking meaningful employment opportunities. Four chapters focus on the workplace, with topics including New Work and meaning orientation, job crafting as a way to increase meaningful work opportunities, development of resilience and meaning-oriented skills in unemployed youth, and the application of a Socratic dialogue exercise among employees at a technology company who are seeking advancement.

The fourth is *connecting and expanding the philosophy and theory of logotherapy*. Four chapters have an expressly philosophical/theoretical orientation toward logotherapy. One connects the fundamental principles of Theravāda Buddhism with those of logotherapy. Next, Sir Francis Galton's theory of nature versus nurture is dissected using Frankl's dimensional ontology. In another chapter, a brief exercise, "The scales of human existence," is presented as a thought experiment, noting the existence of a fourth dimension that is inherent—and noted by Frankl—in the dimensional ontology of logotherapy. The final chapter discusses a Humean approach to the relationship between values and actions.

This volume is rounded out with reviews of two books: The first book connects Frankl's ideas with the Biblical book of Job; the second is an expanded overview of the theory and application of logotherapy, incorporating the works of Frankl, Elisabeth Lukas, and Joseph Fabry, among others.

What stands out to us in reviewing the breadth and depth of these chapters is their variety and scope. Indeed, the reader of this volume is asked to consider a world of ideas—literally—originating from countries across the globe: for example, Brazil, Russia, South Africa, Slovenia, Canada, Israel, Turkey, and Nigeria. In fact, about three-quarters of the manuscripts were written by non-native English speakers, which allows the reader to truly consider Frankl's repeated calls for "unity in spite of diversity."

With such a broad survey of ideas and perspectives, readers are charged with the responsibility for deciding which of these resonate with their own values. Perhaps it is appropriate that Frankl (1979) should have the last word; in the Foreword to *Logotherapy in Action* (Fabry, Bulka, & Sahakian), he wrote:

> I also feel a strong sense of humility as I survey the book while writing my preface. I see an expansion of my own ideas as I formulated them when creating logotherapy. Not every idea in the many chapters finds my full approval but the more the views of unorthodox logotherapists deviate from my own the more justified is its inclusion in this book. Logotherapy is no fixed set of dogmas. It is not a closed system. As I have stated on many occasions, it is open in two directions: open to the cooperation with other scientifically established psychotherapies, and open to its own evolution, to the full development of its own potential.
>
> Ours is an age of pluralism, and we see pluralism also in the field of psychotherapy. Under the circumstances, the co-existence of a variety of schools is appropriate and a sound eclecticism is therefore mandatory. Why, then, shouldn't an "inner" eclecticism be justified—a variety of divergent views within logotherapy?
>
> That is the reason why I grant any logotherapist the right to dissent from what I as the creator of logotherapy believe to be true. On the contrary, I have invited, encouraged, and welcomed criticism of my own teachings because I see in criticism, provided it is earnest and honest, the greatest chance still to learn.

Charlottesville, VA, USA Charles L. McLafferty, Jr.
Baltimore, MD, USA Jay I. Levinson

References

Batthyány, A., & Guttmann, D. (2005). *Empirical research in logotherapy and meaning-oriented psychotherapy: An annotated bibliography*. Zeig, Tucker & Theisen, Inc.

Fabry, J. B., Bulka, R. P., & Sahakian, W. S. (Eds.). (1979). *Logotherapy in action*. J. Aronson.

Frankl, V. E. (1969/2014). *The will to meaning: Foundations and applications of logotherapy* (Expanded ed.). Plume. (Original work published 1969)

Frankl, V. E. (1979). Foreword. In J. Fabry, R. P. Bulka, & W. S. Sahakian (Eds.), *Logotherapy in action*. J. Aronson.

Thir, M., & Batthyány, A. (2016). The state of empirical research on logotherapy and existential analysis. In A. Batthyány (Ed.), *Logotherapy and existential analysis: Proceedings of the Viktor Frankl Institute Vienna* (pp. 53–74). Springer International Publishing.

Acknowledgements

The work of planning and editing this volume over the past few years has required a considerable amount of time and detailed effort, particularly in working with the range of modalities, types of research, and topics involved. Three-quarters of the chapters were written by authors whose first language was not English, which required careful editing to maximize clarity while ensuring that meaning was not lost. I am personally grateful to the coeditor, Jay I. Levinson, for his experience, steady support, and guidance during our regular phone meetings, as well as for his work copyediting manuscripts.

Jay I. Levinson and I are deeply appreciative of the authors for their energy, ideas, and talent in contributing to the extant research on logotherapy and existential analysis—and for their patience as delays emerged in the production process.

We would like to single out the Series Editor, Alexander Batthyány, for placing his trust in us and for his encouragement and fortitude in this prolonged endeavor. We hope that the work contained herein is worthy of his confidence.

Warm thanks go to Olatunde and Tundebola Asagba, the daughter and son of the late Rachel Asagba, for allowing us to present her unpublished manuscript, "Finding meaning in life in a changing world," in this volume. We are also grateful to Maureen Kondrick of Marquette University Press for allowing us to reprint an adaptation of Alexander Batthyány's "Introduction" to *The Feeling of Meaninglessness* as "'For the person is always at work': Viktor Frankl's path to logotherapy and existential analysis," and to the editor of *The International Forum for Logotherapy* for allowing us to include Indiger's chapter on job crafting as well as McLafferty's plenary address and nature-nurture chapters.

A special thanks goes to Sharon Panulla at Springer for her support and encouragement over the past 2 years and to her staff for their persistence and kindness.

Finally, we would like to thank our partners and children, Lori and Gabi (Jay) and Debra and Clair (Charles), for their unflagging support, patience, and sustaining energy as this volume has emerged.

Charles L. McLafferty, Jr.

Contents

Contributors

Bernd Ahrendt FOM University of Applied Sciences, Hanover, Germany

Benjamin D. Aiken Counselling Psychology Program, Adler University Vancouver, Vancouver, BC, Canada

Matti Ameli Private Practice, Valencia, Spain

Andrés Eduardo Aguirre Antúnez Department of Clinical Psychology, Institute of Psychology – University of São Paulo, Lab of Mental Health Multi-Methods – LabSamm, University of São Paulo, São Paulo, Brazil

Pablo Lincoln Sherlock de Aquino Federal University of Paraíba, João Pessoa, Paraíba, Brazil

Thiago A. Avellar de Aquino Federal University of Paraíba, João Pessoa, Paraíba, Brazil

Rachel Bolaji Asagba , Ibadan, Oyo State, Nigeria

Alexander Batthyány Viktor Frankl Research Institute for Theoretical Psychology and Personalist Studies, Viktor Frankl Institute Vienna, Pázmany Péter University, Budapest, Hungary

Clara Benacerraf International College Spain, Madrid, Spain

Jared Bishop Viktor Frankl Institute of Logotherapy, Stamford, TX, USA

Jane Pauley Community Health Center, Indianapolis, IN, USA

Robert S. Brown, Sr. United States Army Reserve (Retired), Charlottesville, VA, USA

Former Clinical Professor, University of Virginia, Charlottesville, VA, USA

Daniele Bruzzone Università Cattolica del Sacro Cuore, Milan, Italy

Italian Association for Logotherapy and Existential Analysis (ALÆF; www.alaef.com), Viktor Frankl Institut, Vienna, Austria

Cynthia M. Evans Liberty University, Lynchburg, VA, USA

William F. Evans James Madison University, Harrisonburg, VA, USA

Valdiney V. Gouveia Federal University of Paraíba, João Pessoa, Paraíba, Brazil

Robert R. Hutzell Retired, Knoxville, IA, USA

Sabine Indinger Ferdinand Porsche Fernfachhochschule/University of Applied Sciences, Wiener Neustadt, Austria

Don Laird Carlow University, Pittsburgh, PA, USA

Dmitry A. Leontiev HSE University, Moscow, Russia

Jay I. Levinson Private Practice, Baltimore, MD, USA

Willem Maas Netherlands Institute for Logotherapy, Wijk bij Duurstede, Netherlands

Edward Marshall Ottawa Institute of Logotherapy, Ottawa, ON, Canada

Maria Marshall Ottawa Institute of Logotherapy, Ottawa, ON, Canada

Charles L. McLafferty, Jr. Purpose Research, Charlottesville, VA, USA

Viktor Frankl Institute of Logotherapy (USA), Stamford, TX, USA

Evgeny N. Osin HSE University, Moscow, Russia

Laboratory LINP2, University of Paris Nanterre, Paris, France

Memduh Nezih Ozmert Viktor Frankl Enstitüsü Türkiye, Ataşehir, Istanbul, Turkey

Aureliano Pacciolla Consorzio Universitario Humanitas, Roma, Italy

Pninit Russo-Netzer Department of Advanced Studies, Achva Academic College, Department of Counseling and Human Development, University of Haifa, Haifa, Israel

Élison Silva Santos Sapiens Institute of Applied Sciences–IPSapiens, Chrysalis Center for Mental Health and Wellness, Washington, DC, USA

Lab of Mental Health Multi-Methods–LabSamm, University of São Paulo, São Paulo, Brazil

Tatjana Schnell Institute of Psychology, University of Innsbruck, Innsbruck, Austria

MF Specialized University, Oslo, Norway

Andreas Schreiber Private Practice, Freiburg, Germany

Teria Shantall Viktor Frankl Institute of Logotherapy of South Africa, Johannesburg, South Africa

David Srakar Private Practice, Ljubljana, Slovenia

Patricia L. Starck The University of Texas Health Science Center at Houston, Houston, TX, USA

Lindsey Umstead James Madison University, Harrisonburg, VA, USA

Alexander Vesely Viktor Frankl Media Archive of the Viktor Frankl Institute Vienna, Vienna, Austria

Bernadette Vötter Institute of Psychology, University of Innsbruck, Innsbruck, Austria

Daniel von Wachter Ludwig-Maximilians-Universität München, Munich, Germany

Cynthia Wimberly Viktor Frankl Institute of Logotherapy, Stamford, TX, USA

Paul T. P. Wong Trent University, Toronto, ON, Canada

Part I
Viktor Frankl's Legacy

"For the Person Is Always at Work": Viktor Frankl's Path to Logotherapy and Existential Analysis

Alexander Batthyány

1923–1927: From Individual Psychology to Logotherapy

In 1926, Viktor Frankl (1926a) employed the term *logotherapy* for the first time in a lecture addressed to the Academic Society for Medical Psychology. In the following 10 years, influenced by his work in the youth counseling centers he helped found and by his specialist training in psychiatry and neurology at the Viennese mental hospitals of Rosenhügel and Maria Theresien-Schössl as well as the psychiatric clinic Steinhoff, Frankl gradually developed logotherapy into the independent therapeutic system that is known today.

During the 1920s, Frankl would not have been able to think of founding his own psychotherapeutic or psychiatric school. In 1926, Frankl (1926a) was mainly interested in the formation of a therapeutic and theoretical program that would complement an understanding of neurosis, based on the framework of Alfred Adler's *individual psychology*. In other words, Frankl (1925) wanted to create an encounter basis for patients whose outlook on life jeopardized the prospects of a successfully conducted therapy:

Excerpts from my Introduction featured in the Marquette University Press edition of *The Feeling of Meaninglessness: A Challenge to Psychotherapy and Philosophy*. Viktor E. Frankl. Edited by Alexander Batthyány ©2010. Reprinted by permission. I would like to thank Marquette University Press for the reprint permission. I would also like to thank Marquette's former senior editor, Andrew Tallon; our joint venture in the compilation of *The Feeling of Meaninglessness* stands as an exemplar of both scholarly rigor and collegial amicability.

A. Batthyány (✉)
Viktor Frankl Research Institute for Theoretical Psychology and Personalist Studies, Viktor Frankl Institute Vienna, Pázmany Péter University, Budapest, Hungary

C. L. McLafferty, Jr., J. I. Levinson (eds.), *Logotherapy and Existential Analysis*, Logotherapy and Existential Analysis: Proceedings of the Viktor Frankl Institute Vienna 2, https://doi.org/10.1007/978-3-031-48922-8_1

> One cannot help a pessimist who is very intelligent and sensible to feed himself and play sports via advice giving, because for that—as for the entirety of his well-being—his philosophy provides him with no reason to do so. Here we must first influence his evaluation in order to provide any grounds for further treatment; namely, his evaluation of the value of discussing neuroses at all! (p. 250)

In the framework of this therapeutic model, Frankl (e.g., 1926a) also worked out a detailed phenomenology and classification system of disturbed world references; he was one of the first within the individual psychology movement to submit a phenomenological research endeavor on neurotic orientations toward life. Interestingly, this classification system did not find its way into modern logotherapy, although Frankl (1949) used a few of his 1926-era thoughts and observations subsequently as excerpts in his *Pathologie des Zeitgeists* (in English, *Pathology of the Times*). While the former was aimed at individually disturbed person–world relationships, the latter collectively described abnormal orientations that were formulated in the context of World War II experiences. As such, these were intended in a narrower sense to serve as diagnostic and therapeutic connecting threads in clinical practice.

There are several reasons why Frankl may have avoided further usage of his classification system: First, within a few years, he had developed *logotherapy and existential analysis* (LTEA) into an independent and complete form of therapy, whereby the classification of neurotic orientations toward life lost its importance relative to the now broader applications of his new theory; second, Frankl recognized the limitations of any typology and diagnostic schematization given the ever-broader applicability of his new form of therapy and increasingly came to place the relationship with the unique person of the patient at the foreground of psychotherapy. Nevertheless, the classification system Frankl worked out presented itself from a differential diagnostic rationale as an enduringly compelling research theme: It is possible, for instance, to look at the thought patterns of the *intellectual neurotic* in the framework of modern-day logotherapy as personality-specific forms of expression of *noögenic neuroses*. This framework provided concrete guidelines that create therapeutic openness, while managing to avoid succumbing to the temptation to place the prevailing typological attribution over the individuality of the patient. In any case, an examination of case studies described by Frankl (1947) in *Die Psychotherapie in der Praxis* (*Psychotherapy in Practice*) suggests that he had quite frequently referred back to his classification system a decade later.

Frankl's recognition that it could be necessary before beginning therapy to make the patient conscious of the value of discussing neuroses reveals a conceptualization of *the person* and of *disease*, in which the successful course of therapy depends entirely upon the motivation and insights of the patient. In and of itself, this was not a fundamentally new insight—every clinician and therapist knows that all patients do not begin their therapy with the same level of motivation. What was new, however, was Frankl's (1926a) attempt to understand the reason for these differences in motivation as an expression of an orientation toward life, as well as to view them as relatively independent of the fundamental neurotic disturbance and to give them due consideration:

> It is, *a priori*, not in the least agreed upon that which we call pathological is actually pathological. It is by no means certain that an intellectual opinion or evaluation, for instance, some view put forward by Individual Psychology, is not in itself incorrect. (p. ix)

In other words, it is by no means a conclusive expression or symptom of a psychological disturbance if a patient doubts the meaning of life. Under certain conditions and particular life philosophies, this can be quite rational and logically consistent. Consequently, there is little hope of altering patients' overall life situation via successful treatment of a physical or mental disease. With this understanding, Frankl uncoupled the neurotic patient's orientation toward life from his mental state of mind. The latter may indicate pathological features, but not the former—at least not necessarily. If this type of symptom is not treated by the therapist, it will persist relatively unchanged during the course of treatment. This is precisely because it is not a symptom of disease as such.

On the other hand, it is more obvious that certain orientations toward life can worsen existing symptoms or undermine the prospects of success in therapy from the outset. Even after successful therapy, certain orientations toward life have a statistically higher risk of relapse. That is why it is necessary in the pre- and postcare phases of therapy to lead the patient into an appropriate person–world relationship or to place before them the possibility of a positive approach to existence. Frankl's earlier teacher and mentor, Rudolf Allers (1963/2006), also defined "the purpose of all psychotherapeutic efforts… as the undertaking of bringing about a reconciliation between Person and World" (p. 12). There is every reason to believe that this does not automatically come to be when the original disease symptomatology is reduced to a tolerable degree or cured entirely. This is due to the fact that, even following successful therapy, the disease leaves its mark on the biography and learning history of the patient, and therefore also alters his philosophy of life.

At the same time, it cannot be the goal of any humane psychiatric or psychotherapeutic treatment to take away the life experience and learning history of the patient: In the first place, it is doubtful whether this is possible at all within the framework of an ethical, justifiable therapy, and even if it were, such an action would contradict the logotherapist's understanding of the dignity of the person. All the more, it remains the task of the logotherapist in the posttreatment phase to lead the patient toward a free and realistic relationship with life, on which basis the patient can go on to prosper and flourish.

Still earlier, in 1923, Frankl (1923) originally observed that there are mistaken and strained manners of existence whose etiology is not confined solely to mental or physical causes, but rather whose reasons lie rooted in the spiritual and philosophical dimensions of the person. At that time, the teenage Frankl (1923) spoke of the possibility of a "spiritual disease in the truest meaning of the word, not in the medical–clinical sense, because I speak of spirit and not of mind" (Frankl, 1923, p. 5). This observation has since been empirically confirmed (e.g., Moomal, 1999; Stewart et al., 1993; Testoni & Zamperini, 1998; McHoskey et al., 1999).

Already as a university student, and even in high school, Frankl's early theories anticipated the developments in psychology that would only be accepted within the scientific community a decade later during the period known as the "cognitive revolution." A broad agreement prevails today on the point that any respectable psychological research program must take into account the variety of human concerns, attitudes, and viewpoints. There are only a few models stubbornly holding out which seek to dismiss the spiritual motives and concerns of humanity as "nothing but" in the context of an ideological reductionism and which seek to replace them with drive-dynamic and behavioral conceptualizations.

We can surmise that Frankl's early orientation toward the spiritual and personal helped to corrode his loyalty to his two first teachers, Freud and Adler. At the same time, it appears that he himself was initially not fully aware of the significance of the delineation between the spiritual and mental. It is also possible that he capitulated for a short time under the influence of his first great teacher, Sigmund Freud: Frankl's (1924) first scientific publication in the *Internationale Zeitschrift für Psychoanalyse* at least truly distinguished the young Frankl as an original thinker: In that article, he attempted an explanation of affirmative and negative facial expressions as continuations of coital and nausea reactions. But even as such, he apparently succumbed to the temptation to trace the problem of fundamental human concerns back to the psychodynamic substrate, explicitly denying that affirmation and negation could have a spiritual element.

> We are not able to search for the origins of the facial affirmation and negation expressions in such a manner that we interpret the relevant head movements as symbols of an intellectual affirmation or negation. We will accordingly refer to the two elementary life instincts—the nourishment instinct and the sexual instinct—for an explanation of the phenomena. (p. 437)

It is not easy to recognize the eventual founder of LTEA in these lines. But soon after the publication of this article, Frankl began to distance himself from Sigmund Freud's psychoanalysis and turn to Alfred Adler's individual psychology. Apart from his unsuccessful attempt to begin *Lehranalyse*[1] under Paul Federn, there were probably several other reasons that led Frankl to turn away from psychoanalysis. The first is perhaps that Frankl's active interest in philosophy and his lively social engagement with the philosophical community were largely ignored in psychoanalysis—indeed Frankl's first postpsychoanalytic publications dedicated themselves to these two themes. Moreover, he may have soon become aware that the psychoanalytic model only described a part of the human psyche, a human nature whose upper portions were continually exposed to danger from psychoanalysis by way of its tendency to pathologize the philosophical and metaphysical concerns of the patient (reductionism), rather than acknowledge them as such and address them in the framework of therapy where judged necessary. These thoughts also found their expression in Frankl's first publication within the school of individual psychology. Only a year after his publication in the *Internationale Zeitschrift für Psychoanalyse*,

[1] *Lehranalyse*, translated roughly as "apprenticeship analysis," is a required part of the training to become a psychoanalyst, whereby the trainee undergoes many hours of psychoanalysis in the role of patient.

Frankl published an article that anticipated many routes of his subsequent life's work. In *Psychotherapie und Weltanschauung* (*Psychotherapy and Worldview*), Frankl (1925) wrote:

> The neurotic patient cannot be happy because he has not grown into life, because he despises it, devalues it, and hates it. It is the task of the psychotherapist to fully give back his love for life and will to community, and while not as empirical proofs, he can easily reinstill these in the course of a critical discussion of the value of living and the value of community. (p. 251)

The contrast between both of these passages, which could hardly be more antithetical, may in part be explained by the three-year gap between their composition; years in which Frankl once again returned to his original notion of the noëtic as its own dimension. He not only returned to it but also attempted to make it therapeutically useful in the framework of individual psychology in a fundamentally expanded and enlarged, deepened form.

In 1926, Frankl was an active Adlerian: among other things, as a regular session participant in individual psychology dialogue rounds at Café Siller and as an editor of a journal "for the proliferation of Individual Psychology" (*Der Mensch im Alltag*; in English, *The Person in Everyday Life*). In September of the same year, he was marked out to present a central position paper at the International Congress for Individual Psychology in Düsseldorf.

At about this time, Frankl had probably met his early mentor Rudolph Allers, who had, like Frankl, recently broken away from Sigmund Freud. From around the beginning of 1925, Frankl associated himself with Adler's circle. Frankl assisted Allers between 1925 and 1926 at the Physiological Institute of the University of Vienna, during which time Allers conducted his sensory and physiological studies on perception of gradations of color. Allers, together with the future founder of psychosomatics Oswald Schwartz, presided over the anthropological wing of the individual psychology union, for whose philosophical concerns he probably took over responsibility in 1924. Meanwhile, content-related conflicts with orthodox individual psychology emerged at the outset of these efforts. There were fundamentally two primary criticisms regarding Adler's theory that were expressed by the anthropological circle of Allers, Schwarz, and Frankl, which can be summarized as a criticism of the one-dimensionality of the picture portrayed by the theory of the human being. First, they argued that Adler presented a mono-causal concept of neuroses, which attempted to derive mental disturbances almost exclusively from conflicts between feelings of belonging, power, and striving after success; second, it seemed to them that the very project of a comprehensive philosophical/anthropological system associated with individual psychology was jeopardized because Adler observed values primarily from the viewpoint of the person's social and psychological utility, failing to draw the distinction between rules and values sharply enough (Allers, 1924, p. 10ff). In an ideal case, a rule described possibilities for the realization of values, without necessarily themselves being such. Over and above that, the emphasis on the compulsory nature of social agreements set forth a concept of norms that occasionally was able to promote nonvalues to values. From the viewpoint of a sound, anthropological epistemology of values, the person is not only responsible to the community but, above all, to his own values—intuition and conscience; this is especially valid whenever these should run counter to prevailing norms or current utility. In a retrospective upon these philosophical discussions later in his career, Allers (1963/2006) wrote:

> No further explanation is required if a statistic is rejected as the basis for a boundary determination. It is obvious that the average only corresponds to normal if it occurs in such a way that the normal phenomena constitute a noticeable majority. This however means that one must be clear with himself about "normal" before one uses statistical data. In a population where 99% exhibit tuberculosis, the remaining one percent still remains representative of normality. This is true of diseases as it is for all other aspects of human existence. Statistics regarding morality are not able to provide evidence for what normal morality is; this must be defined, in order to employ the statistic in a meaningful manner. (p. 123)

In a similar way to Allers and Schwarz, Frankl (2002) first hoped to reform individual psychology from the inside and to be able to place the theory on a firmer philosophical, anthropological foundation (p. 43). After the 1927 Congress for Individual Psychology in Düsseldorf—where Frankl abandoned the grounds for orthodox individual psychology, describing neuroses not only as an arrangement of factors but also as an authentic expression of the person—the rifts between the anthropological wing of the individual psychology section and Adler increased. It came to a public break soon after that, as noted by Frankl:

> Then came… the evening in 1927 at which Allers and Schwarz *coram publico* represented and gave reasons for their already previously announced withdrawal from the Society for Individual Psychology. The meeting took place in the great lecture hall of the Histological Institute of the University of Vienna. In the last few rows sat a few Freudians who gloatingly looked upon the spectacle, as what was now unfolding. Adler was in a position no different from Freud, out of whose Viennese psychoanalytic association Adler, for his part, had likewise left. (p. 42)

In 1927, a few months after Frankl's teachers and mentors, Rudolf Allers and Oswald Schwarz, announced their withdrawal from the Society for Individual Psychology, Frankl was shut out from the society at Adler's personal wish, on account of holding "unorthodox views."

1927–1930: Regarding Adolescent Psychology

For Frankl, the split from individual psychology not only meant the loss of the illusion that what at that time was still the most fundamentally liberal-minded psychotherapeutic school in Vienna could be reformed from the inside but also the loss of an important forum in which he could discuss his ideas and the clinical advancement of individual psychology with Adler and his close associates.

At the same time, the following years brought new challenges for Frankl and the emergence of LTEA. A markedly active time followed his expulsion, during which Frankl collected important experiences in the course of his practical counseling activities. By 1926, Frankl had pointed out the necessity of psychological care for adolescents in numerous publications (e.g., Frankl, 1926b, c). He was stimulated by Wilhelm Börner's founding of prototype counseling centers in Vienna for people who were weary of life. While it is true that comparable facilities were already being coordinated in Vienna by individual psychologists and the first advocates of Austrian social psychiatry, these directed their counseling services primarily toward parents and educators and not to adolescents. Indeed, the concerns and worries of adolescents scarcely found consideration.

After his exodus from the individual psychology union, together with his former colleagues from Adler's circle—among them Rudolph Allers, August Aichorn, Wilhelm Börner, Hugo Lukacs, Erwin Wexberg, Rudolph Dreikurs, and Charlotte Bühler—Frankl answered the request that he himself had initially made in Vienna in 1928, and subsequently in six other European cities after the Vienna Group's model, by organizing youth counseling centers in which adolescents in emotional distress were psychologically attended to, free of charge and anonymously. The counseling took place in the apartment or practice of the volunteer collaborator—and so it was in Frankl's parents' apartment at Czerningasse 6 in Vienna's Leopoldstadt (the apartment identified in all publications and flyers as the contact address) for routing to the youth counseling centers.

In view of the fact that Frankl's initiative filled an important gap in Vienna, it is not surprising that requests for consultation and counseling were many and that the work of the youth counseling centers was extraordinarily successful. Information as to just how successful—and how necessary—came in a later review article of Frankl's, in which he reported retrospectively and summarily on his activity as a youth counselor. In these papers, Frankl (1930, 1935a) referred to approximately 900 counseling cases that he alone had attended to and at the same time took sobering stock of the situation of Viennese adolescents: At least 20% of those who sought counseling exhibited, "enduring weariness of life and thoughts of suicide" (Frankl, 1930, p. 42). From 1930, Frankl paid particular attention to the incidence of student suicide, which had increased considerably in the days immediately preceding and following the distribution of report cards. In the same year, Frankl organized the first special campaign for student counseling, paying particular attention to the critical period of the school year's end.

Already in its first year in 1930, the campaign proved to be a great success; the incidence of suicide attempts among students declined sharply. For the first time in many years, in 1931 no student suicides were recorded in Vienna.

By 1930, Frankl had successfully completed his medical studies; he then took up his specialist training in psychiatry and neurology at four of the most renowned psychiatric clinics and mental hospitals in Vienna at that time. Here, he was able to gain further insights and awareness via direct contact with patients that would fundamentally shape the still-nascent LTEA. For the publication of *Der Mensch im Alltag* (Frankl, 1927) and during his student counseling activities, he had concerned himself up until this point primarily with crisis prophylaxes and psychological hygiene. Now, in the narrower field of psychiatric practice, he expanded his therapy.

Just how mature his theory of motivation was by this time was demonstrated in a work in which Frankl (1933) described the mental and spiritual distress of the unemployed that he interpreted not only socially and economically but, rather significantly, traced back to a lack of a sense of purpose and meaning, i.e., to what he would later call the *existential vacuum*. In the same article, Frankl referred to *attitudinal values* in the face of unavoidable suffering, discussed the concept of *creative values* in the presence of remediable suffering, and also described the application of Socratic dialogue as a therapeutic method for the treatment of the existential vacuum.

With this basic theoretical understanding and equipped with these therapeutic tools, Frankl took up his medical specialist training. Frankl (1933) had already drawn attention to the problem of unavoidable suffering in otherwise psychologically healthy individuals. At the psychiatric clinic of Steinhof, he encountered, in a narrower sense, the psychopathological suffering of psychologically diseased patients (he primarily attended to depressive patients). Here, as well, he was able to observe the effects of the trans-morbid, spiritual resources that he had previously described as a crucial element of treatment during follow-up therapy, as well as for the counseling of unemployed youth.

It appears in hindsight that Frankl's work in psychiatry was the first practical test and possibly even the actual birth of LTEA as we know it today. In order to fully comprehend the magnitude of this development, we must be aware of Frankl's situation at that time: As a young doctor, he discovered what neither of his former teachers (Freud and Adler) were ready to concede—that the noëtic dimension of the human being can make a contribution to the course of counseling and therapy, and this because the spiritual can be taken to be relatively independent of illness and free right up to the last moment despite an oppressive daily existence. In the course of his counseling and therapy activities, he observed that this fundamental principle had an effect across a variety of problem constellations, such as in the treatment of neurotic patients, students at risk of suicide, and unemployed youths. Consequently, his experiences showed him that neither psychological nor social fate could deprive the person of his spiritual freedom. They also demonstrated to him that the spiritual freedom of the person was not only an anthropological fact of experience but could also be quite clinically efficacious due to the fact that it returned autonomy and self-assertiveness to the patient who was being threatened by blows of psychological or social fate.

With this knowledge—along with the methods that arose from efforts aimed at returning freedom of choice to the patient's awareness—Frankl stepped into a patient group in which illness expressed itself biologically while also being socially and psychologically conditioned. Would Frankl's recognition that the noëtic stands relatively independent of fate be confirmed, even here? The answer to this question was, at least at one time, uncertain: The biological component of endogenous depression made discussing neuroses impossible. Moreover, the question presented itself: How would he assess his understanding of the noëtic dimension of the person in his sometimes severely and chronically afflicted depressive patients by making an appeal to personal responsibility and the like, without intensifying the already exaggerated guilt-ideation characteristic of this group?

As a solution to this problem, Frankl proceeded for the time being in a manner more phenomenological than therapeutical. In short, he made careful observations. In a subsequent retrospective, he wrote that during this period, the patients themselves became his teachers; according to his own statement, he attempted at this time "to forget what [he] had learned from Psychoanalysis and Individual Psychology" (Frankl, 2002, p. 52). In place of his academic teachers and mentors, from this point forward, Frankl turned to his patients in order to discover what measures beyond directly psychiatric or psychotherapeutic interventions could contribute to their healing and recovery. Once again, his model of the trans-morbid noëtic proved itself valid, irrespective of the presence of disease. Frankl saw in his recovered patients that the spiritual resources of the person could not only aid the apathetic and neurotic patient, but they could also help the stabilized psychotic patient to accept a self-chosen and responsible stance toward their own illness, which in turn affected the course of the disease itself.

It is in this context that Frankl (1985) subsequently coined the term "*pathoplastic*" (p. 200)—the retained ability of diseased persons to shape (up to a certain point) the nature of their symptoms or to mold an existence that had been overshadowed by a psychological illness. Out of this area of conflict between a fateful illness and one's freely chosen response arose Frankl's enduring concept of freedom, which defined human contingency not as a hindrance, but rather as freedom's impetus. For a freedom that proved itself even or especially when the internal or external circumstances appeared overwhelming was a freedom that persisted not merely as a theoretical ability or philosophical commitment, but rather as a livable reality and persisted, to a clinically relevant extent, even in the face of biological fate.

This model had important consequences for applied therapy: For one, because the attitude of the patient toward the disease influences it and does so particularly in the long term (this has been sufficiently demonstrated, for example, with regard to patients affected by phase-oriented illnesses who take responsibility for their own care in the face of renewed symptomatology) and second, because patients, by way of distancing themselves from events associated with an illness, function not merely as passive bearers of symptoms and seekers of assistance, but to a certain extent become a coworker of the doctor or therapist. However, freedom and responsibility are not guaranteed if the autonomy of individuals so afflicted—even their autonomy toward the doctor/therapist—is not preserved (Frankl, 1985).

Naturally, realistic limits needed to be set regarding these ties to the patient. For example, the collaborative attempt to bring the disease under control presupposed a fundamental understanding of disease that psychotic patients in an acute stage of illness did not, as a rule, possess. Moreover, this collaboration had to be brought to a halt whenever the doctor encountered the patient not as coworker, but as clinician, perhaps prescribing a medicinal (pharmacological) therapy. Frankl (1993) was not concerned with a socially romantic and ill-conceived democratization of therapy, but rather sought to appreciate the personal core of the diseased person and to make this process therapeutically useful, allowing the patient to positively influence the course of disease and therapy. Occasionally—for example, in the case of endogenous depression—this collaboration may not mean any more to the patient for the time being than allowing the doctor to work and supporting therapeutic efforts until the treatment takes effect.

> We have to bring the patient to the place where he does not try to "pull himself together," on the contrary: to where he allows the depression to issue out around himself insofar as it is possible—that he takes it precisely to be endogenous, in a word, that he *objectifies* it and, as such, *distances* himself from it—and this is possible in light to moderate cases. Whether one person *ceteris paribus* distances himself from his endogenous depression while another allows himself to succumb to the depression rests not upon the endogenous depression itself, but rather upon the spiritual person; for the person is always at work, always exerting some effect, always co-forming disease outcomes. (p. 62)

The most important discovery of his training period at Steinhof was the confirmation of the efficacy of spiritual freedom even in the face of biological fate: It was "always co-forming disease outcomes." But how did it co-form and by what criteria? With the posing of this question, Frankl returned from his detour to the dialectic between destiny and freedom back to the question of the value of discussing neuroses at all. In the case of the person with psychotic symptoms, the perception of the value of discussing the illness not in isolation but together with the patient's stance toward the illness proved most efficacious. Also of central importance was the question of whether or not—and if so, to what extent—the patient was ready to make use of their relative freedom. This placed two fundamental concepts of logotherapy before a real-world test: First, the ability of human beings to suffer in the face of an unchangeable fate; and second, the person's *will to meaning*, that is to say, the ability of the person to bear difficult life circumstances because there is a *More* through which suffering becomes bearable.

In his 1933 article on the spiritual distress of the unemployed adolescent, Frankl (1933) had pointed out that the knowledge of a meaning of existence allowed for protection against depression, resignation, and apathy. Frankl (1947) was also able to confirm these observations in his depressive patients who were under suicide watch at Steinhof:

> Now insofar as it is necessary to evaluate precisely to what extent the seriousness of suicide risk a person represents, either when one is determining the advisability and reasonableness of discharging the patient from a closed facility, or else during a patient's initial intake into inpatient institutional care, I myself have created a standard method that proves itself effective without fail. It enables us to provide a diagnosis of continued suicide risk, or rather to make a diagnosis of the dissimulation of suicidal tendencies as such. At first, we pose the question to the respective patient as to whether he still fosters suicidal intentions. In every case—both in the case where he is telling the truth, as well as in the case of mere dissimulation of actual suicidal intentions—he will deny our first question; whereupon we submit to him a second question, which almost sounds brutal: *why* does he no longer wish to take his own life? And now it is shown with regularity, that he who genuinely does not harbour suicidal intentions is immediately ready with a series of reasons and counterarguments that all speak against him throwing his own life away: that he still takes his disease to be curable, that he remains considerate of his family or must think of his professional commitments, that he still has many religious obligations, etc. Meanwhile, the person who has only dissimulated his suicidal intentions will be exposed by our second question, and not having an answer for it, react from a position that is characterized by embarrassment. This is truly simply on account of the fact that he is at a loss for an argument that would speak against suicide. (p. 121)

Frankl developed another central element of logotherapy during his stay at Steinhof. This addressed itself less to the personhood of the patient and more to the doctor's self-perception: Medical actions, as Frankl understood them—especially whenever the doctor was actively conducting research—constituted, among other things, the doctor's attempt to retain his role as scientist while also recognizing the patient not merely as an object of study but also as a unique individual. With this recognition, not only did the doctor and researcher give consideration to Frankl's basic understanding of undetachedly bestowed personal value but also this type of attention to the patient paved the way to new diagnostic and therapeutic findings, making it very important in clinical terms. That Frankl's (1935b) concern was not only for psychotherapy but also for "psychiatry with a humane disposition" (as he often stated in his lectures), it is expressed as the guiding principle of his actions in an exemplary paper, in which he reported of a lively Yom Kippur celebration organized by a colleague and himself at the Steinhof clinic. One must be aware that Frankl set this and similar initiatives in place a decade before any psychiatric reform began in Austria:

> Individual hallucinatory patients continue to quietly lead conversations with themselves and their empty gaze wanders aimlessly about the hall. The rabbi turns himself towards them there—the Service of Men is also the Service of God—and he begins to speak German. He urgently describes to them the meaning of the above... statement—and they attend! It goes on this way through an hour, six hours on the next day. Soon he had achieved what the diseased soul needs accomplished: to snatch him away from the delusional world, to continually draw his attention to something new—to occupy the ill person. Much empathy, adaptability, patience, and interpersonal skill was necessary for this work. (p. 7)

Frankl's fundamental premise that the noëtic dimension of the person is not directly affected by the course of illness, however fully affected they are by the disease of the psycho-physical substrate, has unlimited practical applications for making the patient's estranged experiences at least supportable by recognizing their indestructible dignity and personality. Rather it was Frankl's utmost aim and highest task as a doctor to treat the underlying disease itself under the focal point of the best possible medical care. It is in this context that we recall Frankl's (1933) axiom: "to bear... need, whenever it is necessary, and to remedy it, whenever possible" (p. 45). Those with psychological illness may find the "bearing" to be more possible than "remedy," especially in acute stages of the disease. From Frankl's perspective, it was all the more the task of the doctor to search always for new and better treatment possibilities for psychological illness. Frankl (1939a) described the pharmaceutical support of psychotherapy in a population of neurotic patients and, with the research findings described in this article, took a monumental step forward for modern European psychopharmacology. He subsequently conducted original pioneering work whereby he introduced the common cold medicine Myoscain as a forerunner drug to contemporary antianxiety medications. Credit for his work continues to be found on package inserts included with Myoscain[2] (Sanochemia, n.d.):

[2] [Myoscain is a brand name of a 10% oral solution of guaifenesin, an expectorant medication sold over the counter. –Ed.]

Introduced into therapy by Viktor E. Frankl as the first supplement for the abatement of anxiety in Europe, indicated by anxious arousal in conjunction with depressive conditions, anxiety neuroses (expectations anxiety, test anxiety, etc.), stuttering....

1938–1945: ...Nevertheless, Say "Yes!" to Life (*Man's Search for Meaning*)

In 1938—the year of the Austrian *Anschluss* into Nazi Germany—Frankl (1938) published *Zur gestigen Problematik der Psychotherapie* (*On the spiritual problems of psychotherapy*), in which he not only coined the term *existential analysis* but also applied his theory to a broad range of issues:

> Where is that therapeutically oriented therapy that would include the "higher" strata of human existence in its outline and in this sense, in contrast to the phrase "depth psychology," merit the name "height psychology"? To put it another way, where is that theory of broad mental events and specific neurotic phenomena that, as it regards the domain of the psyche, would sufficiently take into consideration the entirety of human existence and could accordingly be described as Existential Analysis? (p. 36)

In this article, as well as in a subsequent article entitled *Philosophie und Psychotherapie* (*Philosophy and Psychotherapy*), Frankl (1939b) returned to the sources of logotherapy from circa 1933 and issued forth broadly about what he had hitherto published in the field of psychotherapy. For the first time, we find in this work LTEA's theory of motivation—the meaning orientation of the human being—as a fully worked-out concept; we also find here the first mention of the three categorical values, which Frankl later described as the "three avenues to meaning" (p. 45) and here we also encounter for the first time descriptions of a few of its techniques and methods. Also pivotal was Frankl's appeal to psychotherapy, in which he argued that it must with its "*predetermined image of the human being carry over the bodily–mental–spiritual Unity into its view of mentally ill individuals*" (p. 46). After all, Frankl placed so much value on this commitment to the integrity of personality—even of the mentally ill person—that he had this as one of the few passages of his article to be printed in italics.

Frankl wrote these lines precisely at the time when the Nazis were working out the systematic annihilation of mentally ill patients. And here, as already nearly 10 years before on behalf of distressed Viennese adolescents, Frankl made his own plea: At first alone, later with the help of the then-director of the Psychiatry Clinic of the University of Vienna, Otto Pötzl, he managed to protect numerous Jewish psychiatric patients from Hitler and Schirach's euthanasia program using falsified diagnoses (Neugebauer, 1997), to fill the beds of the Jewish nursing home on Vienna's Malzgasse with psychotic patients. It was forbidden for the nursing home to accept mentally ill patients, but:

> I now bypassed this stipulation [the one which forbade the nursing home to accept nursing care cases related to mental illness], as I protected the administrator of the nursing home (whose own head was eventually put into a noose) by issuing medical certifications: one

> with schizophrenia transmuted into aphasia, "thus an organic brain illness," and one with melancholy transmuted into fever-induced delirium, so "no psychosis in the actual meaning of the word." There was once a patient accommodated in a cot in the nursing home who, due to needs associated with schizophrenia, could only be treated in an open section with Metrazol shock therapy, without which there would be a melancholic phase endured without suicide risk. (Frankl, 2002, p. 60)

"Endured without suicide risk"—what Frankl mentioned here in a subordinate clause, represented his final neuro-psychological work before his deportation to Theresienstadt. After he was forced to give up his newly opened first private practice as a psychiatrist and neurologist on the grounds of Nazi race laws, Frankl was appointed from 1939 as the Chief Physician for Neurology at the Rothschildspital of the Israelite Cultural Municipality—a position that guaranteed him and his immediate family members protection against deportation for the time being. At the Rothschild Hospital, Frankl could continue to practice his duties as a doctor, although he would now be confronted with horrors few people would have guessed that were still to descend upon twentieth-century Europe. These set before doctors particular challenges. Within the framework of his certification activities and his duties at the suicide pavilion at the Steinhof Clinic, Frankl had been aware of his obligation as a doctor to protect and save lives, and here again he would fulfill his medical responsibility. Under the degrading living conditions and partly also in the face of looming deportation, numerous Viennese Jews committed suicide. Particularly great was the medical challenge to the hospital: Sometimes up to 10 attempted suicide attempts a day were admitted to the Rothschild Hospital. True to his conviction as expressed in his numerous preceding assignments that, with respect to the suicides, "everything that is therapeutically possible should be done" (Frankl, 1942, p. 59). Frankl developed his own technique with the help of the patients he attempted to save in spite of the most serious poisonings from sleeping pills whereby he circumvented the blood–brain barrier to inject an antidote locally. Patients could be resuscitated for a short time with this method, even though they had already been given up as moribund by the clinic staff. Frankl could not develop this method any further, because in 1942 he was deported with his family and first wife to Theresienstadt (Batthyány, 2006).

Before his deportation, Frankl (1940/1942) completed the first major work of LTEA, *Ärtzliche Seelsorge* (*Medical Ministry*; henceforth referred to by the English title, *The Doctor and the Soul*), although it would not be published until after the liberation. The manuscript of the 1942 original version of this book provides us with insight into Frankl's commitment to hope as the antidote to suicide, even where any hope of a way out is ostensibly hope for a miracle. In fact, this unconditional hope also preserves the argument for the unconditional meaningfulness of existence, including the possibility of retroactively reclaiming meaning from the *tragic triad* of suffering, guilt, and death:

> Even if only one individual from the many who commit suicide under the conviction of the hopelessness of their circumstances proves to be incorrect—namely, if they would have eventually found a way out—then every attempter of suicide is wrong on that point: because the conviction for all of them is equally fixed and no one can know in advance just whether

> his conviction will remain justified, or else be proven a lie through the following events of a missed hour, even though he might not ultimately survive. (p. 83)[3]

A short time after he wrote these lines, Frankl was deported together with his family and first wife to Theresienstadt. Only one sister was able to escape deportation by fleeing to Australia. We know from the autobiographical lectures of Frankl that he strengthened his own argument for unconditional hope in difficult moments of utmost despair by his own stance and, perhaps still more significantly, by trying to help others. Only a short time ago, writings of former cellmates were discovered in private estates documenting that Frankl shared his belief in unconditional meaning with his comrades in the concentration camps, and in that place, even under the most hostile external circumstances, he tried as doctor, friend, and human being to be a comforter to others. ("Comfort ye, comfort ye my people." Isaiah 40:1, King James Version).

Like the majority of doctors there, Frankl was assigned to the section for illness care in Theresienstadt. Here, he encountered the Berlin rabbi and originator of liberal Judaism, Leo Baeck. Baeck, who endeavored to encourage and give heart to camp inmates in Theresienstadt via lectures and sermons, also asked Frankl to give speeches. An announcement card from Frankl's (n.d.) lectures is still preserved—as a motto he noted on the reverse side at that time: "There is nothing in the world that empowers a human being to overcome external difficulties or internal hardships so much as the awareness that one has a task in life."

With the help of the director of medical provisions Erich Munk and his assistant Karel Fleischmann, Frankl erected mobile psychological counseling stations in Theresienstadt. The so-called "Shock Squad" was composed of doctors and volunteer helpers who, wherever possible, dispensed comfort, help, and healing for those inmates affected by psychological distress. The Shock Squad focused their attention above all on the weak and helpless in Theresienstadt: the elderly, the diseased, the psychologically ill, and those who already in the midst of degrading life circumstances stood at the bottom of the camp's social hierarchy. The group of volunteer helpers also prioritized alleviation of the shock of those newly arrived at Theresienstadt. Whenever Frankl and his volunteer collaborators—among them Regina Jonas, the first female rabbi—were referred to a resident of the Theresienstadt Ghetto because of suicide risk, they would seek the person out in order to take the heavy load off of their shoulders, requesting an opportunity for a conversation where they would "return him to life" (ihm dem Leben zurückgegeben.). As in the years before, Frankl's commitment to the suffering person yielded results: The

[3] This quote originates from one of two copies of the original typed manuscript of the first version of *Ärztliche Seelsorge*. As is generally known, Frankl had lost the original in the disinfection chamber at Auschwitz. Two copies remained in Vienna: One was smuggled into the jail cell of Frankl's childhood and climbing friend Hubert Gsur in 1942 as he awaited his execution from a death sentence on account of "subversion of the armed forces and attempted coup." It is not known what happened to Gsur's copy; it was probably destroyed by the prison administration. The other copy found itself in the care of Paul Polak during the war, who gave it back to Frankl after his return to Vienna; it is kept currently in Viktor Frankl's private estate and document archive.

suicide rate in Theresienstadt was able to be significantly reduced (Berkley, 1993, p. 123ff.).

The years in the concentration camps—Frankl would be interned in four concentration camps by the war's end—were stations of farewells for him as well: His father, mother, wife, mother-in-law, and brother—even the manuscript of the first version of *The Doctor and the Soul*—would all be taken from him within a period of months, often only days. On March 5, 1945, Frankl was placed in his final camp, Türkheim. Türkheim, a branch camp of Dachau, was originally erected as a "recuperation camp" for sick camp inmates. Frankl registered himself there voluntarily for service as a doctor and was assigned, among other duties, to the typhus fever barracks. It was only a matter of time until he himself, weakened after a year-long internment, contracted typhus. Stricken by serious illness, Frankl (2002) began to reconstruct the manuscript of *The Doctor and the Soul* that he had lost in Auschwitz:

> What I personally have arrived at—I am convinced that—my determination to reconstruct the lost manuscript contributed not in the least to my own survival. I set out upon it as I took ill with typhus fever and sought to keep myself awake at night so as not to succumb to vascular collapse. A comrade had given me a pencil stub for my 40th birthday and had conjured up a few small SS forms, upon whose backside I now—with high fever—scribbled stenographic notes, with whose help I even thought to reconstruct *The Doctor and the Soul*. (p. 76)

1945–1997: Systematization and Validation

After his liberation from the concentration camp on April 27, 1945 by American troops, Frankl was appointed to the position of camp doctor in the military hospital for displaced persons at the Bavarian health resort of Bad Wörishofen. He worked there for about 2 months as chief doctor until, in the summer of 1945, he finally succeeded in returning to Vienna on the first half-legal transport. Directly after that, he began to reconstruct his first book, *The Doctor and the Soul*, as well as to expand the chapter, "Zur Psychologie des Konzentrationslagers" ("On the Psychology of Concentration Camps") (Frankl, 1946a). In the new edition of the book, Frankl presented LTEA systematically and founded a new independent school of therapy—described after Freud and Adler as the Third Viennese School of Psychotherapy (Soucek, 1948)—one which placed the will to meaning, freedom, dignity, and the responsibility of the human being at the center of its therapeutic efficacy.

Shortly thereafter, Frankl began to work on the transcript of his autobiographical report *...trotzdem Ja zum Leben sagen* (published in English as *Man's Search for Meaning*), which in the spring of 1946 was published originally under the title *Ein Psycholog erlebt das Konzentrationslager* (*A Psychologist Experiences the Concentration Camp*) by the Viennese publishing house Jugend & Folk (Frankl, 1946b). The contemporary title proper *...trotzdem Ja zum Leben sagan* first made the cover a few years later. At first, Frankl planned to publish his autobiographical report using his inmate number as a *nom de plume*; soon afterward he made up his mind to let it be published completely anonymously; he felt a strong aversion toward "psychological exhibitionism" (Frankl, October, 1994), as his autobiographical report incidentally points out. Obviously, the primary point for him was not merely to describe his own fate. In fact, he intended to present an objective text which, along with personal experiences from the concentration camps, would impart the central messages of LTEA: that pain, guilt, and death may not take away the unconditional meaning of our existence; that even in the face of the most adverse life circumstances in the camp, the person can "transform tragedy into triumph"; that even in the most hopeless situation, a final, residual—and decisive—core of existential freedom remained for the human being, a freedom that could come into full force not in spite of, but rather precisely in and through the person's contingency:

> What then is man? We ask again. He is a being who continuously decides what he is: a being who equally harbors the potential to descend to the level of an animal or to ascend to the life of a saint. Man is that being, who, after all, invented the gas chambers; but at the same time he is that being who entered into those same gas chambers with his head held high and with the "Our Father" or the Jewish prayer of the dying on his lips. (Frankl, 1985, p. 112)

While Frankl's (1946a) first postwar publication of the German edition of *The Doctor and the Soul* quickly sold out in the first 3 days after its publication and, on the grounds of enormous demand, five editions were issued between 1946 and 1948, *Ein Psycholog erlebt das Konzentrationslager* sold sluggishly at first. The publishing house launched a second edition in conjunction with the first run of 3000, this time with the author's name on the cover, in an attempt to capitalize on the high degree of popularity of the author of *The Doctor and the Soul* (whose name had even then only been published inside *Ein Psycholog erlebt das Konzentrationslager*). This second edition sold so badly, however, that a good proportion were thrown away, even after Frankl had acquired around a hundred reduced-price copies from the publisher and donated them to the Concentration Camp Association.

There are probably many reasons why the book initially could hardly penetrate the market in postwar Vienna, even though Frankl himself was a much sought-after lecturer and sometimes referred to the book in his discussions and radio presentations. Probably a major reason for the restrained reception of the book may have been his first title, *Ein Psycholog erlebt das Konzentrationslager* (A Psychologist Experiences the Concentration Camp), which Frankl changed, probably not without good reason. This was the first and last time that Frankl altered a book title without at the same time changing the content itself of the corresponding book.

After a decade-long delay, the book's actual impact would unfurl primarily via the American edition, which was promoted by then-President of the American Psychological Association, Gordon W. Allport. The translation was published in 1959 under the title *From Death-Camp to Existentialism* (and after 1963 under the title *Man's Search for Meaning*) by Beacon Press in Boston. It developed quickly into an international bestseller: Since then, 15 million copies of the book have been sold in more than 150 editions. The Library of Congress in Washington nominated it as one of the 10 most influential books in America. It is in this context that Frankl (2002) observed in his memoirs:

> Is it not peculiar, that of all of my books, the one that I wrote assuredly in the mindset that it would be published anonymously and could at no time bring me personal success—that precisely this book advanced into a bestseller, a bestseller even in American terms? (p. 84)

In February of 1946, Frankl was appointed to the post of director of the neurological department of the Vienna Polyclinic. He held this position for 25 years until his retirement. There at the Polyclinic, Frankl met the young dental assistant, Eleonore Schwindt. They married soon after. A year later, Frankl (2000) quoted the eminent American philosopher Jacob Needleman, who referred "to the way in which Elly has been my companion on our lecture tours: 'She is the warmth that accompanies the light'" (p. 111). In 1947, their daughter Gabriele was born.

Many of Frankl's books and articles were published in the following years, among them *Psychotherapie in der Praxis* (*Psychotherapy in practice*) (Frankl, 1947). Next to *The Doctor and the Soul*, this work constitutes one of the most detailed portrayals of LTEA, primarily describing the practice of applied logotherapy by means of diagnostic and therapeutic guidelines. Numerous publications followed, in which Frankl deepened the theory and practice of LTEA and made its area of application relevant to the general public. Altogether Frankl published 32 books over his lifetime, which were translated into 31 languages. Frankl's 33rd book—*Gottsuche und Sinnfrage* (The search for God and the question of meaning; Frankl & Lapide, 2005)—was first discovered in the summer of 2004 among his unpublished writings and has recently been published on the occasion of his 100th birthday. The 34th book was edited and published by Frankl's daughter, Dr. Gabriele Vesely-Frankl, which offers a commentated and edited anthology of Frankl's early writings (appropriately entitled, *Frühen Schriften* (Early Writings); Frankl & Vesely-Frankl, 2005), from 1923 until 1942.

LTEA aroused great interest in German-speaking regions when it first appeared in *The Doctor and the Soul* and found increasing acceptance in international scientific communities from the late 1950s. Frankl was invited worldwide for presentations, seminars, and lectures. Even in America, Frankl became increasingly well known: Guest professorships ensued at Harvard University in Boston and at universities in Dallas and Pittsburgh. The United States International University in California initiated an institute and a professorship for LTEA, specifically on Frankl's behalf. Over 200 universities on five continents invited Frankl for talks and guest lectures.

In the context of the intensified diffusion of Frankl's scientific work within university campuses, practitioners and researchers developed more methodological branches of research: Numerous scientific studies were carried out to investigate empirically the basic principles, concepts, and clinical efficacy of LTEA. Over the last 40 years, over 600 empirical contributions validating Frankl's psychological model and his therapeutic applications have been published in psychological and psychiatric professional journals (Batthyány & Guttmann, 2006). These stand alongside an approximately similar number of further publications investigating the theoretical foundations and numerous areas of application (Vesely & Fizzotti, 2005).

Next to his work for and on LTEA in the narrower sense, Frankl published further in the area of neurology and psychopharmacology: His neuropsychological research works after 1945 returned to the theme of the somatic substrate of mentally disturbed character structures—in this way he was able, among other things, to show that certain forms of anxiety and depersonalization disturbances are co-induced by endocrinal factors (Frankl, 1993, p. 84ff.) and to achieve with that discovery a meaningful contribution to the differential diagnosis and therapy of these diseases.

Frankl's model held body, mind, and spirit in the human being to be aspects of a single entity, whose component parts needed to be distinguished qualitatively in order to be able to appropriately describe or treat the whole with a single method. Frankl had also anticipated something that a decade later, sometime after his death, would enter the scientific arena for the first time: The trend toward varying methodologies reflects itself today in the increasing interdisciplinary interdependence of the empirical behavioral sciences. There are calls from many factions within the field of scientific psychology for a systematic focusing of the research activities of different subject disciplines. It remains to be seen whether these calls will be heard and what concrete form their realization will assume. In any case, however, we can already see an acceptance that there is not one but numerous sciences of humanity, which was a fundamental creed of Frankl's conceptualization of the human being. His differentiated etiological model of mental disturbances has met with empirical confirmation in the last few decades: For one, modern cognitive psychology schematics increasingly afford insight today into the cognitive mechanisms of numerous psychological disturbances as, for example, anxiety and compulsive illnesses. Two of the central techniques of logotherapy—*dereflection* and *paradoxical intention*—have also been shown to be useful in nonclinical settings. For the first time, a contemporary theoretical model is emerging that is able to explain what happens on the cognitive level whenever patients lose conscious monitoring of their experiences (e.g., during panic attacks) or will (e.g., in compulsive disorders [Wenzlaff et al., 1988; Wegner, 1989; Anderson & Green, 2001]). Many of these models express with only slightly different language what Frankl—long before the cognitive revolution period of psychology—proposed to be co-etiological in the emergence of disturbed states of experience and behavior and made successfully treatable through the development of his therapeutic methods.

His model of the bodily contribution to the disease etiology of a whole series of mental disorders—a subject that during Frankl's lifetime remained particularly prone to conflict, primarily within humanistic psychotherapy and the psychiatric movement—has found empirical validation in the course of the last decade. And here again, the ideas of Frankl emerge—with logotherapy at the center—as pioneering concepts: In the course of refined diagnostic methods and the development of imaging techniques, it is becoming increasingly clear that there is no mental condition that occurs that is not capable of being linked to a neuronal correlate. The recognition of the neuronal–mental covariance represents the standard for empirical behavioral science today. Frankl described this model in the formation of the *somatopsychic parallelism* in a day when front-line psychotherapy sought to validate early childhood and psychodynamic causes of mental disorders and was, as a rule, inclined either to devalue or completely deny the somatic component of their etiology. In contrast, Frankl endeavored over his lifetime to abandon the essence of various (spiritual, mental, and bodily) phenomena to their wholeness and then to conceive of them in their collaborative impact upon the unity of the human person. To abandon them to their wholeness meant to recognize the proper dimension of each of the phenomena, without classifying it in an inferior category of phenomena. Meanwhile, to conceive of them in their wholeness and unity meant to understand them within the interplay of the totality of being embodied by each person. Frankl (1965) summarized this sophisticated ontology and methodology in the dictum of *Der Pluralismus der Wissenschaften und der Einheit des Menschen* (*The pluralism of the sciences and the unity of man*).

Frankl developed this model at a time when psychotherapy as a science still fell within the discipline of classical medicine, but when it was at the same time largely speculative (Robinson 1985, p. 3ff.; 1995, p. 149ff). It is true that he himself argued that the noëtic dimension—on the grounds of its ontological independence—is in and of itself an aspect of the human being that exists beyond the purview of every sort of empiricism, but given this it is surely all the more noteworthy that it was Frankl who, to a much greater degree than both of his early mentors Freud and Adler, was interested in LTEA as a branch of research to be empirically validated. In actual fact, logotherapy has undergone further developments since its fundamental principles were initially formulated, primarily in dialogue with its neighboring academic disciplines.

Future Prospects: The Challenges of the Future

Until 1997, the developmental process of LTEA was primarily tied to the person of Frankl and the first generation of students to be acquainted with logotherapy. But Frankl (in Fabry, 1978) supported the connection and dialogue between logotherapy and science among future logotherapists as well:

> You cannot turn the wheel back and you won't get a hearing unless you try to satisfy the preferences of present-time Western thinking, which means the scientific orientation or, to put it in more concrete terms, our test- and statistics-mindedness. So why should we lose, unnecessarily and undeservedly, whole segments of the academic community, precluding them a priori from understanding how much logotherapy "speaks to the needs of the hour"? Why should we give up, right from the beginning, getting a hearing from the modern researchers by considering ourselves above tests and statistics? We have no reason not to admit our need to find our discoveries supported by strictly empirical research....
>
> That's why I welcome all sober and solid empirical research in logotherapy. (p. 5–6)

This retrospective also offers the opportunity to honor one of the youngest deceased pioneers of empirical logotherapy: James Crumbaugh. LTEA have him and his coauthor Leonard Maholick to thank for one of the first large-scale empirical works. Crumbaugh and Maholick (1964) were the first to attempt to capture the logotherapeutic construct of *meaning fulfillment* psychometrically, with the help of the *Purpose in Life* (PIL) tests. Their paper was published in 1964 in the *Journal of Clinical Psychology* under the revealing title: "An experimental investigation in existentialism." This was an unusual choice for a title at that time, as it is today—one does not bring existentialism in direct connection with empirical studies. However, it is precisely this tension between fundamental philosophical research, on the one hand, and, on the other, the readiness to submit to empirical scrutiny outside of the protected realm of philosophy that illustrates the unique position of logotherapy within psychiatry and psychotherapy and moreover its attempt to be accepted there as an anthropological branch of research. Crumbaugh and Maholick's study marked the beginning of the scientific-empirical tradition within logotherapy: The PIL was the first of what would prove to be 20 test instruments that have been developed in the framework of logotherapy (Guttmann, 1996).

It is against this background that logotherapy is recognized in Austria and Switzerland by the state as an independent school of psychotherapy, as well as in the United States by the American Psychological Association. Recognition in Germany is still due, although there is still cause for hope that the deepening of the empirical foundations of logotherapy can help to change this. Worldwide, there are approximately 140 institutes and training programs.[4] Moreover, logotherapy seems to have withstood its most important real-world tests. It is an independent school of therapy and research, which has grown into an integral part of the nonreductionist tradition in the clinical, theoretical, and empirical behavioral, social, and human sciences and, as such, can no longer be casually dismissed.

References

Allers, R. (1924). Die Gemeinschaft als Idee und Erlebnis. *Internationale Zeitschrift für Individualpsychologie, 2*, 7–10.

Allers, R. (1963/2006). *Abnorme Welten. Ein phänomenologischer Versuch zur Psychiatrie. Herausgegeben und kommentiert von Alexander Batthyány*. Beltz.

Anderson, M. C., & Green, C. (2001). Suppressing unwanted memories by executive control. *Nature, 410*, 366–369.

Batthyány, A. (2006). Mythos Frankl? Entgegnung auf Timothy Pytell. *Sonderbeilage noos* 12.

Batthyány, A., & Guttmann, D. (2006). *Empirical research in logotherapy and meaning-oriented psychotherapy*. Zeig, Tucker & Theisen.

Berkley, G. (1993). *Hitler's gift: The story of Theresienstadt*. Branden Books.

Crumbaugh, J. C., & Maholick, L. T. (1964). An experimental study in existentialism: The psychometric approach to Frankl's concept of noögenic neurosis. *Journal of Clinical Psychology, 20*, 200–207.

Fabry, J. B. (1978). Aspects and prospects of logotherapy: A dialogue with Viktor Frankl. *The International Forum for Logotherapy, 1*, 3–6.

Frankl, V. E. (1923). Geistversportlichung. *Der Tag*, 4.3.1923.

[4] For a list of these institutes, see https://www.viktorfrankl.org/institutes_wwE.html

Frankl, V. E. (1924). Zur mimischen Bejahung und Verneinung. *Internationale Zeitschrift für Psychoanalyse, 10*, 437–438.
Frankl, V. E. (1925). Psychotherapie und Weltanschauung. Zur grundsätzlichen Kritik ihrer Beziehungen. *Internationale Zeitschrift für Individualpsychologie, III*, 250–252.
Frankl, V. E. (1926a). Zur Psychologie des Intellektualismus. *Internationale Zeitschrift für Individualpsychologie*, IX–XII.
Frankl, V. E. (1926b). Schafft Jugendberatungsstellen! *Die Mutter*, 31.8.1926.
Frankl, V. E. (1926c). Gründet Jugendberatungsstellen! *Der Abend*, 31.8.1926.
Frankl, V. E. (1927). Vom Sinn des Alltags. *Der Mensch im Alltag* Vol. I, Bd. 3, S. 3.
Frankl, V. E. (1930). Jugendberatung. In: *Enzyklopädisches Handbuch der Jugendfürsorge*. o.O.
Frankl, V. E. (1933). Wirtschaftskrise und Seelenleben vom Standpunkt des Jugendberaters. *Sozialärztliche Rundschau, 4*, 43–46.
Frankl, V. E. (1935a). Aus der Praxis der Jugendberatung. *Psychotherapeutische Praxis*, VII.
Frankl, V. E. (1935b). Kol nidre auf dem Steinhof. *Mitteilungsblatt der Vereinigung jüdischer Ärzte* II (1935), *22*, 6–7.
Frankl, V. E. (1938). Zur geistigen Problematik der Psychotherapie. *Zentralblatt für Psychotherapie, 10*, 33–75.
Frankl, V. E. (1939a). Zur medikamentösen Unterstützung der Psychotherapie bei Neurosen. *Schweizer Archiv für Neurologie und Psychiatrie, 43*, 26–31.
Frankl, V. E. (1939b). Philosophie und Psychotherapie. Zur Grundlegung einer Existenzanalyse. *Schweizerische Medizinische Wochenschrift, LXIX*, 707–709.
Frankl, V. E. (ca. 1940/1942). *Ärztliche Seelsorge*. Urfassung. Viktor Frankl Institut (unveröffentlicht).
Frankl, V. E. (1942). Pervitin intrazisternal. *Ars Medici (Schweiz), 32*(1), 58–60.
Frankl, V. E. (1946a). *Ärztliche Seelsorge. Grundlagen der Logotherapie und Existenzanalyse*. Deuticke.
Frankl, V. E. (1946b). *Ein Psycholog erlebt das Konzentrationslager*. Verlag für Jugend und Volk.
Frankl, V. E. (1947). *Die Psychotherapie in der Praxis*. Deuticke.
Frankl, V. E. (1949). Aus der Krankengeschichte des Zeitgeistes. *Wiener Universitäts-Zeitung*. I/7.
Frankl, V. E. (1965). Der Pluralismus der Wissenschaften und die Einheit des Menschen. In *Die Sechshundertjahrfeier der Universität Wien. Festbericht*. Selbstverlag der Universität Wien.
Frankl, V. E. (1985). *Psychotherapy and existentialism*. Washington Square Press. (Original work published 1967)
Frankl, V. E. (1993). *Theorie und Therapie der Neurosen*. Reinhardt bei UTB.
Frankl, V. E. (1994, October). *Erlebte Geschichte*. Lecture at the Community College, Leopoldstadt, Wien.
Frankl, V. E. (2000). *Recollections: An autobiography* (J. B. Fabry & J. Fabry, Trans.). Basic Books. (Original work published in German as *Was nicht in meinen Büchem steht*)
Frankl, V. E. (2002). *Was nicht in meinen Büchern steht. Lebenserinnerungen*. Beltz.
Frankl, V. E. (n.d.). *Announcement card from Frankl's lectures at Theresienstadt*. Unpublished material, Frankl Archives, Vienna.
Frankl, V. E., & Lapide, P. (2005). *Gottsuche und Sinnfrage. Ein Gespräch*. Gütersloher Verlagshaus.
Frankl, V. E., & Vesely-Frankl, G. (2005). *Frühe Schriften. Herausgegeben und kommentiert von Gabriele Vesely-Frankl*. Maudrich.
Guttmann, D. (1996). *Logotherapy for the helping professional. Meaningful social work*. Springer.
McHoskey, J. W., Betris, T., Worzel, W., Szyarto, C., Kelly, K., Eggert, T., et al. (1999). Relativism, nihilism, and quest. *Journal of Social Behavior and Personality, 14*(3), 445.
Moomal, Z. (1999). The relationship between meaning in life and mental well-being. *South African Journal of Psychology, 29*(1), 36–41.
Neugebauer, W. (1997). Wiener Psychiatrie und NS-Verbrechen. In: *Die Wiener Psychiatrie im 20. Jahrhundert*. Tagungsbericht, Institut für Wissenschaft und Kunst, 20./21. Juni 1997.
Robinson, D. N. (1985). *Philosophy of psychology*. Columbia University Press.

Robinson, D. N. (1995). *An intellectual history of psychology*. Wisconsin University Press.
Sanochemia. (n.d.). *Package insert for Myoscain*.
Soucek, W. (1948). Die Existenzanalyse Frankls, die dritte Richtung der Wiener Psychotherapeutischen Schule. *Deutsche Medizinische Wochenschrift, 73*, 594–595.
Stewart, J. W., Mercier, M. A., Quitkin, F. M., McGrath, P. J., Nunes, E., Young, J., et al. (1993). Demoralization predicts nonresponse to cognitive therapy in depressed outpatients. *Journal of Cognitive Psychotherapy, 7*(2), 105–116.
Testoni, I., & Zamperini, A. (1998). Nihilism, drug addiction and representation of death. *Giornale Italiano di Suicidologia, 8*(1), 13–21.
Vesely, F., & Fizzotti, E. (2005). *Internationale bibliographie der logotherapie und existenzanalyse*. Internationales Dokumentationszentrum für Logotherapie und Existenzanalyse. (www.viktorfrankl.org)
Wegner, D. (1989). *White bears and other unwanted thoughts: Suppression, obsession and the psychology of mental control*. Viking.
Wenzlaff, R. M., Wegner, D. M., & Roper, D. W. (1988). Depression and mental control: The resurgence of unwanted negative thoughts. *Journal of Personality and Social Psychology, 55*(6), 882–892.

Prof. Alexander Batthyány, PhD, holds the Chair of the Research Institute for Theoretical Psychology and Personalist Studies at Pázmány Péter Catholic University in Budapest, Hungary. Since 2012, Batthyány has served as Visiting Professor for Existential Psychotherapy at the Moscow University Institute of Psychoanalysis, Russia.

So Much to Learn: Keynote Address at the Third Future of Logotherapy World Congress, Vienna, Austria

Jay I. Levinson

Guten morgen meine damen und herren und willkommen sur Logotherapie Konference.

Unfortunately, that is the extent of my German. Dr. Batthyány, Elly and the Frankl family, and distinguished guests, when Dr. Batthyány first called me about the possibility of being the keynote speaker, he asked me if I believed in free speech. I said, "Well, of course, Alex, I'm an American, free speech is a tenet of our democracy." He said, "Good, because I have one that I want you to give." In truth, I was very moved by his request and truly consider it an honor to give this keynote address.

Logotherapy is not just a clinical treatment for mental illness. Rather, it is a philosophy of life combining common-sense brilliance, poignant humor, and an enduring message of hope and human potential. Though Dr. Frankl reserves a special respect for the many clinicians among us who help people deal with the challenges of both physical and mental health, his ideas also appeal to philosophers, theologians, educators, and the "person in the street," as they all struggle to find meanings and make a difference in the world. The transcultural quality of his work is unique to the field of psychology. This is proven by the 38 languages into which his work has been translated. His work has been translated into Japanese, Persian, Tagalog, Chinese, Korean, Swahili, all the Western Romance languages, and of course Spanish and English, to name a few. This is unique to the world of psychotherapy, where many prior theorists such as Freud and Adler have no relevance in some other cultures.

There are those, of course, who question Dr. Frankl's theories, worldview, optimism, and even his relevance in our field. But I can tell you one thing with absolute certainty, there is no question about the number of people worldwide, from every different culture, who benefit from his wisdom.

J. I. Levinson (✉)
Private Practice, Baltimore, MD, USA

C. L. McLafferty, Jr., J. I. Levinson (eds.), *Logotherapy and Existential Analysis*, Logotherapy and Existential Analysis: Proceedings of the Viktor Frankl Institute Vienna 2, https://doi.org/10.1007/978-3-031-48922-8_2

Forty years of clinical practice has left me with a humbling and healthy realization of just how little I know. The psychologist across the hall from my office in Baltimore, who does educational testing, hangs the following sign on his wall, "Hire a teenager while they still know everything." When I was a typical teenager, I was sure that I knew it all. When I graduated from college, I was certain that there was no more to learn. But as I earned my master's and doctoral degrees and began to practice therapy, I began to realize just how little I knew—despite the best efforts of some great teachers.

However, none compared to the experience of working with Dr. Frankl for over 20 years. He was, arguably, the greatest mind of the twentieth century and why he chose me I will never know. I will only say that it was an unbelievably challenging, enlightening, and humbling, once-in-a-lifetime experience. I cherished my time with Dr. Frankl and miss him tremendously.

Of course, I was never his personal or intellectual equal. I also know that I missed a lot of learning opportunities. But I am eternally grateful for the kindness and opportunities that I was given. Getting to know Dr. Frankl, both inside and outside of the classroom, was a gift beyond words. He was not only an intellectual giant, but a human being of the highest quality. In fact, Dr. Frankl would have been very unhappy with the part of this presentation that praises his contributions to mankind. He was a very private and humble man despite his fame. He resisted praise, only focusing on his desire to help his fellow human beings. However, I believe that credit is long overdue for his many unselfish contributions to humanity.

Recently, three events occurred that publicly reinforced Dr. Frankl's influence and relevance even today, 60 years after *Man's Search for Meaning* was first published. When Jimmy Fallon, a late-night television host in the United States, returned to his television show after suffering a very serious hand injury in an accident, he held up a copy of *Man's Search for Meaning* on national television to explain how he was able to cope with the pain, grow as a person, and return to his work. Shortly thereafter, on June 24, 2016, *The New York Times* (Crouse, 2016) published an interview with Michael Phelps, the record-breaking Olympian and Baltimore native, as he prepared for the forthcoming games in Rio de Janeiro. At one point, the reporter asked Mr. Phelps what turned his life around. After all, the reporter pointed out, he had transformed himself within the last year from a substance-abusing, undedicated, selfish teammate and person into a truly fine human being and very dedicated athlete. Phelps agreed with the reporter and even shared that he was in substance abuse and mental health treatment several times. He stated that during his last inpatient stay, he read three books that changed his life; *Man's Search for Meaning* was the first one that he named. At least partially due to their fame, and all the fine work done by logotherapists throughout the world, *Man's Search for Meaning* was the eighth bestselling book on Amazon.com in July 2016. This is an amazing 60 years after its first publication.

Before I share the rest of my presentation, I would like to offer a heartfelt disclaimer. I am not trying, as we say in English, "to toot my own horn," because I was fortunate enough to work for Dr. Frankl. Nor do I believe that I have mastered all the lessons that I will discuss today. Rather, I view these lessons as ongoing personal challenges. Since I am often asked how I met Dr. Frankl, what it was like to work with him, and what he was like as a person, I thought that today I would share some of my good fortune with you. As I share these reflections of a grateful student, I hope that you will find it useful in your own quest to make the world a better place.

Lesson 1: There Is No Substitute for Luck

I would rather be lucky than good. There is no substitute for luck. Although I usually make this comment when I make a lucky tennis shot, it applies to almost everything in life. Personally, I know that I have had my share of good luck, some of which I will share with you shortly. I am also aware that good luck alone is not enough to help us achieve our goals. Rather, we also need hard work, diligence, the right attitude, and opportunity. In fact, one must be lucky and good to succeed.

Perhaps the most luck any of us are blessed with is the luck of the genetic draw. It is so easy to take for granted all the blessings that come along with where we are born, including the parents we are born to and innate abilities. In addition, opportunities for education, multicultural exposure, resources to help us pursue our goals and survive illness and political trauma (such as a concentration camp) are also taken for granted. For example, in my case, I was initially a mediocre student. However, my mother was focused on the importance of education. I was actually 18 years old before I found out that one is not required to go to college. I thought it was mandatory, like high school (though high school is only mandatory in the United States until the age of 16 years). Due to my mother's focus on education, when I struggled as a high-school student and was asked "not to return" to my high school for my senior year, my family was fortunate enough to have the resources to send me to a private school. That school rekindled my focus and restored my confidence in my academic abilities. It was only then that I could pursue a higher education.

Sometimes luck is disguised as a challenging situation. Often, what appears as unlucky is an opportunity in disguise to deal with unavoidable suffering. Physical and mental illness, poverty, deaths of loved ones, and even racism, as Frankl reminds us by example, are opportunities to make us better people. Most Holocaust survivors agree that one had to be extraordinarily lucky to survive the random scepter of death in the concentration camps. Without such luck, perhaps none of us would be here today celebrating the work of Dr. Frankl. So appreciate how fortunate you are and the blessings you have been given, and of course, give back to the world.

Lesson 2: Embrace the Journey

One never knows what the future holds. We plan, study, save our money, set goals, etc., but life often has a way of messing with us. I have a t-shirt that says, "Life is what happens after you make your plans."

As I said earlier, I am often asked how I got to know Dr. Frankl. In order to reinforce this particular lesson of embracing one's journey, I thought this would be the appropriate time to share my story. In past presentations, I have always limited my talks to the more academic aspects of logotherapy.

When my father, with whom I worked in our family business and to whom I was very close, died in 1974 of his first heart attack at the age of 49 years, I was devastated. He was my hero, my role model, and the person who tried to teach me to be a mensch. "Mensch" in this case is not German, but a Yiddish word that is used to describe the right kind of man. My family and I could not imagine life without him when he died. I was working for my father at the time, along with his brother and two cousins, who were his partners. As a result of his death and my overwhelming grief, as my daughter's kindergarten teacher might say, I did not "work and play well with others." My relationships with my new partners deteriorated to the point that I found life with them unbearable. As a result, I decided to change professions. It was not an easy decision for me due to the security and money that I would have to give up. There would also be potential family consequences because I was the only one to leave the family business in 115 years. In fact, it did cause a rift in our family.

When I was accepted to graduate school for my doctorate at United States International University (USIU) in San Diego, I had already completed my master's degree (MS) at Johns Hopkins University. I had never really heard of this small and progressive school until someone gave me a book for my birthday written by one of its faculty members. Though small and unknown, the faculty was superb. It included Viktor Frankl, Carl Rogers, Rollo May, Everett Shostrom, Max Lerner, and other greats in our field. It was also fully accredited and would provide me with the necessary requisites to apply for a psychology license when I completed the program.

When I arrived to register for my classes, I was told that, due to the fact that my master's degree was in education, I had to earn a master's degree in psychology. This was upsetting since I had visited the school just 3 months prior and talked with the registrar. The registrar had never mentioned to me that I would have to make up a master's degree. Nevertheless, the counselor was adamant, I would not be allowed to begin the doctoral program until I finished an MS in psychology.

As an older student, at 30 years old, with a lot of business and life experience, and with my usual stubbornness, I decided to speak with a supervisor. When I asked for a supervisor, I was informed that I was speaking to the head counselor. I asked him to whom I should appeal his decision, and was told no one. I then sarcastically asked him if he was the President of the university. He then referred me to the Dean of the School of Human Behavior, Dr. W. Ray Rucker.

I had to wait 7 hours to see Dr. Rucker. As one might imagine, the day before school started there were many students who had questions, concerns, and complaints that had to be addressed. I returned at the appointed time and was shown into Dr. Rucker's office. Dr. Rucker was Harvard trained with a doctorate in education, so I figured he would be a stickler for rules. As we spoke, however, he turned out to be a wonderful human being. The conversation started with me arguing like a lawyer about my acceptance letter being a "contract" to enter the doctoral program. In fact, I had only one semester of law school behind me, but that empowered me to give him a hard time for several minutes. He listened patiently and then asked a few questions. He then began to look at my transcript from my master's program in education at Johns Hopkins University.

Suddenly, he started to write on it, and my anticipatory anxiety told me he was documenting why he was going to ask me to leave the program. I began to have flashbacks about my problems in high school. A few minutes later, he informed me that he was quite familiar with the Johns Hopkins University program and knew that it was one that allowed me to take virtually all of the academic requirements for a master's in psychology through the school of education. He then showed me he had scratched out the education prefixes on my transcript and replaced them with a "PSY" prefix, allowing me to enter the doctoral program. The only caveat was that I had to make up one class. I quickly thanked him, and he walked me out of his office. I was certain that he had had quite enough of me.

As we walked out the door, his secretary was on the phone. She turned to him and told him that his graduate assistant had a family problem and he needed to take this semester off from school at the last minute. It was the end of the day and classes were starting the next day. The office was empty and the rest of the staff and students had gone home. Dr. Rucker, thinking out loud said, "What will I do for a graduate assistant?" Though I had given him a very hard time, and with all the courage that I could muster, I said, "I could really use the money," and I promised to work hard for him. I then asked for the job. He shrugged his shoulders, looked around the empty office, and hired me.

Interestingly, a few weeks later I had another dilemma. I was admitted off the waiting list to a different, more prestigious university. I asked the caller to give me 24 hours to decide whether I would go there or stay at USIU. Since I had a nice apartment, a job, liked the school, and loved San Diego, I turned the other school down and stayed at USIU, a fortuitous decision.

I worked hard for Dr. Rucker that first semester. At the end of the semester, we met to go over grades, etc. Afterward, he reminded me that he was not teaching a course the next semester and asked me if I had found another professor to work for. I told him that I had not yet had time. He asked me if I knew that Dr. Frankl was coming to teach his course on logotherapy the next semester. I said that I did, in fact, know and had registered for his course. He then asked me why I didn't apply to be Dr. Frankl's graduate assistant. I told him I didn't think I was qualified. I had heard that there were dozens of applicants for the job, all of them third- and fourth-year students. He then said the words that changed my life forever, "I think Dr. Frankl would really like you" and offered me the job. That took a while to sink into my brain, and for the first time in my life I was speechless. But when he asked again, I eagerly accepted.

At the end of that first semester with Dr. Frankl, he asked me to be his assistant the following year, when he returned to teach his course. I was delighted. At the end of that second year, Dr. Frankl knew that I was going back to Baltimore to do my residency and write my dissertation. He asked me if he could call upon me from time to time for whatever assistance he might need in the United States. This was before personal computers and email would have made my services irrelevant. I gladly accepted and thus began a fulfilling 21-year relationship with him and a wonderful 40-plus year relationship with his family.

I never really knew why I was chosen by either Dr. Rucker or Dr. Frankl. Of course, I knew that I was a driven perfectionist having come from a whole family of them. I also suspected that Dr. Rucker felt that being Jewish would be a plus for Dr. Frankl, though I doubt that it mattered to him. I was just immensely grateful to continue my relationship with Dr. Frankl. It was then that I first learned to embrace my journey and appreciate my good fortune.

I also learned from that experience that Dr. Frankl was right about another aspect of one's journey. One never knows where one's path is leading and it's the process, not the outcome, that counts. We must learn from our experiences, good and bad, personal and professional, and, as George Santayana (1905) once said, "Those who cannot remember the past are doomed to repeat it" (p. 284).

So be your authentic self, be self-accepting, warts and all. Know your strengths and weaknesses. Build on your strengths and grow from your failures. We all fail at something and most of us learn from the hardest lessons. Embrace your journey!

Lesson 3: Discover the Meanings

Any discussion on Frankl and learning must, of course, include his most fundamental concept: Life unconditionally holds meaning under any and all circumstances. It is a lesson obvious to all of us here today. As I stated earlier, logotherapy is not just a clinical theory but a philosophy of life. Finding true meaning is not about money, power, and/or pleasure. It is about discovering the myriad of potential meanings available to us in any situation. Dr. Frankl (1973) told us "We must accept our destiny as we accept the ground on which we stand, the ground which is the springboard for our freedom" (p. 75). In other words, he encouraged people to accept their reality and use their challenging life situations to grow beyond themselves, to transcend their predicaments and empower themselves to find reasons to be resilient and find their inner strength when life overwhelms them.

In the concentration camps, Dr. Frankl often reminded himself of his own reasons to survive the unbelievable suffering of this great human tragedy. When I asked, he said he had four meanings. First, he wanted to see his family again. He wanted to see his parents until he heard that they had died, his siblings and, of course, his beloved first wife, Tilly. Second, he wanted to reconstruct the manuscript of his life's work, *The Doctor and the Soul*, which had been ripped away from him when he entered the camps. Perhaps some of you have been fortunate enough to see the pictures of his notes, scribbled on folded scraps of paper stolen by those who worked in the concentration camp administrative offices, and hidden between the boards of the various huts in which he lived in the concentration camps. He hoped that they would survive, even if he did not. Third, Dr. Frankl wanted to return to climb the beautiful Rax Mountains again. This was a place of peace, physical and mental challenge, and sheer beauty, a place that nurtured his soul. And finally, while in the camps, he found tremendous meaning in risking his own life to help other inmates using his logotherapeutic principles in the hope that he might alleviate some of their suffering under those horrendous conditions. However, he knew full well that every time he snuck out of his hut to help others, he was subject to immediate execution. But his commitment to serving his fellow man was more meaningful to him than the value of his own life.

Many of us use these principles for personal growth and many other meaningful causes that change mankind for the better. People like Nelson Mandela and Gandhi come immediately to mind. When one reads their biographies, it is certainly clear that they embraced a logotherapeutic philosophy, though they may not have learned them from Frankl. Others such as Jerry Long, with whom I am sure most of you are familiar, and who Dr. Frankl often referred to as a living example of logotherapy lived, clearly started their journey was directly influenced by Frankl. As Dr. Frankl often reminded us, "It is not what we expect from life, but what life expects from us." This is a mandate that years later was reinforced by the great United States President John Fitzgerald Kennedy (1961) when he said, "Ask not what your country can do for you, ask what you can do for your country."

Of course, not all meanings available to us have such a grand influence. Many sources of meaning are very personal to those involved. But they are part of the myriad of meanings available to us in any situation. They, too, are just as meaningful to those who discover them.

In clinical use, helping patients to discover meaning in their lives is key to their therapy and motivation, as well helping them transcend their symptoms and challenges. As therapists, we don't just chip away at a patient's unhealthy defenses. After all, they have a function, that is, to "protect" the patient by helping them cope with their problems, albeit in an unhealthy way. People often adopt whatever defenses are available to them to protect themselves. Sometimes they are overly aggressive or too passive, which turns challenges into burdens. As logotherapists, we do help them give up their dysfunctional coping styles. But, more importantly, we encourage them to go toward something meaningful so they can transcend their problematic patterns. It is a daunting task to give up one's internalized dysfunctional coping styles without something better to aspire to. Just ask Michael Phelps.

In a recent article in *The Baltimore Sun* (Santora, August 19, 2016), my hometown newspaper, the writer was praising a new program to reduce the large percentage of welfare recipients in our city. The key to the success of the program was teaching these food stamp recipients job skills. Then they could make a decent living and support their families. In the past, many of them said they did not even try to get off welfare because the minimum wage jobs that were available to them did not even cover the cost of childcare, transportation, etc. So why work when there wasn't anything to gain? This new program offered them a way out of poverty.

In other programs, such as at the University of Mississippi, logotherapy colleagues, such as Rosemary Henrion, James Crumbaugh, and Stefan Schulenberg, have done amazing work with individuals who abuse substances, tremendously increasing long-term abstinence rates. As many of us were privileged to hear at the

2014 Future of Logotherapy conference, Dr. Breitbart's use of a logotherapy-based program at Sloan Kettering Memorial Hospital in New York greatly enhanced the quality of life of those undergoing cancer treatment.

From my own work, treating people who survive the death of loved ones, especially grieving parents, helping them discover the meanings available to them and motivating them to rebuild their lives after this devastating life event is of paramount importance.

Lastly in this section, I remind you that Frankl (2000) said that happiness is a by-product of leading a meaningful life. It is not something that one can pursue directly. We all know that money, drugs, and power do not equate with life satisfaction. In fact, in a recent article in the *APA Monitor* ("By the numbers," July/August 2016), a researcher for the World Happiness Report, in a study conducted by Gallop for the Sustainable Development Solutions Network, found that the mean "happiness level" in the world is a 5.43 on a scale of 10. They listed the following variables as significant to facilitating happiness: GNP per capita (not wealth, but national productivity), health, perceptions of conditions (attitudes), social support (relationships), freedom to make life choices, and generosity (what we give to others). Certainly, almost all of these are grounded in logotherapeutic philosophy.

Lesson 4: Don't Worship Money

This first-world problem haunts wealthier societies. As we discussed earlier, the addiction to compulsive consumerism does not buy happiness. My private practice is in a wealthy suburb of Baltimore, yet so many of my patients suffer from an existential vacuum and low quality of life.

Those companies that manufacture products that further the feeding frenzy of modern consumerism often do so at the expense of their personal, societal, and political consciences. They exploit third-world workers and have little regard for the greater good. Pope Francis, in a recent address in Poland, "decried a modern escapism into consumerism and computers that isolate people" ("Pope Francis to world's youth," July 30, 2016). Instead, he encouraged us to focus our energies on the greater good.

The number of handgun murders committed each year in my home state of Maryland, with approximately 2 million residents, far exceeds the number of nonterrorist-related murders in Japan, Austria, Israel, and England combined. In these countries, gun control is strictly regulated. Yet, in the United States, where "cash is king," we continue to encourage production and international sales of guns. This is not a constitutional issue, as gun advocates argue. The United States Constitution never intended for every citizen to carry a gun for public safety. Its intention was to allow defense forces to be formed to protect the country against imperial British rule. In reality, this is an infamous example of pure greed meant to maximize profits for people who value money over common sense and human life.

As a final example of how money does not equate with quality of life, let's look at the week of September 2, 1997, the week of Dr. Frankl's death. That same week, two other well-known people died: Princess Diana and Mother Teresa. Princess Diana had all the wealth and influence that money could buy. Yet, she was a tragically unhappy figure who never discovered the meanings available to her. On the other hand, Mother Teresa, a nun who lived in abject poverty, found great satisfaction in life administering to the sick and downtrodden in her world, for which she was recently canonized. And, of course, our own Dr. Frankl was never concerned with money and material things. Rather he was always focused on healing and teaching others to heal. He travelled the world to address audiences he deemed worthy, sometimes without even earning an honorarium for his efforts. It is also widely known that the first edition of *Man's Search for Meaning* was published anonymously because he did not believe that he should benefit from any fame or fortune that might come his way when his true purpose was just to help those who were suffering after the war. What is less widely known is the paltry sum he received for the English rights to *Man's Search for Meaning*. When I found out, I was appalled at how he had been cheated. In fact, I told him that I thought he was taken advantage of and that I knew lawyers in the United States who could reopen negotiations with Simon and Schuster to get him a fair price for a book that has sold approximately 16 million copies in English to date. He looked confused by what I was saying and began to wave his hand at me and said, "Nein, nein, nein, I'll hear no more about this." That was the end of my efforts to get him a fair settlement for this brilliant and influential work.

Lesson 5: Be a Sponge (to a Mentor)

The Talmudic scholar Gambliel once said, "Find for yourself a mentor," sage advice. However, in my personal experience, it is more likely that a mentor will find you. Our job, as students in need, is to take advantage of the opportunities that come our way. Throughout the years, I have been fortunate enough to meet some amazing people, many of whom I consider to be secondary mentors to me. People such as Elisabeth Kübler-Ross, Harold Kushner, and Jerry Long have all given generously of their time and energy to help me. I am, and will always be, grateful beyond words for their kindness.

When asked, I tell students two things: (1) absorb everything your teachers do, on and off the "playing field"; and (2) God gave us two ears, two eyes and one mouth, use them in that proportion. Pay close attention in the classroom, but observe just as closely how they conduct their daily lives. How do your teachers treat their family, strangers, subordinates, and those in authority? What are their passions, hobbies, strengths, and weaknesses? How do they face adversity and deal with difficult people?

Working with Dr. Frankl was a once-in-a-lifetime experience. He was both a genius and an exemplary human being. He often thought in paradigms and models that had never been explored, and he had an uncanny ability to see many sides of issues and integrate them into his ideas. However, what made him so outstanding as a mentor was his desire to pass on his knowledge. He was open with me about so many things, which was somewhat contrary to his very humble and private nature. I was not only accepted into his academic life, but into some of his home life as well. He was clearly committed to my development, in much the same way as I was determined to learn from him and help him in any way I could.

Dr. Frankl was extremely patient with me when I did not understand something, or when I asked endless questions about something we had discussed, violating my own rule about listening twice as much as talking. In truth, this was never my strongest quality. He also accepted and forgave my shortcomings even when I did not. Once, when I was consumed with self-doubt over my lack of publications, and was certain that he was disappointed that I chose to emphasize clinical work over writing, I told him this. He reassured me and encouraged me to do what my heart prescribed. This, of course, inspired me to write a little more.

I was also in awe of his ability to balance his professional and personal life. Dr. Frankl not only wrote about the three ways to discover meaning, but lived them. While he wrote prolifically and traveled the world teaching and practicing psychiatry, he somehow found time to make his family a priority. No two people were more dedicated to each other than Viktor and Elly Frankl.

Elly was truly "the woman behind the great man," an American expression that recognizes that no man becomes great without a loving and committed spouse. She was his caretaker, secretary, conscience, confidant, colleague, and best friend. Without her, his life would have been very different. She is a kind, loving, humble, and brilliant person in her own right.

Her importance to Dr. Frankl cannot be overstated. He expressed it best himself when he inscribed a copy of the book *Homo Patiens* to her, which she discovered only after he died. It read, "For Elly, who succeeded in changing a suffering man into a loving man. Viktor." In fact, one of the proudest moments of his life was when Dr. Hadden Klingberg, without telling Elly, had arranged for her to be awarded an honorary doctorate recognizing her extraordinary contributions to Dr. Frankl, logotherapy, and humankind.

If it takes a village to raise a child, it takes a loving family to make a great man. His love and commitment to his daughter, Gabi, son-in-law Franz, and grandchildren Alex and Katia was unwavering, as was their dedication to him. He was a tremendous role model as a family man, one from whom I learned so much. Clearly, Elly, I also consider you a mentor, as well as a friend, and I will forever be in your debt.

Perhaps the best advice Dr. Frankl ever gave me was when I visited him shortly before his death. I had traveled to Vienna to help him complete his last book, *Man's Search for Ultimate Meaning*. Due to his failing eyesight and his desire to "Americanize" his writing, he had asked me to help edit the manuscript. This was the highest compliment that he ever bestowed on me. After we finished our work, I stopped by his home before leaving Vienna. I suspected it would be the last time I'd see him. I asked for some private time and tearfully told him how much he meant to me and how much I valued our relationship. When I finished, he got up and wrote a brief letter to me. It said the following: "When one enters a helping profession such as psychology, one should set before himself a three-fold goal: 1. Be a psychologist. 2. Be a good psychologist. 3. Remain a human being." Those words still hang on my office wall as a profound reminder to me always.

Albert Schweitzer (cited in Burke & Tumbleson, 2019) once said, "Sometimes our light goes out, but is blown again into instant flame by an encounter with another human being. Each of us owes the deepest thanks to those who have rekindled this inner light" (p. 1). So cherish your mentors, then be one for others!

Lesson 6: Work Hard

There is no substitute for hard work. As I said earlier, I was raised by a family of compulsive, perfectionistic workaholics, so I was never afraid of hard work. Work hard, study hard, and most importantly learn hard. In Judaism, when Jewish youth study to become rabbis, they do not say that they are "studying." Rather, as they discuss things with their mentors and teachers, they say they are "learning." The difference is subtle, but reflects a tremendous commitment to what they are doing. Expect a lot from others and seek your potential, a fundamental tenet of logotherapy.

Dr. Frankl himself kept an exceptionally busy schedule teaching, writing prolifically, and lecturing all over the world. I once shared with him that I sometimes had so much to do that I didn't know where to start. His response? "Do your most unpleasant task first and the rest of the day will be easier." This solid advice has become part of my routine.

As I mentioned a few minutes ago, Dr. Frankl was a superb role model at balancing his work and family life, another important lesson. It is ever true: "Nobody ever died wishing they had spent more time at the office."

Lesson 7: One Size Does Not Fit All

Dr. Frankl was the first eclectic therapist, at least to admit it! Modestly, he said he used logotherapy with just 20% of patients. In my almost 40 years of clinical practice, I find I use logotherapy with virtually 100% of my patients. That is not to say that I use logotherapy exclusively in these situations, but as part of what I do. Like Dr. Frankl, I have no loyalty to one school of thought or one set of techniques. Rather, I consider everything I know that I think might help the patient. I then combine them with everything the patient knows to facilitate a good outcome.

In fact, Frankl (1969) put it quite succinctly with the following equation:

$$\Psi = X + Y\left(\text{p.}163\right).$$

In this equation, X is what the patient knows, notice that that comes first. Y is everything the therapist knows, and Ψ is the optimum outcome. Clearly, only when both patient and therapist work together, with an open mind, can they achieve a synergic relationship and realize therapeutic goals.

That said, I obviously have great respect for logotherapy. I find it motivational for virtually all the patients I see. Many patients have difficulty accepting their need for help as well as finding reasons to face the challenges necessary for a successful therapy. In reading and discussing the messages of *Man's Search for Meaning*, they can often then engage in a more productive therapy.

Of course, certain therapeutic issues respond particularly well to logotherapy. Those dealing with the unavoidable suffering of chronic and/or life-threatening illnesses, death of loved ones, and toxic life situations benefit greatly from the lessons of logotherapy.

It is also paramount to remember that the "techniques" of logotherapy (or for that matter the techniques of any therapy) are but a small part of a successful treatment. As Frankl emphasized, there is absolutely no substitute for the truly human connection between patient and therapist. All the techniques in the world do not replace a sympathetic understanding of the human beings we aspire to help. This is what connects with patients, helps them trust us, and creates a safe environment in which they can do their difficult and challenging therapeutic work.

When I do clinical supervision with students who wish to learn about working with terminally ill patients, or those grieving the death of loved ones, I often find myself helping them unlearn some of the rigid teachings of graduate school. I teach them that one should not always avoid countertransference. Rather, there are many times when it has tremendous therapeutic value. For example, in my opinion, a therapist who does not get teary-eyed hearing the stories and suffering of grieving parents will be of little therapeutic value.

Today we see the foundations of modern psychotherapy in much of Frankl's writings. Socratic dialogue, paradoxical intention, dereflection, and other aspects of logotherapy obviously led to some of the modern schools of therapy, such as cognitive therapy, behavior therapy, mindfulness, positive psychology, etc. One need only read some of the wonderful work by many of our logotherapeutic colleagues such as Paul Wong, Elizabeth Lukas, Bianca Hirsch, Matti Ameli, Teria Shantall, etc., to see the connection. This is diametrically opposed to what many early (and even later) theorists taught.

Freud clearly said that any deviation from his prescribed methods of psychoanalysis were unacceptable. In fact, Freud also once said that if one, as an analyst, could not figure out a proper interpretation of a patient's dreams, thoughts, or behavior, that analyst should ask his analyst. If his analyst didn't know, he should then ask his analyst, and so forth until the chain of authority went back to Freud himself. Freud would then make the correct interpretation!

Though I have great respect for Freud and his pioneering efforts in psychotherapy, it is clear to me that in this regard his ego has confused his judgment. No one is the ultimate authority on everything.

Albert Ellis, the father of rational-emotive therapy, was well known for his huge ego and adherence to rigid techniques. His often-inappropriate rants directed at anyone who disagreed with his ideas are legendary. As a graduate student at the United States International University, I saw Ellis debate Sidney Smith, from the Menninger Clinic, a psychoanalytically oriented, world-famous treatment facility. After Smith did his 20-minute presentation, Ellis got up and said, "Are you going to believe that bullshit? If you listen to that, you'll know nothing and never be able to help patients." He then stormed out of the room, so the audience then listened to Smith's rebuttal. A few minutes later, Ellis came back into the room, cursed again about the irrelevance of Smith's theories, and said, "I have a plane to catch" and left the room. In this example, he deprived many people of the valuable lessons he had the potential to teach us. His message was lost due to his poor style.

On a broader scale, the intolerance of so many violent political and religious groups has plagued civilization throughout history. It is like the bumper sticker that says, "Why can't we all just get along?"

One last thought regarding the idea that one size does not fit all. When I was trained as a psychologist, there was tremendous bias against the use of medication for many illnesses. Of course, everyone recognized the importance of medication for the severely mentally ill, i.e., schizophrenia, severe bipolar disease, and other psychoses. But as nonprescribers, the emphasis in training psychologists was on psychotherapeutic interventions. On the other hand, in many modern psychiatry residency programs, there is far too much emphasis on medication as a cure-all. In fact, most researchers agree that it is the combination of medication and psychotherapy that is most effective in treating most mental illness.

So be open minded, listen to your patients, and remember that one way of thinking does not work for everyone. Or, as I like to say, one size does not fit all.

Lesson 8: Challenge the Status Quo

In a world full of misfortune, injustice, and many other challenges, it is precisely these challenges that hold the potential for a meaningful life. If not for pioneers like Sigmund Freud, Elisabeth Kübler-Ross, Albert Ellis, and, of course, Viktor Frankl, modern psychology would be much different. Their courage to challenge the traditional thinking of their time opened the door to contemporary treatment. Without their creativity and courage, our ability to help others would be significantly limited.

In addition, the many brave people who trust us to be their therapists, and help them challenge the way they think, are perhaps the bravest of all. Most of you know the story of Jerry Long (1982) and his dogged determination to challenge and transcend the limitations of his physical body. He tried to become a role model and healer, which led to Frankl calling him the "living embodiment of logotherapy," perhaps the highest of compliments. So, ask lots of questions, don't stop advocating for your ideas, and respect others' points of view. In my work with Frankl, I was so grateful for his limitless patience and tolerance for my inquiries, something I cherish to this very day and try to do for others.

Lesson 9: Degurufy Logotherapy: Do Creative Research and Help Others

Viktor Frankl always encouraged people to build on his work. He would often deflect those who tried to make him the guru, not only of logotherapy, but of all things therapeutic, by asking others what they thought. He understood the challenges of measuring existential concepts and encouraged others to find empirical answers. People such as James Crumbaugh, Elisabeth Lukas, and other early pioneers were very special to him.

In fact, his often-stated mantra to "degurufy logotherapy" (Frankl, 1969) was a tenet of his personal and professional philosophy; he wanted others to find answers beyond his own writings through creative and critical thinking (p. 158ff). He truly valued the many books, articles, and dissertations building on his work. He kept them in his archives as cherished keepsakes. In fact, one of the most meaningful moments of his life was when the American Psychological Association recognized the importance of logotherapy and accredited the U.S. Viktor Frankl Institute of Logotherapy as an American Psychological Association-approved provider of research and continuing education.

I am certain that he would agree completely with Pope Francis (July 30, 2016), who, while dedicating a shrine to Pope John Paul II in Poland said, "Dear young people, we didn't come into this world to vegetate, take it easy, to make our lives a comfortable sofa to fall asleep on. No, we came for another reason, to leave a mark."

If Dr. Frankl were here today to witness this wonderful conference, dedicated not only to advancing his work but also to the general welfare of humankind, he would be extremely pleased. What better legacy to this great man?

Lesson 10: Be Humble

For me, this has always been a challenging lesson. Though as I said earlier, the more I studied and the more experience I gained, the less I realized I know. The upside of realizing my limitations is that it has inspired a lifelong thirst for more knowledge.

One of the first things I understood as I began working as a graduate assistant is that the best way to gain knowledge was to do to whatever my teachers needed me to do, whether it was grading papers, monitoring exams, or setting up the classroom. My goal was to make myself a valuable team member. No job was too small and that philosophy often led to opportunities of much greater significance. When I first started working for Dr. Frankl, there were many small tasks that I provided, whether it was picking him up at the airport, carrying his classroom materials, or bringing him the many cups of coffee he drank when he traveled; no job was too small. I also sent things to him that were not available at the time in Vienna; for example, I mailed him his favorite breakfast cereal, Post Raisin Bran. I never classified these tasks as unimportant. For me, they were ways to make him more comfortable to do his very important work. I also saw them as ways to demonstrate my abilities and earn his trust, hoping that when the need arose on more important matters, he would see me as a resource.

I was rewarded for my efforts as I progressed from graduate assistant to trusted colleague and friend. When, due to his failing eyesight, he asked me to edit his last book, *Man's Search for Ultimate Meaning*, I felt extremely honored. Even so, I was once again reminded of the inequality of our knowledge as our editorial discussions progressed. It was humbling to learn that most of my suggested edits were due to my lack of understanding of his theses and that his command of written English was better than mine!

As I spent more and more time working with Dr. Frankl, I also noticed how little he was concerned with the many accolades he received. He was never interested in credit or praise for his work, just that it helped others. Frankl (1973) often described himself with a quote from the German philosopher Stekel who said that even "a dwarf standing on the shoulders of a giant can see farther than the giant himself" (p. 3). He truly believed that he was that dwarf, building on the work of the giants who came before him; we all know that, he too, was a giant in his own right.

If I needed any more proof of his humility, I observed it again on a visit to Vienna. I had recently revised his vita because I had been contacted by a group of people who were putting his name in nomination for a Nobel Prize. I had to do this without his knowledge because the nominating process does not allow the nominee to know he is being nominated until he actually receives an official nomination. So I told him that I was preparing the vita for a group who was going to sponsor a lecture he was scheduled to give in the United States. I said they needed the material to get continuing education credits for their members.

As I put together the section of the vita describing the many awards and honors he received, I was amazed by the number of very high-level awards and honors that had been bestowed on him. As we were chatting one day toward the end of my visit to Vienna, it struck me that none of these awards were displayed in his office or apartment. I asked him about this, so he led me to a closet in the apartment and opened it. There on the walls of the closet, and on temporary steel shelving, were stacks and stacks of awards and honors. Since I displayed all my degrees and the few awards that I had received proudly on my office walls, I wondered out loud why he did not. With a wave of his hand, he dismissed the thought of displaying his accolades as irrelevant to the true purpose of his work.

Another time, when we were riding in a taxi to a presentation that he was about to give in San Jose, California, I was vaguely aware that he was having a conversation with the taxi driver. I paid little attention as we rode, enjoying the scenery. When we arrived at our destination, he excitedly explained how much he had learned from the driver, a man of very limited education. It once again reminded me of how much more I had to learn from him.

Dr. Frankl adamantly respected the rights of others to express their opinions. The only caveat was that they be socially responsible. This was true even if their views disparaged him personally. He never defended himself against his critics, even if he found it hurtful, stating they were entitled to their opinions. He focused only on offering his own views and trusted people to decide for themselves. He lived by a philosophy best expressed by Benjamin Franklin who once advised us that we should doubt our own infallibility.

A few years after his death, an article was published by a somewhat sociopathic professor of history in Florida. It accused Dr. Frankl of being a collaborator with the Nazis. The article said that Dr. Frankl abused his fellow concentration camp inmates by using them for horrible medical experiments on behalf of the Nazis.

When this article was brought to my attention, I was outraged. Not only were these allegations preposterous, but they were contrary to the compassion he demonstrated in the camps by risking his own life to administer to the emotional needs of his fellow prisoners. I knew I had to write a response to these absurd allegations. I simply could not allow this kind of injustice. I also knew that if I told Elly and his family of my intention to write a rebuttal, they would, like Dr. Frankl, not allow it. And I would never have done something that they directly forbade me to do. Therefore, I wrote my response to these terrible accusations, and it was published by the same journal a few months later. Only then did I tell Elly what I had done.

Dr. Frankl also humbly understood that it was the patient who did the most important work in therapy, not the therapist. He knew that restructuring their worldview, and asking them to give up their unhealthy and protective defenses, required courage and hard work. Change is always hard. He knew that it was a privilege to help others heal and that what they needed from the therapist was hope, guidance, and a truly human encounter.

Dr. Frankl also knew that his ideas were useless unless they could be understood by "the person in the street." He was dedicated to the idea that complex and sophisticated ideas must be understood by those who need them most, the average person. He did not feel these things should be limited to the ivory towers of academia. Of course, he also wrote many things that were challenging for even the most learned of people, but this did not deter him from his commitment to the "person in the street."

In addition to those examples, Dr. Frankl displayed his humility in his interactions with others. He was welcoming and charming when meeting new people. He accepted their inquiries graciously and was appreciative of their interest. And, he was always so grateful to me for any little thing I did for him, making me even more eager to be of service.

Lesson 11: Have a Sense of Humor

How many psychologists does it take to change a light bulb? Answer: Just one, but it really has to want to change. Dr. Frankl was the first therapist to incorporate humor into psychotherapy. His use of paradoxical intention, Socratic dialogue, and asking patients questions whose answers turned out to be humorous is well documented. Dr. Frankl knew that if patients could see the humor in their circumstances and laugh at themselves, they could transcend their symptoms. It also helped patients to accept themselves and their strengths and weaknesses and to put negative traits and behaviors into perspective. This allowed them to dereflect negative self-judgment, maintain self-esteem, and fulfill their potential meanings.

In my own patients, I have seen how an individual's superego is often their own worst enemy. Patients who set standards ridiculously high evoke nothing but self-dissatisfaction. This occurs even in the most accomplished and respected people. People who see anything less than perfection as failure get stuck in the paralysis of anticipatory anxiety, leading to low self-worth and depriving themselves and the world of their goodness. The French philosopher Voltaire (1772) once said, "Le mieux est l'ennemi du bien" (The perfect is the enemy of the good, p. 50), meaning that good behavior is often overlooked when the focus is on perfection as the only acceptable standard. A healthy sense of humor encourages people to not take themselves and their failures too seriously, allowing them to learn from their mistakes and fulfill the potentials and meanings available to them.

Having a sense of humor about others is also very important. Everyone has certain personality traits that are challenging for others to deal with. For example, if someone is continuously dealing with a critical parent, boss, or colleague, the use of paradoxical intention can be very comforting. Anticipating and even counting critical remarks, telling oneself that perhaps this time their parent may establish a personal record for the number of critical remarks they will make, is a great way to prepare oneself for a forthcoming encounter. And of course, one must have a sense of humor about a world that inevitably throws challenge after challenge our way. One can be overwhelmed by these challenges or transcend them through the use of humor as one of their attitudinal values.

Prior to Frankl legitimizing humor as an acceptable therapeutic tool, humor was interpreted by Freud and others as an unhealthy defense against the painful work of psychotherapy. However, both Freud and Frankl were correct. Freud, who by all accounts did not have much of a sense of humor, missed its transcendent healing value. Often people need to protect themselves from the rigors of an intensive therapy like psychoanalysis and ease into painful insights before they are ready to take on the difficult work of change. They need to be able to laugh at their struggles and see them as opportunities to grow.

Dr. Frankl's own sense of humor is well documented. He loved puns, paradoxes, and being silly when it was called for. If you've seen the film, "Viktor and I," by his grandson Alexander Vesely, you've seen his playfulness with his grandchildren when they were young as he played with sock puppets or talked to them with his feet. This demonstrates his own ability to enjoy humor as a meaningful experience and as a way to connect with others.

So have fun, don't take yourself too seriously, and recognize and make time for the joys of life.

Lesson 12: Talk with Others

There is no substitute for direct, in-person conversation. Good communication is defined as communication that fosters understanding in an effective manner. That does not mean that we always get our way. It means that we gain a deeper understanding of another person. Hopefully, this will also lead to resolution of difficult issues, whether it leads to agreement, agreeing to disagree, or is the basis for further dialogue.

I would like to share with you a communication model that I developed for my patients to help them become more effective communicators (Fig. 1).

When teaching communication, I often use a quote often attributed to Henry James: "Three things in human life are important: the first is to be kind. The second is to be kind. And the third is to be kind." A good process goes a long way toward achieving synergic relationships.

In the above picture, we see the four possible kinds of communication. *Good positive communication* is fairly easy to understand. One says something that people want to hear, the positive content, in a nice way, a good process. In *bad negative communication*, one says something people don't want to hear, negative content, in a poor process. Those two are relatively easy to understand. *Bad positive communication* is a little more difficult to understand. If fact, bad positive communication is telling another person something they may want to hear, positive content, but in a bad way. This is most often manifested as sarcasm, or as a "left-handed compliment." It is *good negative communication* that is the true art in both psychotherapy and life. In this form of communication, one communicates something that another might not want to hear: negative content in a good process. This will allow the person to hear the feedback in a productive way and make choices for the future about their behavior.

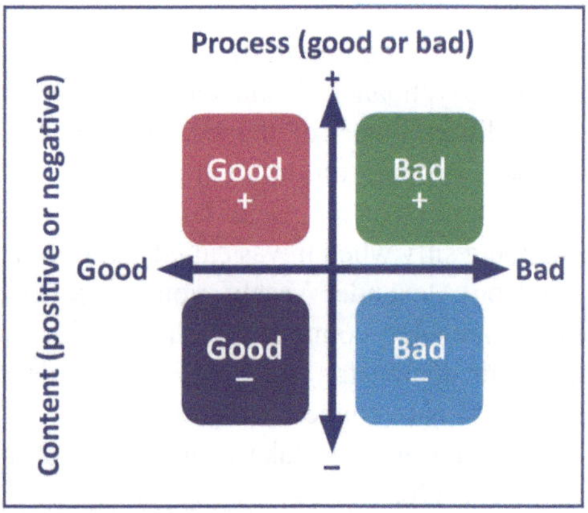

Fig. 1 Four kinds of feedback

The importance of talking to others in person cannot be overemphasized. One need only sit down to dinner with others to see how society's obsession with electronic media has interfered with the quality of interpersonal relationships. The constant attention to emails, texts, smartphones, and other electronic media stifle meaningful communication. When you sit down to dinner with your friends, family, and especially your children, collect the cellphones and talk with them in a truly human encounter.

I recently saw a TV ad espousing the virtues of using iPhones as multitasking time savers, on the surface a very good idea. However, this ad shows a father bottle-feeding his infant, a very special bonding experience for both parent and child. In one hand, he holds the infant, in the other he holds the bottle. While feeding the infant he is also talking on his cell phone, which is lodged between his ear and his shoulder. The voice over the picture says that this particular phone, "allows you to complete life's tasks without losing valuable time to other demands." Do we really want parents to be distracted from this all-important bonding experience so they can do more business or talk with friends? While this ad may sell a lot of iPhones, I wonder what effect it will have on father and child.

Letter writing is a lost art. Cryptic and abbreviated electronic communication creates vague and stunted communication that is open to misinterpretation. On the other hand, well-thought-out and organized letter writing affords one the opportunity for clear and concise communication. Though this can be done via email, it is rarely the case. In my many letters to and from Dr. Frankl over 20+ years, I saw the benefit of this type of communication. Dr. Frankl often thought in complex models difficult to understand. However, he had an uncanny ability to communicate these to the "person in the street" and it is part of what makes his work so effective. I wonder how today's cryptic email writers will develop these skills. As clinicians, it is imperative for us to rehumanize psychotherapy and preserve this authentic and unique relationship.

Lesson 13: Master the Art of Forgiveness

Much attention in the psychological literature in recent years has been given to the concept of forgiveness. In addition, all true religions have preached the importance of forgiveness for thousands of years. Pope Francis is often pictured not only giving absolution during confession but asking for absolution himself in his own confession. He is a great role model.

Several authors have discussed the importance of forgiveness. Yet, even today, when the challenges to survival are greatest, we struggle with this all-important concept. Revenge and punishment take precedence over common sense and peaceful coexistence.

Dr. Frankl (1967) was one of the loudest voices for forgiveness following World War II and the Holocaust. In fact, "In Memoriam," an essay in *Psychotherapy and Existentialism*, discussed the importance of forgiveness so that victims of Nazi atrocities will be able to rebuild meaningful lives. We are all human, he argued, while recognizing that to err is human and to forgive divine.

I'd like to share a discussion I had with Dr. Frankl during my second year of graduate school that demonstrates his commitment to this concept. I come from a long line of Eastern European and then-modern American Jews. My father was a World War II veteran who saw combat in Europe. As a result, he was not only anti-Nazi, but anti-German as well. Our family was not allowed to buy German or Japanese products, even when the only car I could afford to buy in high school was a Volkswagen Beetle. Though he said he would match whatever money I saved for a car, he insisted I wait until I had enough money to buy an American car, which took me 4 more years. Of course, like most children who love and respect their parents, if my father thought it was important to hold this grudge against all Germans, then I agreed completely.

At the end of my second year as Dr. Frankl's graduate assistant, he took my first wife and me out to dinner to thank me for helping during the semester. By coincidence (or was it fate?), I had just finished reading "In Memoriam." Over dinner that night, I began to discuss it with him. It was so difficult for me to differentiate between war criminals and the average Reich citizen who was required to join the Nazi party in order to work or serve in the Army, something most saw as their patriotic duty. After all, the following idea (often attributed to the Irish philosopher Edmond Burke) is relevant here: "The only thing necessary for the triumph of evil is for good men to do nothing."

Over our two-hour dinner, I badgered him with the tenacity of a pit bull, challenging his lack of insight and understanding. This continued for two more hours in the hotel lounge after dinner. After all, I argued, did not the average German elect Hitler? How could they stand by while witnessing the injustices of the Nuremberg Laws and the atrocities of Hitler's "Final Solution," his codename for genocide. I was belligerent and rude to the teacher I admired most.

As Dr. Frankl patiently let me complete my rant against the Reich, I finally ran out of energy and allowed him to speak, without trying to think of a way to contradict his views.

Finally, his reasons for forgiveness began to take hold in my hateful, unforgiving brain. He carefully explained that by the time the average citizen understood the extent of the "Final Solution" there was little they could do. Once Hitler was elected and then seized absolute power, there was no democratic dissent tolerated. This was not the United States that encouraged and allowed free speech. Those who did so in Nazi Germany were systematically executed as treasonous or, worse yet, deported to the concentration camps themselves. The time for political solutions had long passed.

Though he vehemently advocated for the accountability of war criminals who actually carried out these heinous acts, he could not, he explained, expect superhuman self-sacrifice from the average person. To illustrate this point, he turned to Elly, who had been sitting there quietly and was hanging on every word. He then asked me if I would insist on her execution or punishment as she was an unwitting witness to history. After all, he argued, she worked in a dental clinic in Vienna during the war working on many party members and perhaps some relatives of Hitler himself. What good would it do to imprison or execute her, he asked? Would I deprive him of all that she meant to him?

Since I have always respected Elly as a person, and am grateful for the love and kindness she always showed me, I could not imagine punishing her. In fact, I felt that she, too, was a victim of the Nazis. At that point, I thought that my head would explode from my conflicting feelings. Who was right, Dr. Frankl or my beloved father? Could they both be right to some degree? Both agreed that war criminals who perpetrated genocide should be prosecuted to the fullest extent of the law. But what of the average citizen?

Dr. Frankl then explained that, having been a "hero" himself, that is, meaning that he had been forced to endure the hardships of the camps, he could not expect the average person to voluntarily put themselves in a position to suffer the same fate. It was too much to ask the average person to sacrifice their lives and families to take a public stand against the Holocaust, especially since most of them had no personal connections to the victims. Life in Nazi-occupied Europe was tenuous enough without becoming a self-sacrificing "hero." However, he held in the highest esteem those few "righteous Christians," as they are now called by Jews worldwide who, at great personal risk, assisted thousands of Nazi victims.

I finally understood what he was saying, though true understanding of this kind of forgiveness took me much longer. As we rode home that night, my ex-wife was aghast at my behavior toward Dr. Frankl. She chastised me for my rude behavior and reminded me that I was "just a snot-nosed graduate student" with limited understanding but a big mouth, who had no right to be so disrespectful to Dr. Frankl, whom we agreed was one of the greatest minds of our century. She was right, of course! I should have listened with an open mind to what he had to offer, rather than rudely push my own agenda of ethnic racism. I felt terrible and slept little that night. My conscience was screaming at me with remorse.

When I arrived at their hotel the next day to take them to the airport for their return trip to Vienna, I immediately blurted out a lengthy and heartfelt apology. Dr. Frankl looked at me, seemingly confused. He then walked over to me, grabbed me by the arms, and said, "Jay, you challenged Viktor Frankl. Don't ever stop." He went on to let me know that he had enjoyed the lively debate from the night before and that I should never be afraid to debate with him. I then experienced firsthand the power of forgiveness and its potential for personal growth.

As the great statesman Mahatma Gandhi (1953) once said, "The weak can never forgive. Forgiveness is the attribute of the strong" (p. 258).

Lesson 14: Social Responsibility

There is so much to learn that it is hard to single out a most important lesson. Dr. Frankl's concept of finding meaning in life is often considered his most important concept and certainly the most well-known. However, his thoughts on social responsibility are arguably the most important for the survival of humankind. In this blink of an eye we call life, it is the very finiteness of life that inspires us to impact the world for truly meaningful endeavors. However, those who impose their rules on society without regard for the greater good are not acting in a truly meaningful way. Only those goals that seek to improve the general welfare can truly be classified as meaningful. Those who throughout history have exploited others for their sociopathic needs are not searching for meanings.

Modern-day businesses that spend millions of dollars producing weapons of mass destruction, exploiting workers, or wasting precious natural resources in the name of profits are also not pursuing meaningful endeavors.

In a world gone mad with greed and political and personal narcissism, logotherapy is the voice of reason and hope. All of us who understand the principles of logotherapy must be the guiding light for the survival of humankind. It is imperative that we, as future world leaders, nurture human potential toward a synergistic society—one that maintains individual identity while using its collective knowledge and strengths for the greater good.

As I look at this audience today, I see so many creative, dedicated, and brilliant people who are committed to making the world a better place. It is an honor to be a small part of this conference and this community of logotherapists.

In closing, I would like to, once again, quote Dr. Frankl, when he addressed the Washington Hebrew Congregation in 1986 on the overwhelming importance of social responsibility: "Since Auschwitz we know what man is capable of. And since Hiroshima we know what is at stake" (cf. Frankl, 2006, p. 154).

Thank you.

References

Burke, J. J., & Tumbleson, B. E. (2019). Mentoring in academic libraries. *Library Leadership & Management, 33*(4). https://doi.org/10.5860/llm.v33i4.7348

"By the numbers." (2016, July/August). By the numbers: Happiness around the world. *Monitor on Psychology, 47*(7), 11. Retrieved from https://www.apa.org/monitor/2016/07-08/numbers

Frankl, V. E. (1967). *Psychotherapy and existentialism*. Washington Square Press.

Frankl, V. E. (1969). *The will to meaning*. World Publishing Company.

Frankl, V. E. (1973). *The doctor and the soul* (R. Winston & C. Winston, Trans.). Penguin Books. (Original work published 1946 as *Ärztliche Seelsorge*. Franz Deuticke)

Frankl, V. E. (2000). *Man's search for ultimate meaning*. Perseus. (Original work published *Der Unbewusste Gott, 1948 and English translation, The Unconscious God, 1975)*

Frankl, V. E. (2006). *Man's search for meaning*. Beacon Press. (Original work published 1946)

Gandhi, M. (1953). *All men are brothers: Life and thoughts of mahatma Gandhi as told in his own words*. Columbia University Press.

Kennedy, J. F. (1961). Inaugural address, January 20, 1961. Retrieved from https://www.jfklibrary.org/learn/about-jfk/historic-speeches/inaugural-address

Long, J. L. (1982). A journey into meaning. *International Forum for Logotherapy, 5*(1), 57–58.

Pope Francis. (2016, July 30). *Prayer vigil with the young people: Address of the Holy Father*. Retrieved from https://www.vatican.va/content/francesco/en/speeches/2016/july/documents/papa-francesco_20160730_polonia-veglia-giovani.html

"Pope Francis to world's youth." (2016, July 30). *Pope Francis to world's youth: Don't be a couch potato, try activism*. Retrieved from https://www.cbsnews.com/news/pope-francis-to-worlds-youth-dont-be-a-couch-potato-try-activism/

Santayana, G. (1905). *Life of reason, Volume 1: Reason in common sense*. Charles Scribner & Sons.

Santora, K. (2016, August 19). Adults head back to school in Harford County. *The Baltimore Sun*.

Voltaire. (1772). *Contes en vers*. Retrieved from https://fr.wikisource.org/wiki/Contes_en_vers_(Voltaire)/La_B%C3%A9gueule

Dr. Jay I. Levinson, is a licensed psychologist in private practice in Baltimore, Maryland. He has lectured internationally and served on the faculties of both the Johns Hopkins University and the University of Maryland School of Medicine. He is the only person to publish research integrating the work of Dr. Viktor Frankl (meaning in life) and Dr. Elisabeth Kubler-Ross (meaning in death). He was privileged to serve as a special assistant, colleague, and friend to Dr. Frankl for over 20 years and edited his last book, *Man's Search for Ultimate Meaning*. In addition, *Existential Psychotherapy of Meaning*, coedited by Dr. Alexander Batthyány and Dr. Levinson, is a compilation of the next generation of work in logotherapy. Dr. Levinson was recently honored by the Vienna Institute of Logotherapy with its Lifetime Achievement Award and made an honorary member of the Austrian Medical Society. In an effort to give back to his community, he has served on boards of several charitable foundations, including the Vienna Institute of Logotherapy, and was a founder of the Baltimore Ronald McDonald House.

Building the Viktor Frankl Archives

Alexander Vesely

The Beginnings

Earlier in my life, my interest in Viktor Frankl's work was limited. This only changed in the summer of 1993 when my sister and I were invited to speak at The World Congress of Logotherapy in Toronto, Canada. I was fresh out of high school and had not read *Man's Search for Meaning* (Frankl, 1985a). Mainly in order not to embarrass myself, I read it on the plane to Toronto. This—plus the experience at the World Congress of first-hand reports of people whose lives had been changed by my grandfather's work—sparked my interest in logotherapy.

Viktor's archival room in his apartment in Mariannengasse, or "Geist-Stall" ("mental barn") as he jokingly referred to it, contained more than 1200 tapes in various formats, such as reel-to-reel audiotapes, compact cassette tapes, long-forgotten video tape formats from the 1970s and 1980s, and a few 16 mm films dating back to the 1950s. In the early 1990s, I noticed the layer of dust on the tapes getting thicker and the tiny labels with numbers falling off as the glue started losing its stickiness over the years. The information identifying these tapes was contained in a loose stack of papers typed through the decades by my grandmother—a list about 100 typewritten pages long that was becoming increasingly faded and brittle. When I asked Viktor about his plan was for these recordings, he told me he had none. I realized that, unless something was done soon, these recordings were in danger of becoming unidentifiable and eventually, as more time passed, lost. Without my grandfather's knowledge (or permission), I made a copy of the list at a nearby copy shop. A new and affordable digital audio format, the Sony MiniDisc had just been introduced to the world, and it proved to be a reliable and robust medium.

A. Vesely (✉)
Viktor Frankl Media Archive of the Viktor Frankl Institute Vienna, Vienna, Austria
e-mail: alex@viktorfranklamerica.com

C. L. McLafferty, Jr., J. I. Levinson (eds.), *Logotherapy and Existential Analysis*, Logotherapy and Existential Analysis: Proceedings of the Viktor Frankl Institute Vienna 2, https://doi.org/10.1007/978-3-031-48922-8_3

Using a borrowed reel-to-reel machine, I started transferring the oldest tapes onto MiniDiscs. The reels had been recorded at different speeds and had different sizes, and some reels were too big for the tape machine, a problem that could easily be fixed with pencils, cardboard, and scotch tape.

Reel-to-Reel Treasures

Despite being stored in a room where temperatures fluctuated with the seasons, most recordings were in good shape, especially when they had been wrapped in an extra layer of plastic. Many recordings had been made at the Vienna Policlinic and included live therapy sessions. Some cases were described in Viktor's books, such as the famous case of Mrs. Kotek, her reflections and subsequent change of attitude about her life just before dying (see Frankl, 1969/1988, pp. 120–124; 1978, pp. 106–109; 1985b, pp. 95–98). Many live therapy sessions demonstrated the successful application of paradoxical intention; for example, in the cases of washing compulsion and stuttering. On one tape, the patient suffering from a washing compulsion is heard reporting how another psychiatrist told her that if her condition did not improve, she would have to undergo a lobotomy—still a common practice in the early 1960s. Fortunately, her symptoms completely disappeared after a single session in which paradoxical intention was applied.

Among those early recordings is a radio feature about Viktor going on a lecture tour to South and North America. This was the first of many times he lectured in the United States. Another highlight is a recording of a lecture given at the San Quentin prison in the mid-1960s. Viktor was invited to speak there several times because his words resonated particularly well with the audience.

Compact Cassette: The World Through Viktor's Ears

I thought my task would get easier from a technical point of view once I got to the recordings from the late 1960s, when cassette tapes became the norm. However, the opposite was the case, mostly because smaller parts mean more things can break. The number of recordings also increased dramatically by the late 1960s, as Viktor began to bring a portable tape recorder with him when he traveled and spoke around the world.

There are complete lecture series that he captured in this way. While the content is often similar, he had a habit of frequently going off script. He would react to current world events or questions from the audience, weaving in personal experiences or a new joke he had just heard. Viktor must have been aware of the value of these fleeting spur-of-the-moment comments, which according to him varied in quality depending on the quality of the coffee he had consumed beforehand. He made sure to have his tape recorder with him to save them for posterity. He was accustomed to being frequently misquoted and misunderstood, so having a recording from which a transcription could be made later was of great use to him.

He also recorded a number of nonlogotherapy-related moments, many of which document his humorous side. One recording is that of a wrestling match at Vienna's Heumarkt and documents uniquely "raw" expressions from members of the audience. A couple of lecture recordings are graced with songs by Kermit the Frog captured from a hotel's TV set. (Viktor was a fan of Jim Henson's work.) Another recording he made of himself imitating the fictional characters "Bof" and "Nebof," (a Jewish version of a Laurel-and-Hardy-like duo) which he created to entertain my sister and me when we were kids. Viktor's love of both humor and music came together in a recording in which he sang the different voices of an old tune, recorded, overdubbed, and synchronized using two tape recorders. The tune, performed by the (remarkably accurate) "Viktor Frankl choir," ends as Viktor himself fails to hold back his laughter.

"Groovy" Formats

The Frankl Archive also received contributions from other collections, such as the Viktor Frankl Collection and memorabilia at GTU in Berkeley, once founded by Randolph Sasnett and Robert Leslie. They had accompanied Viktor on his first lecture tours in the United States and recorded some of it. One of the recordings presented a major technical challenge because it was recorded in a short-lived system called "Soundwriter." This system did not use magnetic tape but instead etched sound mechanically on a thin plastic foil, technically similar to an LP record, but the groove is much thinner than that of a regular LP, allowing for up to 30 minutes of audio on each side of a single plastic sheet. Some research and asking around led me to find out about the existence of a new technology which was able to extract the sound from photographic scans of shellac records and Edison cylinders without the necessity of touching the original brittle medium. This revolutionary technology is named "IRENE," which stands for "Image, Reconstruct, Erase Noise, Etc." ("Project IRENE," 2019); it provides access to many vintage recordings that would otherwise never be heard. It also provided access to these 1957 recordings, consisting of two-and-a-half hours of Frankl lecturing followed by a fascinating Q&A session, whose quality in content compensates for the mediocre sound quality.

Moving Images

Digitizing video recordings presented an equally interesting challenge. From the 1970s through much of the 1990s, a multitude of different tape and recording formats came and went. The process of preserving them became a long journey from electronics repair shops to television archives and various places in different countries housing fascinating vintage video equipment. Timing was also an issue. Deterioration of video recordings results in damage that is harder to fix than just added hissing sounds. Today the quality of many video recordings from the 1970s has become unusable. One videotape from 1972 of a live television interview went from one company to the next, and even was temporarily lost, before it finally ended up in a place that had the right equipment to play it. Another "lost and found" video that stands out is a mid-1970s studio interview by the Austrian Broadcasting Company, which for some reason had no entry in their own archives. In this live studio interview, Viktor answered questions sent in by viewers of the program. The coffee must have been good as well. Fortunately, Viktor himself had captured it on a bulky video "VCR" cassette, a remarkably good early home video system introduced by Philips in 1972. I was able to get Viktor's original player fixed and digitize the recording from it. The video stands out for the quality of both the technical aspects and the content as one of the best interviews in existence.

The last video in Viktor's archive was a Hi-8 mm video cassette with a message recorded by his longtime friend Jerry Long, who was suffering from quadriplegia after a diving accident and famously wrote the words: "I broke my neck, it did not break me," which Viktor quoted time and again. Viktor was in the hospital when Jerry's tape arrived in the mail in August of 1997. Unfortunately, he did not live to see it. Jerry died a few months later. It was quite a moving experience to watch this video letter in which Jerry gives detailed insights into his daily life.

Still Photographs

An easier format to work with is that of film and photographs. The archive contained several 16 mm and 8 mm films and countless negatives and slides, which—thanks to ever-evolving digital technology—can now be scanned with ultrahigh resolution. This allows for details to become visible that would otherwise go unnoticed. Such was the case with photographs donated by David Lisak, whose mother, Thea Kissmann, had been a friend of Viktor before the war. He found one of the few photographs showing Viktor and his team during wartime—presumably at the Rothschild hospital, Vienna's Jewish hospital, which was later completely destroyed. By way of magnifying a high-resolution scan of the tiny photograph and comparing it to a historic photograph of the Rothschild hospital building, the exact location where the picture had been taken could be determined.

Present and Future

By 2022, I had digitized the last audio recording. In total, the archive now contains about 2000 hours of digitized audio material and well over 100 hours of video. However, archival work is never completely finished. Once items are in digital form, they are not entirely safe from loss or deterioration. Even if digital information is stored under perfect conditions, the programs that interpret this vast number of zeros and ones, turning them into analog pictures and sounds, are constantly changing; tomorrow's software may not be able to decipher their meaning. Therefore, it is necessary to keep copying and converting all the material into different formats.

But the purpose of an archive is not only to find and preserve recordings but also to make them accessible. For that purpose, the Frankl Archives established a partnership with distributors Auditorium Netzwerk; photographs are available through Brandstaetter images. Besides that, many video clips are available on YouTube and are today enjoyed by tens of thousands of viewers. When Viktor and I first talked about the idea of making some of his recordings public, neither of us could anticipate the technical possibilities of today. I had to promise him to keep the prices at a level at which "nobody would have to think twice if they could afford one or not."

I am grateful to all who contributed through the years in one way or another. The archive received a large number of recordings from institutions and individuals around the world, such as Wolfgang Kocourek, Alexander Brehm, Jon Kent, David Lisak, Otto-Suel Hintz, Dr. Patricia Starck, Dr. Teria Shantal, the Jewish Learning Center, the Graduate Theological Union in Berkeley, Dr. Lilia Suchocka, and David Stiver, just to mention a few.

Recently Dr. Haddon Klingberg (2001) generously donated much of his original material recorded for his 2001 biography *When Life Calls Out to Us: The Love and Lifework of Viktor and Elly Frankl* to the archives. The support from my parents, who helped with the transfer of material, research, and database building, was integral to the successful completion of this project.

I hope and believe that this vast pool of information will allow anyone who is interested to fill existing gaps of information on logotherapy and to gain deeper insights and a more complete picture of my grandfather and his life work.

References

Frankl, V. E. (1969/1988). *The will to meaning: Foundations and applications of logotherapy*. Meridian. (Original work published 1969)

Frankl, V. E. (1978). *The unheard cry for meaning: Psychotherapy and humanism*. Simon and Schuster.

Frankl, V. E. (1985a). *Man's search for meaning* (3rd ed.). Washington Square Press/Pocket Books. (Original work published 1946)

Frankl, V. E. (1985b). *Psychotherapy and existentialism*. Washington Square Press. (Original work published 1967)

Klingberg, H. (2001). *When life calls out to us: The love and lifework of Viktor and Elly Frankl*. Doubleday Books.

"Project IRENE." (2019). *Website of the Lawrence Berkeley National Laboratory*. Retrieved from https://tay.rhp.mybluehost.me/

Alexander Vesely, MS, Dr hc, is a documentary film maker, licensed psychotherapist, and cofounder of the Viktor Frankl Institute of America. As well, he passionately imparts knowledge as a logotherapy teacher at the Online Academy for Logotherapy in Bamberg, Germany and is head of the Viktor Frankl Media Archives in Vienna. The intersection of psychology and cinema has been a constant theme in Vesely's career. Initially entering the field of TV and film, he later pursued studies in psychology, becoming a tutor at the University of Vienna and a guest lecturer at the Hochschule fuer Fernsehen und Film (HFF) in Munich, Germany. Vesely collaborated with dramaturg Christian Mikunda at CommEnt Production Group. Subsequently, he cofounded the production company Clipwerk and continued his impactful work with Noetic Films and StraightUp Entertainment in Los Angeles, California. His 2019 documentary *Viktor* & I has won several awards internationally. Vesely traverses the world as a speaker, addressing audiences on logotherapy, the meaning-centered school of psychotherapy founded by his grandfather, Viktor Frankl, author of Man's Search for Meaning.

Part II
Prevention and Amelioration of Suffering, Fostering Hope

Human Suffering

Patricia L. Starck

The alleviation of suffering is the aim of all who work in the health and helping professions. Indeed, the Latin origin of the word "patient" is "one who suffers" (Adil, 2010). Yet, this topic is rarely found in curricula of caring professions or in general medical and health care literature; rather, it seems confined to palliative care and religious literature. And of the existing literature, it seems that much is concerned with measuring suffering, assessing its characteristics, quantifying its extent, but with little insight for the front-line helper who comes face-to-face with the sufferer. What to say? What to do that is helpful? But, alas, confronting human suffering is part of the daily work of a wide variety of those whose life is dedicated to caring for others. It is an important but understudied domain. Providers of care need knowledge and wisdom beyond the biomedical paradigm in order to respond to existential issues being experienced by suffering patients. In the *Diagnostic and Statistical Manual of Mental Disorders (DSM-5)* (American Psychiatric Association, 2013), there is no diagnostic category for suffering as there is for depression and anxiety disorders. There is no 0–10 scale for assessing suffering. There are no scientific, evidence-based practice guidelines for managing suffering.

The purpose of this chapter is to discuss how logotherapy can support the response to human suffering. An understanding of spiritual/existential distress through the framework of logotherapy and its application will be discussed as a way of coping with unavoidable suffering.

P. L. Starck (✉)
The University of Texas Health Science Center at Houston, Houston, TX, USA

C. L. McLafferty, Jr., J. I. Levinson (eds.), *Logotherapy and Existential Analysis*, Logotherapy and Existential Analysis: Proceedings of the Viktor Frankl Institute Vienna 2, https://doi.org/10.1007/978-3-031-48922-8_4

Definitions and Descriptions of Suffering

In spite of the fact that it has been a topic of concern through the ages and a matter of scholarly discourse for at least 25 decades, there is no standardized definition of suffering. Human suffering, according to Travelbee (1971), is a subjective experience unique to the individual, varying from simple, transitory discomfort to extreme anguish, despair, or apathetic indifference. No matter the extent, it is an all-encompassing experience. Suffering is thus unique to the individual, and not to be compared with previous suffering or the suffering of others. Furthermore, suffering fills the entire person. Because Frankl's (1973) concept of the human included three dimensions—body (soma), mind (psyche), and spirit (noös)—suffering affects the whole person. He held firm to the belief that meaning can be found in spite of suffering through the meaning of the moment within the values of creativity, experience, and one's chosen attitude.

Eric Cassell (1982, 1983, 1992) defined suffering as a state of severe distress associated with events that threaten the intactness or wholeness of a person. Cassell emphasized the effect that suffering had on a person's perception of their integrity; in fact, suffering disrupted one's view of oneself as an intact person. This theme was carried forward by Kahn and Steeves (1986), who simply described suffering as an individual's experience of threat to the self. A similar definition was proposed by Cherny et al. (1994) as "an aversive emotional experience characterized by the perception of personal distress that is generated by adverse factors undermining the quality of life" (p. 57).

A protégée of Frankl's, psychologist Elisabeth Lukas (2020), defined suffering as representing loss. Likewise, Starck (1992) in a qualitative study of elderly nursing home residents found suffering to be conceptualized as multiple losses, which could be categorized in various human dimensions. In the physical dimension, there was loss of strength, mobility, sensory, and memory. Psychosocially, there was loss of friends, family, and activities. Economic losses included those of one's home, possessions, and often loss of resources sufficient to last for care and burial expenses. However, the greatest number of losses were those of the human spirit—loss of autonomy, one's authority, usefulness, choice, the sense of masculinity/femininity, privacy, self-worth, and purpose in life.

In palliative care, Kirkorian and Limonero (2012) defined suffering as a multidimensional and dynamic experience of severe stress that occurs when there is a significant threat to the whole person and regulatory processes are insufficient, leading to exhaustion.

VanderWeele (2019) described the concept of suffering as the undesired experience, of considerable intensity or duration, of a negative physical or affective state. He acknowledged the subjective nature of suffering and the perception of some perceived good that needs to be regained, mourned, dealt with, compensated for, or overcome. He further offered that suffering involves some inability to control the scope of suffering.

Edwards and Van Tongeren (2020), in their study of how people understand the relationship between suffering and meaning, defined suffering as "a prolonged experience of psychological or emotional pain that may follow an unexpected negative event" (p. 722). They used the term *meaning* as having three features: purpose, significance, and coherence. Asking subjects to focus on past and current sufferings, the authors concluded that as more time passes after suffering, overall meaning is greater.

Boston et al. (2011) in an integrated literature review on existential suffering found some 56 definitions, some of which were linked to spirituality. Themes included finding meaning, the loss of meaning or purpose in life, wanting to find answers to ultimate questions, connectedness, hope/hopelessness, loneliness, isolation, and fears of being a burden to others and of dying.

As depicted in Fig. 1, the concept of suffering is complex. An analysis of various definitions would conclude there are four commonalities about suffering, that it is (a) universal, (b) subjective, (c) unique to the individual, and (d) results in loss. The areas of differences have to do with several factors. VanderWeele (2019) specified the necessity of intensity or considerable duration; whereas Travelbee (1971) allowed for a range of human experience, from simple, transitory ailments to extreme anguish or apathetic indifference. Cassell (1983) as well as Kahn and Steeves (1986) included the requisite of loss of intactness of the person. However, a

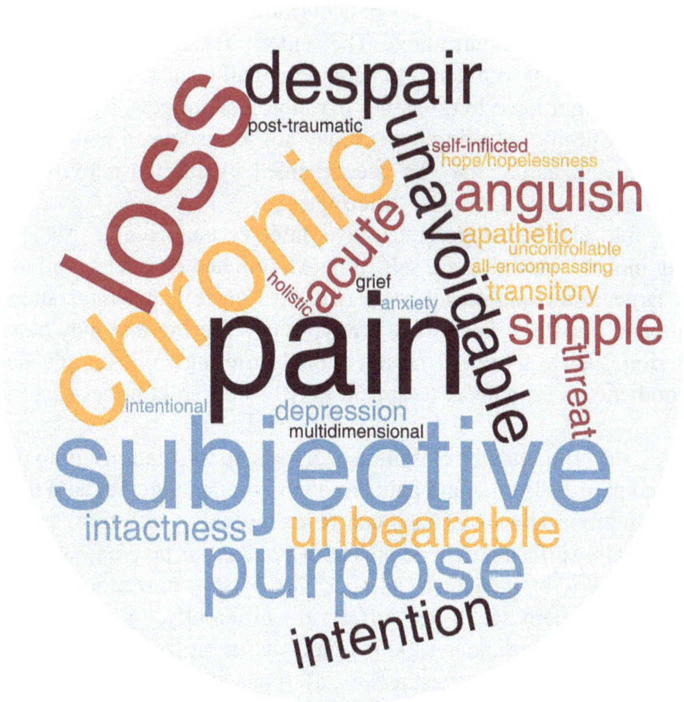

Fig. 1 The definition of suffering is complex

logotherapist might challenge this assertion, e.g., "Does the value of one's life depend on having two limbs?" Cherny et al. (1994) defined suffering as experiences that undermine quality of life, but Frankl's (1946/1984) definition allowed for attitude modification and finding greater meaning. Likewise, they also specified that suffering was the inability to control the scope of suffering, yet Frankl's assertion that everything can be lost except the ability to control one's own attitude would refute loss of control as a defining characteristic.

Thus, to date, the understanding of human or existential suffering is inconsistently defined and understood. Lack of conceptual clarity is no doubt at the root of the paucity of research and lack of consistent clinical training, much less guidelines and protocols. It would seem that Travelbee's (1971) definition, outlined earlier, is broader and less limiting, allowing for individual uniqueness. Therefore, it will be used as the preferred definition in this article in designing interventions.

Characteristics of Suffering

There are various ways to categorize suffering; considering all of them helps to develop a broader understanding of the concept of suffering. Suffering may be acute or chronic. Acute suffering may be temporary or short-lived. Respiratory distress and heart arrythmias can be examples of acute suffering which, with proper medical treatment, are intense but controllable. The acute suffering of maternal labor, while usually very unpleasant, soon leads to happiness if all goes well. On the other hand, acute suffering might have long-lasting psychological effects, e.g., post-traumatic stress disorder. Chronic suffering may or may not be associated with pain. Diseases that are chronic in nature may be accompanied by limited activity and forced changes in lifestyle, thus adding to suffering.

Suffering may also be categorized as avoidable vs. unavoidable. Avoidable types of suffering include those that are self-inflicted, inflicted by others, and inflicted by society at large. Unavoidable suffering may be chance happenings such as man-made or natural disasters. Then there are types of suffering that may be hard to fit either criterion, such as iatrogenic or intentional suffering. For example, deciding to have chemotherapy or a painful treatment may be chosen in hopes of an improved outcome.

Moreover, suffering may be classified according to its relationship to physical or psychological pain. Suffering and pain are often grouped together as if they are one concept or symptom. However, there can be pain without suffering; suffering may be caused by pain; suffering may be present when there is no pain; and indeed, suffering may be caused by the pain of another. Two persons may report the same level of pain on a 0–10 pain scale, yet suffer very differently. In a study of hospice patients, Baines and Norlander (2000) found that more respondents experienced suffering than pain, but the highest mean suffering scores occurred in patients with severe pain. Although they may accompany suffering, depression, loss, and grief are separate concepts.

Ruijs et al. (2009) described a unique category as *unbearable suffering*, which they defined as "a subjective experience of suffering that is so serious and uncontrollable that it overwhelms ones [sic] bearing capacity" (p. 5). This team developed a quantitative instrument to measure unbearable suffering in end-stage cancer patients. In the Netherlands, each year there are an estimated 8400 explicit requests for euthanasia from patients who consider their suffering unbearable. The researchers found that quality of life was not a determining factor with those who found life unbearable. This finding confirms the basic belief of Frankl and others that perspectives on suffering are very individual.

Unbearable suffering is not unlike Frankl's (1946/1984, 1969) description of the *existential vacuum*, which is a loss of meaning in one's life, the worst of suffering and utter despair. Before reaching this stage, one experiences *existential frustration*, a state in which one is searching for meaning, but without success.

Suffering from Selected Religious Perspectives

Frankl (1969) specified that logotherapy is a secular approach to clinical problems, but "when a patient stands on the firm ground of religious belief, there can be no objection to making use of the therapeutic effect of his religious convictions and thereby drawing upon his spiritual resources" (pp. 120–121). Therefore, in the study of suffering, it seems prudent to reflect on various religious perspectives.

Fitzpatrick et al. (2016) reported discussion from experts in the world's six major faith traditions (Jewish, Roman Catholic, Hindu, Buddhist, Evangelical Anglican, and Islamic) around questions of suffering. Various religious traditions have a long history of interest in the topic of human suffering and, while there are commonalities among different faiths, there are also unique differences. A thorough discussion is beyond the scope of this chapter, especially since there is much variation even within a particular faith or denomination. However, there seem to be three common beliefs among all religions regarding suffering: (a) suffering is an inevitable part of human existence, (b) individual suffering affects others around, and (c) suffering is a disruption or disharmony. Traditions vary in the view of causation of suffering, whether it is random, the result of present or past behaviors, or external evils. In general, no faith tradition claims that suffering itself has value, but traditions vary in the understanding of value to be derived from suffering; for example, sharing in Christ's suffering, bearing one's suffering, testing one's faith, becoming more compassionate, or repairing past karma. All traditions agree that suffering should be eliminated by all ethical means.

The following discussion is given to present a brief overview of how various religions perceive human suffering. It should be understood that believers may differ from the main tenets of any one religion and beliefs and traditions may differ within a religious category. A religious perspective should certainly be acknowledged by anyone responding to another's suffering.

Jewish Perspective

Suffering is understood within the Jewish perspective as a characteristic of physical existence, to be expected in life. The primary challenge is the response within an ethical framework. Suffering is not to be accepted, but always calls for a response. Jewish literature is replete with dialogue about suffering. Can suffering be atonement for sinful behavior? Can suffering be called chastisements of love? Can suffering be welcomed? On the whole, suffering is understood as a disorder without spiritual value, and not a way to transformation via a spiritual journey. The response to suffering is an act of justice. In clinical contexts, there is a strong focus on alleviating and eliminating suffering. Doing so is a primary duty within Jewish ethics (Fitzpatrick et al., 2016).

Roman Catholic Perspective

Catholics consider the entire world to be broken as a consequence of Adam's fall. Suffering may have a purpose, value, or meaning but remains somewhat mysterious and beyond our earthly comprehension. Even though suffering may not be understood, God will bring good out of all evils. The life of Christ was aimed at redeeming all suffering; followers of Christ can share in this redemptive work through good deeds and prayer. Suffering is a state of disharmony and often includes feelings of alienation, abandonment, loss, and the absence of wholeness. The approach is to search for the root cause and do the work of repair, while also recognizing that some forms of disharmony are beyond repair, likely to end in despair. Christians are called to see suffering as not meaningless, but rather a way to share in Christ's work (Fitzpatrick et al., 2016).

Hindu Perspective

Suffering is thought to be an inherent part of the cycle of living and rebirth and is the unfolding of karma from current or past inappropriate actions. It is not random. Thus, acceptance and endurance of suffering helps to satisfy the debt of past negative behavior. By accepting one's suffering, one becomes less attached to changing it. Suffering is influenced by attachment to this world and wanting things to be different. Pain and suffering can be seen as leading to progress on one's spiritual path by learning from a difficult experience. The spiritual goal is detachment from things of this world in order to focus on God/The Ultimate as the primary goal of the Hindu traditions (Whitman, 2007).

With the conviction that people are accountable for their suffering and must accept their responsibility, in the Hindu tradition is relief of suffering acceptable or even desirable? According to Fitzpatrick et al. (2016), alleviation is acceptable within a limited context and for a greater good. For example, relief of suffering would be acceptable so that a person could go to a temple to worship.

Buddhist Perspective

The perspective of Buddhists is based on the doctrine of the Four Noble Truths, which are that suffering, pain, and misery exist in life; that suffering is caused by selfish craving and personal desire; that this craving can be overcome; and that the way to overcome suffering is through the Eightfold Path. The way to eliminate suffering is through right view, right intention, right speech, right action, right effort, right livelihood, right mindfulness, and right concentration (Kurtus, 2022).

The general term for all types of suffering is *dukkha* and its liberation is known as *nirvana*. Buddhists believe that the ultimate source of suffering is within our own minds as the reaction to difficult situations. Buddhists also believe that suffering can be a great teacher, giving insight about the true nature of the human condition, avoiding future suffering, and generating compassion for others (Fitzgerald et al., 2016).

Evangelical Anglican Perspective

Trials and tribulations are an inevitable part of life. Suffering is a disruption of how things should be and suffering entered the world because of a disruption between the Creator and human beings. The suffering of Jesus Christ is God's plan for rescuing humankind and reconciliation. Suffering can produce positive growth—perseverance, character, and hope. Christians believe that suffering should be prevented and relieved whenever possible. Indeed, the early Christians were noted for their efforts in alleviating the suffering of the sick. Jesus and his apostles had compassion for the sufferer and spent much effort in healing. Suffering may sometimes enhance human dignity (Fitzpatrick et al., 2016).

Islamic Perspective

Muslims treat suffering as an inevitable aspect of human experience and believe that suffering occurs within the context of God's will even though a person may be responsible for the cause. Therefore, human beings should endure what befalls them. This attitude of passiveness generates patience based on the belief that the suffering is in some way purposeful. It calls for the discipline of a person and the submission to God's will. However, Muslim traditions believe that illness needs to be cured by every possible legitimate means, as God has also created its treatment (Fitzpatrick et al., 2016).

Assessment of Suffering

Much of the scholarly work in the area of human suffering has been in the area of assessing suffering—attempting to measure the extent of this subjective experience. The clinical interview is considered essential to assess individual suffering.

Many psychometric tests to quantify suffering have been devised within the specialty of palliative care. Krikorian et al. (2013) conducted a wide search of such available instruments. Using criteria for validity, reproducibility, responsiveness, interpretability, and minimum clinically important difference, the authors found 10 such instruments used in caring for advanced or terminally ill patients. These instruments are used for research purposes as well as to evaluate patients, monitor progress, and guide treatment decisions.

Not surprisingly, many of the instruments were based on the definition of suffering by Cassell (1992). The Initial Assessment of Suffering (MacAdam & Smith, 1987) is administered as part of a semi-structured interview. Instruments developed subsequently, such as The Suffering Scales (Schulz et al., 2010) and Pictorial Representation of Illness and Self Measure (PRISM; Mühleisen et al., 2009), may be self-administered. Nine of the 10 instruments reviewed by Krikorian et al. use a discrete numeric score, with either a Likert-scale or visual-analogue score ratings from 0 to 10. One would conclude that this is an attempt to measure the extent of suffering in the same way that pain is measured on a 1–10 scale. (For a thorough discussion of the characteristics of the instruments, the reader is referred to the original article by Krikorian et al.)

It would seem that these instruments address only the preliminary step of assisting with suffering—that of seeking to quantify or describe the intensity or experience of suffering. Another instrument, the Meaning in Suffering Test (MIST; Starck, 1985), was developed to assess the beliefs one has about suffering, and particularly those that help or hinder one to cope with suffering. This instrument has two parts: Part 1 has 20 items answered on a seven-point Likert scale measuring the extent to which the sufferer has found meaning; Part 2 asks a single question to quantify suffering and 15 other questions with multiple-choice answers that indicate ways of coping with suffering. Answers for multiple-choice items were formulated based on qualitative responses from hospitalized patients participating in a study (Starck, 1983). The final question asks about religious preference.

Starck (1983) used the MIST in a study of 99 hospitalized patients. On the first part, scores ranged from 61 to 140 with a mean score of 101.48. The three most frequent diagnoses were psychiatric, cardiovascular-medical, and gastrointestinal disorders. Respondents with cancer were the most optimistic; those with medical breathing problems perceived themselves as suffering more; patients undergoing surgery perceived their suffering as most meaningful; and individuals with psychiatric problems had the highest scores on suffering without meaning. On the second part of the test, respondents offered answers to the question of how they cope with suffering. Their responses were then categorized as to Frankl's (1973, p. xiii) three value categories of finding meaning: *creative values*—talk to family, pray, read, do something for someone else; *experiential values*—listen to music, fantasize, remain calm and alone, watch a sunset; *attitudinal values*—try to see the good in a situation, think about blessings, take an interest in others.

Finally, these patients indicated they had a positive reaction to discussing the suffering experiences with the nurse researchers. Likewise, Ruijs et al. (2009), while constructing the SOS-V instrument, found that patients appreciated the opportunity to talk about their disease and its impact on their lives. This finding should encourage other researchers on this topic and also help to assure members of Institutional Review Boards that these types of instruments are not emotionally harmful to patients.

Frankl's Tenets

As espoused by Frankl (1969, 1973), the following tenets may be considered relevant to human suffering and prove useful as a guide to clinical practice:

- Suffering is a universal human experience and an inevitable part of life.
- Suffering is holistic; it affects all dimensions of the human—body, mind, and spirit.
- Life is potentially meaningful under all conditions, even the most miserable.
- There is no meaning in suffering, but meaning can be found in spite of suffering.
- As a teacher, suffering can prompt a search for meaning.
- Choice and responsibility are available to every sufferer—the freedom to choose a response and attitude toward our suffering.
- The way one bears suffering is like a monument that endures.
- Suffering can activate the defiant power of the human spirit.
- Meaning can be found in self-transcendence—getting outside the self for the benefit of others.
- Humans must accept their inability to grasp ultimate meaning.

Logotherapeutic Applications to Suffering

Frankl (1946/1984) maintained that there is always the potential for meaning in life experiences:

> There are situations in which one is cut off from the opportunity to do one's work or to enjoy one's life; but what never can be ruled out is the unavoidability of suffering. In accepting this challenge to suffer bravely, life has a meaning up to the last moment, and it retains this meaning literally to the end. In other words, life's meaning is an unconditional one, for it even includes the potential meaning of unavoidable suffering. (p. 137)

Elsewhere, Frankl (1969) noted:

> Life never ceases to hold a meaning, for even a person deprived of both creative and experiential values is still challenged by a meaning to fulfill, that is, by the meaning inherent in the right, in an upright way of suffering. (p. 70)

Logotherapy is a meaning-centered approach to facing one's problems and deciding upon appropriate action.

Although Frankl (1973) argued against rigid techniques for clinical practice, requiring creativity of the logotherapist while being guided by the interaction with the patient, it may be helpful to offer a general framework in assisting patients who are suffering. Remembering that suffering is subjective and unique to each individual, the therapist must be guided by the patient and respond accordingly. The model offered in Table 1 is a framework for a plan of care. It consists of three stages:

Taking stock: Assess and Acknowledge
Prompting: Plan, Seek, Explore
Actualizing: Act, Fulfill, Evaluate

Table 1 A logotherapeutic model to address unavoidable suffering

1. *Taking stock*	*Assess and acknowledge*
Clinical interview	Illness stories
Describing suffering	Level? Acute or chronic? Temporary or permanent? Pain? Depression? Onset? Religious implications? What helps? Attitude, Past coping, Expected outcome
2. *Prompting*	*Plan, explore, seek*
Paradoxical intention	Detaching from symptoms
Dereflection	Reducing focus
Attitude modulation	Proving, challenging
Socratic dialogue	Questioning assumptions
Exploring values	New insights, parallel vs pyramidal values
Parables	Morals, life mottos
Fate vs freedom chart	Choosing areas of freedom
Self-distancing	Activating defiant power of the human spirit
3. *Actualizing*	*Act, fulfill, and evaluate*
New meanings	Creative, experiential, and attitude
Personal responsibility	Actualizing potential
Self-transcendence	Getting outside the self
Track achievements	Monitor change
Celebrate changes	Maintain change

Taking Stock

The first stage would be assessment of the individual and acknowledgment of the suffering involved. Precisely because suffering for each individual is unique, the therapist needs to understand the suffering experience of the patient in the patient's own words. The therapist then needs to express acknowledgment.

Assessment. An instrument(s) to quantify the level of suffering previously described may be helpful, but it should be remembered that the clinical interview is considered the basic method of assessing suffering. Dialogue with the patient might be: "Tell me about your suffering—when did it start and how has it progressed?" Egnew (2018) encouraged illness stories and offers examples of questions to explore suffering, such as "What is it like to live with ___________?"

Caregivers need skills in communication to draw out the illness stories of the past. Telling the illness story serves three purposes: (a) to gain distance by putting the occurrence in the past, (b) to gain affirmation of a changed self, and (c) to foster transcendence beyond the suffering.

Another step in the assessment is to clarify the categorization of the suffering—is it temporary or permanent? Acute or chronic? Accompanied by pain, depression, etc.? How did it happen? Is it expected to be progressive? Are there religious implications? Is it considered bearable or unbearable at this time? What helps? What is the patient's attitude toward the suffering? How has the patient dealt with past sufferings? What is the expected outcome—recovery, chronic state, terminal?

It is hoped that at some point the assessment of suffering might become a standardized part of the patient's clinical chart—just as temperature, pain level, and other vital signs are recorded. This would ensure that every member of the clinical team had some understanding of the level of distress being experienced by the patient.

Acknowledgment of the patient's suffering simply by listening can be very therapeutic. Spending time in the initial assessment will possibly create a bond that will have lasting therapeutic effects. Acknowledgement can take the form of verbal validation, e.g., "I recognize that you have suffered greatly." Frankl acknowledged one's ability to bear suffering as a lasting achievement that could not be erased from the granaries of life.

Prompting

Suffering can be a teacher, and the second step of the intervention model is to guide the patient in the exploration of what suffering has to teach. This is the stage to plan, explore, and seek new pathways. Frankl (1969) emphasized that suffering is not necessary to find meaning; it is certainly not indispensable to achieve a meaningful life. But since hardly anyone will escape an earthly existence without some kind of suffering, it is prudent to consider how suffering might be put to some use for a more fulfilling life. Suffering may then become an opportunity to actualize potentialities and to realize creative, experiential, or attitudinal values. One might even say that human beings have a responsibility to seek such values in times of suffering. As Frankl cautioned, this is the time to remember that it is not we who should question life or suffering, but rather it is life that questions us: How will we respond? Indeed, he believed that suffering offers a rich opportunity to find meaning. "The meaning of suffering—unavoidable and inescapable suffering alone, of course—is the deepest possible meaning" (p. 75).

Frankl (1946/1984) explained that when one is suffering from a condition that ought not to be, there is a tension between what is, the current situation, and what ought to be. The defiant or dynamic power is that inner resource that one uses to overcome limitations. This *defiant power of the human spirit* takes a stand against restrictions—whether biological, psychological, or social. Suffering shows us the deficit of the current situation so that a better one can be imagined. "Meaning orientation enhances our ability to endure suffering because even a life darkened by suffering does not lose its meaning" (Lukas, 2020, p. 98).

Techniques, Tools, and Exercises

Paradoxical intention and dereflection are two techniques often used in logotherapy to detach the person from troubling symptoms. Paradoxical intention is used to educate the individual that, rather than running away from fear, one should wish for what is feared, even to the point of exaggeration. The image becomes even humorous. This visualization paradoxically creates distance from the fear and frees one from the fear. Dereflection counteracts hyperreflection and focuses on other values, turning attention to something else.

These techniques were described by Frankl (1946/1984); Lukas (1986/2014) articulated them as follows: "Paradoxical intention helps in cases where the suffering is caused by feeling trapped in a vicious cycle…; dereflection aims at reducing unnecessary suffering…" (p. 30). Lukas (2020) explained that, in dereflection, "participants first learn to raise their heads and stop tensely watching their own steps" (p. 131).

Attitude modulation is helpful when suffering is unalterable, based on Frankl's tenet that attitude is not determined by the situation or circumstances, but can be chosen. The overall approach for a logotherapist when supporting a person who is suffering, regardless of cause, is to prompt the engagement of the human spirit. Often this can be done by quoting a sentence and asking the person to comment on its meaning. Some examples from Frankl are: "If there is a meaning in life at all, then there must be a meaning in suffering" (Frankl, 1946/1984, p. 88) and "The destiny a person suffers therefore has a twofold meaning: to be shaped where possible, and to be endured where necessary" (Frankl, 1973, pp. 111–112).

Socratic dialogue is used in probing, challenging, and questioning so that the patient can gain new insights. Logotherapists often use Socratic dialogue to pose questions that are meant to evoke reflection and attitude change. Caring for the human spirit of an individual who is suffering is challenging. Socratic dialogue can activate the defiant power of the human spirit, assisting the individual to cope with present circumstances and to discover meaning regardless of the suffering. Suggestions for dialogue that calls forth positive memories in each of the categorical values are:

Creative values—What we give to life: "Was there a time in your life when there was something you thought you could not do, but you did?" "What are the thing(s) you are most proud of accomplishing in your life?"

Experiential values—What we take from the world: "What are the things you have treasured most in life?" "What was the happiest experience you remember?" "What was the most memorable birthday you ever had?"

Attitudinal Values—The stance we take toward our uncontrollable fate: "What has been your motto in life?" "Have you ever had a time you have been faced with events that you had no control over?" "What principles do you live by?" "Even in your suffering, are you able to do anything for others?"

An example of the last question can be found in the person with an intractable disease; she was bedridden with multiple sclerosis. She expressed how she hated being a burden to others, not being capable of doing anything for herself. The therapist reminded her that she did do something for others. She gave them the opportunity to do a good deed, to express their love with human kindness.

With this change in attitude, Frankl (1973, p. 102) illustrated what he called a "Copernican revolution" (p. 102). He pointed out that it is not we who should question life, but rather, it is life that questions us, with questions such as "How will you respond to this challenge life has given you?" The choice and responsibility are ours. Things happen to us that are undeserved, unexplained, unjustified, and unavoidable. Meaning comes from the stance we take toward suffering.

Attitude modulation can be triggered by asking the "What if" question. "What if it had been the other way around?" "What if you had died before your husband?" "If you could give this condition to someone else in your family, who would you give it to?" (In one case where this was asked, the patient thought, but finally said, "I would keep it myself," which brought about an attitude change.)

"What if you could choose between not having this disease but having your children not turn out well or having the disease but your children turned out well?" This question was used by Elisabeth Lukas (1986) in a demonstration session with patients with chronic respiratory problems whose two highest values were their children and their health. She then asked them to hypothetically rank order these two values.

Helping the patient verbalize positive versus negative thoughts can lead to a shift in attitude. "You have suffered a great deal. What has helped you through it? Have you learned anything during this journey? Has anything positive come about in spite of the suffering?"

Parables can be used as another way to engage and prompt the human spirit specifically to bring about an attitude change, again asking the patient to interpret the meaning in light of his own personal situation. Although Frankl (1969) referred to this as the "parable method" (p. 118), it might also be called therapeutic storytelling.

The Buddhist parable of the mustard seed (Burtt, 1955) tells how a young mother, Kisa Gotami, pleaded with the Buddha to bring her dead baby son back to life. She was told to bring a mustard seed from a house where there had been no death and suffering to the Buddha and he would restore life to the child. As the story goes, in house after house, she learned of deaths in each one with the clear lesson that suffering and death comes to everyone. Such a thought-provoking story can help a person change an attitude of "Why me?" to "Why not me?" We can be the victim—or the master—of our thoughts and attitudes.

Values clarification is a helpful exercise at the prompting stage and involves a review of what is held most sacred in one's life. Logotherapy teaches the importance of having parallel values rather than a pyramid of values with one thing far more important than other values. "It is dangerous to cling to a single value in life and to place it at the peak of a pyramid of values; the peak breaks off all too easily and leaves behind a pile of ruins" (Lukas, 2020, p. 126). The patient may need prompting to develop parallel values.

Fate vs freedom chart. Making a fate vs. freedom chart is a useful tool and can help one see the choices that are still available. On the Fate side, the patient is asked to list things that have happened in the past, losses that cannot be regained, a medical diagnosis that has been confirmed—things over which one has no control. The Freedom column, on the other hand, requires thinking about the possible choices, prominent among these choices is what attitude one will choose to take. It is also prudent to think of assets/abilities remaining: things you could do; things that are possible to do. In the case of patients with spinal cord injuries, many paraplegics realized they had the use of their arms even though on the Fate side they must list the inability to walk. By strengthening their arms, they can learn to transfer, operate a wheelchair, compete in sports, engage in manual and intellectual activities, and maximize independence with daily activities. Instead of "the world owes me a living," they are able to choose to prepare themselves for a career using the abilities they had.

Self-distancing is a uniquely human ability; Frankl (1969) emphasized its importance in a meaningful life and in coping with suffering. Self-distancing requires that one does not identify with the illness; rather than "I am a paraplegic," there is a possibility of "I am a bright young man who has paraplegia." And not, "Hi, my name is Bill and I am an alcoholic," rather, "Hi, my name is Bill. I am suffering from alcoholism, but it is not me. It is like a bag of rocks I am carrying, and I am working on putting it down."

Actualization

The third phase of a logotherapeutic approach to suffering involves actualizing new meanings that have been discovered despite suffering that cannot be changed. Personal responsibility is a vital factor in success. Frankl (1969) pointed out that one is responsible for what to do, whom to love, and how to suffer.

Meaning can be found even when facing a helpless situation. Frankl (1969) stated, "For what matters is to bear witness to the uniquely human potential at its best, which is to transform a personal tragedy into a triumph, to turn one's predicament into a human achievement" (p. 135). In relaying the words of a patient who had survived the Nazi concentration camp, Frankl noted, "I really understood the meaning of suffering. It can have a meaning if it changes *you* for the better" (p. 79). Finding meaning effectively mediates the relationship between suffering, well-being, and satisfaction with life (Edwards & Van Tongeren, 2020).

Self-transcendence. A key tool in the actualization stage is self-transcendence. The general literature on suffering often speaks of transcendence, as in transcending, going to a different mental plane, or distracting oneself from the suffering experience. An example would be a sufferer who takes up a paintbrush and canvas to live in another world temporarily. Such activities may be helpful to some extent. However, Frankl's (1969) concept of self-transcendence is different. In the practice of logotherapy, self-transcendence is recommended as getting outside the self, being concerned with something larger than the self, doing something that benefits others in the world. Such an occurrence was seen in a young girl who at age 15 had been injured in a drive-by shooting, leaving her with quadriplegia. She was totally dependent on others, and she bemoaned the fact that she could not even take a sip of water from the glass nearby unless someone helped her. Yet her determination to find meaning in spite of her situation led her to the following practice: Each day she would scan the news and find at least one story of tragedy—a family almost drowned at sea, a house fire with all possessions lost, a child injured with a gun. She would then, using a mouth stick, type a letter of condolence and encouragement to the party. Acknowledging that many people did not have the time or would take the time, she used the asset that she had plenty of time as well as a personal knowledge of such suffering to do her bit to make the world a better, kinder place. This is self-transcendence.

Other Models

Wong (2015) has built upon basic principles of logotherapy and integrated other types of therapies to develop what he terms *meaning therapy*. Wong offers a number of assessment instruments regarding the quest for meaning as well as intervention strategies that might be useful with patients who are suffering.

Meaning-centered therapy was the treatment used in a randomized controlled trial with patients who had advanced cancer, defined as stage III or IV solid tumors (Breitbart et al., 2010). Patients who participated in the eight-week meaning-centered group psychotherapy protocol with weekly topics on meaning demonstrated significant improvements in spiritual well-being and a sense of meaning. These findings remained even 2 months after the therapy. Frankl's three ways of finding meaning—creativity, experiences, and attitude—were parts of the sessions. More of these randomized, control trials are needed.

In hospice or palliative care, logotherapy can assist in bringing peaceful closure and fulfillment. For such patients, questions such as the following may be confronted: "What has my life been about?" "What legacy will I leave behind?" "How will I respond to the challenges as I face death?"

Individuals need support when they are in the process of actualizing new meanings in a life that has undergone many changes and abundant suffering. More education for a different career may be needed, new resources may be required. It is important to continue encouragement until a new normal has been achieved. At that time, it is wise to evaluate by looking at the before and after, to determine goals still in progress, and to celebrate changes achieved. Frankl (1969) also made it clear that what we have achieved and the meaning we have found have lasting values, even beyond our death. "In the past nothing is lost, but everything is stored as though it was safely deposited in a storehouse" (p. 120).

Suffering of Caregivers

Finally, something must be said of those who attend the suffering—the caregivers, both professionals and non-professionals. Witnessing the suffering of others can be very stressful to the body, mind, and spirit of the caregiver.

In the words of one caregiver working in a nursing home:

> This is a depressing job. I often cry. I feel sorry for them. I am crying and praying, and giving of myself so that sometimes I neglect myself.... At work, I forget to take my medicine; I don't take time to drink water like I should. ("Ms. B.," cited in Starck, 1992, p. 145)

The caregiver suffers along with the care recipient. Indeed, Schulz et al. (2010) concluded that caregivers overestimate the magnitude of suffering of the care recipient almost twice as high as the recipient self-reports. The giving of self and willingness to sacrifice for others are sure to take a toll. The caregiver may feel helpless to stop the inevitable progression. The caregiver may see ahead to more suffering to come, yet try to keep an optimistic outlook with the sufferer. Attention should be given to the needs of caregivers while they are sacrificing for the benefit of others; they may need encouragement to take care of themselves without guilt. Socratic Dialogue may help in maintaining a healthy sense of self. Certainly, the feeling of having met one's responsibilities and building treasured memories during a job well done can be an enormous source of meaning for the caregiver.

Future Research

VanderWeele (2019) has laid out directions for empirical research in the study of suffering and response. Such empirical research would lead to an "epidemiology" of suffering, followed by empirical studies of the effectiveness of responses to suffering so that it "can also lead to personal and character growth and spiritual and religious transformation which itself may lead to, and constitute, a yet greater flourishing" (p. 65).

Conclusion

A standardized definition of human suffering is needed, and Travelbee's definition is the clearest and most comprehensive: a subjective experience unique to the individual, varying from simple transitory discomfort to extreme anguish, despair, or apathetic indifference which is all-encompassing. Categorizing one's suffering is part of an overall assessment. Suffering seen through a person's religious perspective may be helpful to the caregiver. Various instruments have been developed to assess suffering, but the clinical interview remains of central importance.

A logotherapeutic model consisting of three phases—taking stock, prompting, and actualizing—with suggested tools and exercises may prove helpful to caregivers. More research is needed to develop an epidemiology of suffering and to test models to alleviate suffering from the whole person perspective.

References

Adil, J. (2010). Ancient origins of the term patient. *The Psychiatrist, 34*(3), 117–118. https://doi.org/10.1192/pb.34.3.117b

American Psychiatric Association. (2013). *Diagnostic and statistical manual of mental disorders: DSM-5* (5th ed.). American Psychiatric Association.

Baines, B. K., & Norlander, L. (2000). The relationship of pain and suffering in a hospice population. *American Journal of Hospice & Palliative Medicine, 17*(5), 319–326. https://doi.org/10.1177/104990910001700509

Boston, P., Bruce, A., & Schreiber, R. (2011). Existential suffering in the palliative care setting: An integrated literature review. *Journal of Pain and Symptom Management, 41*(3), 604–618. https://doi.org/10.1016/j.jpainsymman.2010.05.010

Breitbart, W., Rosenfeld, B., Gibson, C., Pessin, H., Poppito, S., Nelson, C., et al. (2010). Meaning-centered group psychotherapy for patients with advanced cancer: A pilot randomized controlled trial. *Psycho-Oncology, 19*(1), 21–28.

Burtt, E. A. (Ed.). (1955). *The teachings of the compassionate Buddha*. New American Library.

Cassell, E. J. (1982). The nature of suffering and the goals of medicine. *New England Journal of Medicine, 306*(11), 639–645. https://doi.org/10.1056/nejm198203183061104

Cassell, E. J. (1983). The relief of suffering. *Archives of Internal Medicine, 143*(3), 522–523. https://doi.org/10.1001/archinte.1983.00350030136022

Cassell, E. J. (1992). The nature of suffering: Physical, psychological, social, and spiritual aspects. In P. L. Starck & J. P. McGovern (Eds.), *The hidden dimension of illness: Human suffering* (pp. 1–10). National League for Nursing Press.

Cherny, N. I., Coyle, N., & Foley, K. M. (1994). Suffering in the advanced cancer patient: A definition and taxonomy. *Journal of Palliative Care, 10*(2), 57–70. https://doi.org/10.1177/082585979401000

Edwards, M. E., & Van Tongeren, D. R. (2020). Meaning mediates the association between suffering and well-being. *The Journal of Positive Psychology, 15*(6), 722–733. https://doi.org/10.1080/17439760.2019.1651890

Egnew, T. R. (2018). A narrative approach to healing chronic illness. *The Annals of Family Medicine, 16*(2), 160–165. https://doi.org/10.1370/afm.2182

Fitzpatrick, S. J., Kerridge, I. H., Jordens, C. F., Zoloth, L., Tollefsen, C., Tsomo, K. L., et al. (2016). Religious perspectives on human suffering: Implications for medicine and bioethics. *Journal of Religion and Health, 55*, 159–173. https://doi.org/10.1007/s10943-015-0014-9

Frankl, V. E. (1969). *The will to meaning*. World Publishing Company.

Frankl, V. E. (1973). *The doctor and the soul (Original work published 1946 as Ärztliche Seelsorge; Vienna: Franz Deuticke.)* (R. Winston, & C. Winston, Trans.). Penguin Books.

Frankl, V. E. (1984). *Man's search for meaning* (3rd ed.). Pocket Books. (Original work published 1946)

Kahn, D. L., & Steeves, R. H. (1986). The experience of suffering: Conceptual clarification and theoretical definition. *Journal of Advanced Nursing, 11*(6), 623–631. https://doi.org/10.1111/j.1365-2648.1986.tb03379.x

Krikorian, A., & Limonero, J. T. (2012). An integrated view of suffering in palliative care. *Journal of Palliative Care, 28*(1), 41–49. https://doi.org/10.1177/08258597120280010

Krikorian, A., Limonero, J. T., & Corey, M. T. (2013). Suffering assessment: A review of available instruments for use in palliative care. *Journal of Palliative Medicine, 16*(2), 130–142. https://doi.org/10.1089/jpm.2012.0370

Kurtus, R. (2022). *Four noble truths of Buddhism*. Retrieved from https://www.school-for-champions.com/religion/buddhism_four_noble_truths.htm

Lukas, E. (1986). *Logotherapy life: End of life counceling at 5th Worldcongress in Toronto, Kanada*. Retrieved from https://www.youtube.com/watch?v=d6CzHIlD5UI

Lukas, E. (2014). *Meaning in suffering: Comfort in crisis through logotherapy*. Purpose Research. (Original work published 1986)

Lukas, E. (2020). *Understanding* Man's Search for Meaning: *Reflections on Viktor Frankl's logotherapy* (J. B. Fabry, H. T. Smith, B. Z. Hirsch, & J. O'Meara, Trans., C. L. McLafferty, Jr., Ed.). Purpose Research.

MacAdam, D. B., & Smith, M. (1987). An initial assessment of suffering in terminal illness. *Palliative Medicine, 1*(1), 37–47. https://doi.org/10.1177/026921638700100105

Mühleisen, B., Büchi, S., Schmidhauser, S., Jenewein, J., French, L. E., & Hofbauer, G. F. (2009). Pictorial Representation of Illness and Self Measure (PRISM): A novel visual instrument to measure quality of life in dermatological inpatients. *Archives of Dermatology, 145*(7), 774–780. https://doi.org/10.1001/archdermatol.2009.121

Ruijs, C. D., Onwuteaka-Philipsen, B. D., van der Wal, G., & Kerkhof, A. J. (2009). Unbearability of suffering at the end of life: The development of a new measuring device, the SOS-V. *BMC Palliative Care, 8*, 1–10. https://doi.org/10.1186/1472-684X-8-16

Schulz, R., Monin, J. K., Czaja, S. J., Lingler, J. H., Beach, S. R., Martire, L. M., et al. (2010). Measuring the experience and perception of suffering. *The Gerontologist, 50*(6), 774–784. https://doi.org/10.1093/geront/gnq033

Starck, P. L. (1983). Patients' perceptions of the meaning of suffering. *International Forum for Logotherapy, 6*(2), 110–116.

Starck, P. L. (1985). *Guidelines: Meaning in Suffering test*. Viktor Frankl Institute of Logotherapy.

Starck, P. L. (1992). The management of suffering in a nursing home: An ethnographic study. In *The hidden dimension of illness: Human suffering* (pp. 127–153). National League for Nursing Press.

Travelbee, J. (1971). *Interpersonal aspects of nursing* (2nd ed.). F.A. Davis Company.
VanderWeele, T. J. (2019). Suffering and response: Directions in empirical research. *Social Science & Medicine, 224*, 58–66. https://doi.org/10.1016/j.socscimed.2019.01.041
Whitman, S. M. (2007). Pain and suffering as viewed by the Hindu religion. *The Journal of Pain, 8*(8), 607–613. https://doi.org/10.1016/j.jpain.2007.02.430
Wong, P. T. P. (2015). Meaning therapy: Assessments and interventions. *Existential Analysis, 26*(1), 154–167.

Patricia L. Starck, PhD, is dean emerita of the School of Nursing at the University of Texas Health Science Center at Houston and a long-time member of the international board of the Viktor Frankl Institute for Logotherapy. She is recipient of both the Lifetime Achievement Award and the Presidential Award for Distinguished Contributions and Sterling Leadership from the Institute. Starck earned a master's in rehabilitation nursing from Emory University and a PhD in community mental health from the University of Alabama in Birmingham. She has published extensively in The International Forum for Logotherapy as well as other professional journals. Her research has focused on pain and suffering, especially the role of the human spirit in these experiences.

Management of Moral Injury in Healthcare Workers During the COVID-19 Pandemic: Contribution of Viktor E. Frankl's Logotherapy and Existential Analysis

Edward Marshall and Maria Marshall

The original definition of moral injury (MI) referred "to the psychological, social and spiritual impact of events in high-stakes situations that involve the betrayal or transgression of an individual's deeply held personal moral beliefs and values" (Phoenix Australia Centre for Posttraumatic Mental Health, 2020, p. 6). It was initially described in the military field, where it was characterized as a betrayal of personal values in high-stakes situations by a person in authority (Shay, 1994, 2003, 2014). It is understood that MI presents as an existential struggle resulting from values transgressions in extreme situations as a consequence of actions, or lack thereof, which violate a personal code of ethics (Hossain & Clatty, 2021; Williamson et al., 2020).

Over the years, the understanding of the circumstances that can lead to MI has been expanded to include the following: (a) actions committed by oneself or by others; (b) not living up to personal ethical principles; and/or (c) the psychological, social, and spiritual impact of events involving betrayal by those in legitimate power in high-stakes situations that breached ethical principles (King's College London, 2020; Phoenix Australia Centre for Posttraumatic Mental Health, 2020).

The primary symptoms of MI are "guilt, shame, feelings of betrayal, difficulty forgiving, loss of meaning, loss of trust, self-blame, spiritual struggle, and feelings of inner conflict about the moral implications of those transgressions" (Koenig et al., 2019, p. 2). These symptoms can vary in intensity and can be divided into the following categories (Pearce et al., 2018; Yeterian et al., 2019):

E. Marshall (✉) · M. Marshall
Ottawa Institute of Logotherapy, Ottawa, ON, Canada
e-mail: edward.marshall@ltea.ca; maria.marshall@ltea.ca

C. L. McLafferty, Jr., J. I. Levinson (eds.), *Logotherapy and Existential Analysis*, Logotherapy and Existential Analysis: Proceedings of the Viktor Frankl Institute Vienna 2, https://doi.org/10.1007/978-3-031-48922-8_5

- Intrapersonal feelings, such as guilt, remorse, shame, anger, sadness, anxiety, disgust, contempt, low self-esteem, high self-criticism, convictions of being powerless, weak, ineffective, or unworthy, nightmares, avoidance, detachment from feelings, reduced empathy, and self-injurious behaviors.
- Interpersonal symptoms, such as loss of faith in others, loss of trust in authority figures, and avoidance of intimacy.
- Spiritual consequences, such as loss of faith in religious beliefs, loss of confidence in goodness and a just world.

The symptoms of MI indicate the scale and spectrum of outcomes that can result from morally injurious events that confront us with human fragility, vulnerability, and fallibility (Litz & Kerig, 2019). Apart from personnel in the armed forces, MI can affect other professionals, such as healthcare workers, social workers, educators, lawyers, judges, law enforcement officers, first aid providers, firefighters, chaplains, and volunteers (Asken & Goldman, 2021; Talbot & Dean, 2019).

Given the great complexity and frequency of ethical challenges that confront healthcare professionals, especially in high-stakes emergency situations, it has been suggested that with regard to the levels of stress and potential for trauma experienced, the distinctions between medical care and military conflict have become blurred (Asken, 2020). It is likely that, despite the differences in the environments and contexts, there are common factors that contribute to the development of MI, both in the military field and in civilian healthcare (American Psychiatric Association Committee on the Psychiatric Dimensions of Disaster and COVID-19, 2020; Williamson et al., 2020).

The recognition, identification, and management of MI in healthcare workers has gained significant attention in recent years, especially since the start of the COVID-19 pandemic (Dean et al., 2019; Greenberg et al., 2020; Hines et al., 2020, 2021; Kopacz et al., 2019; Williamson et al., 2020). Keeping with this momentum, it is urgent and relevant to address the management of MI in healthcare workers from an existential and meaning-centered point of view (Marshall & Marshall, 2021).

Moral Injury in Healthcare Workers

According to the American Psychiatric Association Committee on the Psychiatric Dimensions of Disaster and COVID-19 (2020), MI occurs in situations in which physicians, nurses, and other healthcare workers are required to make decisions that violate their professional commitment, inherently related to the curing and caring for the sick, in the course of providing healthcare services. Another working definition states that MI occurs when heathcare workers are unable to live up to, or to defend, their values or moral beliefs (Hossain & Clatty, 2021).

In an online survey of 114 physicians conducted in Romania during the COVID-19 pandemic in April 2020, Maftei and Holman (2021) found that 50% of these clinicians were exposed to morally injurious events. Almost half of the physicians worked in COVID-19 treatment clinics. The researchers did not find significant associations between morally injurious events and the physician's specialization, medical experience, gender, and whether or not they were working in a unit that cared for COVID-19 patients. However, significant correlations were reported between morally injurious events and the physicians' self-reported impact on their physical and emotional well-being. Adverse health and mental health outcomes were reported in relation to exposure to morally injurious events.

In a sample of 181 healthcare professionals (71% physicians) Mantri et al. (2020) validated the Moral Injury Symptom Scale for Health Professionals (MISS-HP) to examine the prevalence and predictors of MI; the study was conducted from mid-November, 2019 to mid-March, 2020, just before the COVID-19 pandemic. Mantri et al. (2021a) also found from these data that 7.8% of the participants reported severe symptoms of MI. A strong correlation was found between the symptoms of MI and the severity of clinician burnout ($r = 0.57$). Small-to-moderate correlations were observed between symptoms of MI and both depression ($r = 0.25$) and anxiety ($r = 0.37$). About a quarter of the participants (23.9%) showed moderate levels of functional impairment due to symptoms related to MI. Higher scores on the MI scale were associated with younger age, shorter time in practice, committing medical errors, greater depressive or anxiety symptoms, greater clinician burnout, no religious affiliation, and lower reported religiosity. Functionally limiting symptoms of MI were found to be significantly associated with medical errors and clinician burnout.

A follow-up study by Mantri et al. (2021b) during the initial surge of COVID-19 in the United States between April and October 2020 with 1831 health professionals taking the MISS-HP reported that means on the symptom scale increased from 27.4 ($SD = 11.6$) in April to 36.4 ($SD = 13.8$) in October, 2020 ($p < 0.001$). In April, 26.7% of all respondents reported at least moderate functional impairment due to symptoms of MI; this number increased to 45.7% in October ($p < 0.001$). Greater functional impairment was associated with direct experience caring for patients with COVID-19 symptoms, and among widowed, divorced, or never married clinicians. MI scores increased during the pandemic while burnout scores remained unchanged. The researchers differentiated between burnout and MI; they speculated that MI may be a predisposing factor for burnout. Healthcare professionals may benefit from interventions intended to reduce the delayed consequences of MI, such as depression and post-traumatic stress disorder (PTSD).

Wang et al. (2020) assessed psychometric properties of a Chinese translation of the MISS-HP (Mantri et al., 2020) to assess symptoms of MI among physicians and other health professionals across mainland China in March and April, 2020. A total of 583 nurses and 2423 physicians were surveyed. Wang et al. (2020) also found from these data that MI was reported by 41.3% of the participants. The prevalence of severe symptoms of MI was found to be 20.4%. Healthcare professionals who worked in COVID-19 care clinics had a 28% greater risk of MI than those providing care to patients without COVID. MI symptoms were strongly correlated with clinician burnout, psychological distress in the form of anxiety and depression, and a deterioration of social and occupational functioning with reported poor health and well-being.

The MI guide of the Phoenix Australia Centre for Posttraumatic Mental Health (2020) listed the following as among the morally injurious events that can contribute to the development of MI symptoms in healthcare workers: (a) having to make difficult decisions when resources are scarce to provide potentially life-saving care, (b) discharging patients from the hospital before they are sufficiently recovered from their ailments to avoid the risk of infection, and (c) not being able to offer quality care to all patients.

There is evidence that healthcare workers around the world experience ethically challenging situations as cognitive-emotive dissonance—and moral distress as an existential struggle—when they are directed to participate in practices contrary to their professional ethics and feel compelled to act against their own beliefs and values (American Psychiatric Association Committee on the Psychiatric Dimensions of Disaster and COVID-19, 2020; Asken & Goldman, 2021; Berger, 2014).

Moral Injury and Trauma

Some individuals are more likely to develop PTSD after being exposed to traumatic events than others. Unlike PTSD, MI is a syndrome related to morally injurious events (Bélanger et al., 2018; Koenig et al., 2020). Some people will develop MI after being exposed to morally injurious events. MI can coexist with PTSD in situations in which a person has been exposed to a traumatic event (Bélanger et al., 2018; Currier et al., 2013, 2017, 2019; Koenig et al., 2020; Litz & Kerig, 2019) and/or a morally injurious event (American Psychiatric Association Committee on the Psychiatric Dimensions of Disaster and COVID-19, 2020; Koenig et al., 2019).

MI has an adverse impact on mental health. If a morally injurious event is not managed correctly, it can become a traumatic event and give rise to PTSD, accompanied by symptoms of depression, anxiety, and suicidal behaviors (American Medical Association, 2019; American Psychiatric Association Committee on the Psychiatric Dimensions of Disaster and COVID-19, 2020; Bryan et al., 2018; King's College London, 2020; Koenig et al., 2019; Mantri et al., 2020; Volk & Koenig, 2018). Thus, MI can occur separately or concomitantly with PTSD, or it can lead to PTSD (Drescher et al., 2011; King's College London, 2020; Litz et al., 2019; Phoenix Australia Centre for Posttraumatic Mental Health, 2020).

According to *The Diagnostic and Statistical Manual of Mental Disorders* (5th ed., American Psychiatric Association, 2013), the diagnosis of PTSD is based on the following trauma-related criteria, which cause significant distress or impairment for more than a month:

1. Direct or indirect exposure to a traumatic event (Criterion A).
2. Presence of one or more of the following intrusion symptoms: Distressing memories, distressing dreams, dissociative reactions, psychological distress at exposure of cues that symbolize the traumatic event, and physiological reaction to cues that resemble an aspect of the traumatic event (Criterion B).

3. Persistent avoidance of stimuli associated with the traumatic event (Criterion C).
4. Negative alterations in cognition and mood associated with the traumatic event (Criterion D).
5. Marked alteration in arousal and reactivity associated with the traumatic event (Criterion E). (pp. 271–272)

Norman and Maguen (2021) compared and contrasted MI and PTSD: MI shares several core symptoms of PTSD, although they remain two different entities. Guilt and shame are core symptoms of both MI and PTSD. Betrayal and loss of trust occur in both MI and PTSD. Disgust and anger are some of the hallmarks of MI. In regard to the differences between the MI and PTSD, the latter includes hyperarousal, which has not been linked with MI.

Although the core symptoms overlap, it is possible to have MI that does not meet the criteria for PTSD (Norman & Maguen, 2021). Having MI in addition to PTSD, on the other hand, is associated with greater PTSD and depression severity and greater likelihood of self-harming and suicidal behavior (Bryan et al., 2018; Currier et al., 2019; Koenig et al., 2018). Studies that have evaluated the core features of MI, such as trauma-related guilt and shame, have also found these to be associated with more severe depression, PTSD, and functional impairment (Browne et al., 2015; Norman et al., 2018).

Studies on resilience following traumatic events have emphasized the role of meaning in modulating the stress response and opening the possibility for post-traumatic growth (Southwick & Charney, 2018; Southwick et al., 2016). In a similar vein, we have postulated that, following morally injurious events that give rise to existential struggles, meaning can modulate the amount of toxic stress generated, and mitigate the clinical and social outcomes of MI (Marshall & Marshall, 2021).

From an existential point of view, suffering occurs not only as a result of physical or psychological causes, but simultaneously has a root cause in the question of meaning. Suffering in the presence of meaning helps to avoid despair. Alternatively, as Frankl (2000) noted, "despair equals suffering minus meaning" (p. 133).

Existential Conceptualization of Moral Injury

MI can be conceptualized as a transgression of personal values that gives rise to existential struggles, resulting in a sensation of loss of meaning, accompanied by existential suffering (Marshall & Marshall, 2021). The deep sense of loss of meaning that occurs after a morally injurious event undermines confidence, hope, and optimism, affecting a person's vision of themselves and the world. Following a morally injurious event there is a value transgression, and a person's internal compass becomes disoriented. Beliefs and expectations are shaken; there is a feeling that the world, as it used to be known, does not exist.

The experience of loss of meaning that arises following the transgression of values gives rise to an existential struggle. Some people try to ameliorate existential struggles by seeking pleasure or power. The manifestation of these efforts to seek pleasure and power can be through addiction and violence. Eventually, failing to find meaning, a person sinks into despair. On the other hand, some people do not experience despair after a morally injurious event. These people do not repress or deny the impact of the value transgression on their lives, but they do not become victims of it (Marshall & Marshall, 2021).

Erik Erikson (1980) spoke about a basic trust that develops in early childhood and can be easily lost. According to Frankl, "basic trust is, ultimately, a belief in the meaning of life that we can choose to embrace. Among other things, it means becoming aware of our irreplaceable uniqueness" (as cited in Schechner & Zürner, 2013, p. 150). Thus, trust based on this more encompassing and deeper notion of trust in life's meaningfulness can be gained and regained following a morally injurious event. Basic trust is based on the belief that life is ultimately meaningful rather than meaningless. Embracing this basic trust implies that we are valuable and expected in the world and unconditionally loved as a new and irreplaceable creation. Inherent in this view is an appreciation of what is good, true, and beautiful, and also gratitude for the wonder of life and creation. The loss of this basic trust can lead to an over-reliance on success, happiness, power, self-worth, and seeking the approval of others. These experiences and expectations give rise to existential struggles manifested by insatiable restlessness (cf Lukas, 2022).

Basic trust brings about an inner recognition and change of heart and mind to be free from the approval of the world and of others and to be self-determined, free, and responsible in the pursuit of meaning. Having a sense of basic trust helps the person to overcome avoidance and a kind of "anxiety motivation" with a "love motivation" and intention toward purposeful goals (cf Lukas, 2020, 2022). It can be fostered in the following ways: (a) by opening our eyes to possibilities of the ability to do good, by inviting us to experience something beautiful, and by allowing us to transform suffering into something meaningful; (b) by opening our eyes to the wonder and gift of every moment; (c) by activating a sense of gratitude and kindness; (d) by developing culture, art, and one's own personhood; (e) by nurturing a healthy image of God as loving and forgiving; and (f) by being willing to open oneself to the wonders of the world and inner changes through gaining new experiences and insights (Schechner & Zürner, 2013).

Joseph Fabry (1988/2021) noted that the foundation of trust can be a fertile ground for fostering meaning by following the guideposts to its recovery through realizing one's own: (a) uniqueness, (b) capacity to make choices, (c) capacity for self-distancing, (d) self-transcendence, (e) responsibility, and (f) response-ability. In several studies, meaning has been associated with several positive health and mental health outcomes (i.e., Boyle et al., 2010; Breitbart, 2017; Breitbart & Masterson, 2016; Breitbart & Poppito, 2014; Case & Deaton, 2015; Chen et al., 2020; Kaplin & Anzaldi, 2015; Koizumi et al., 2008; Southwick & Charney, 2021; Southwick & Southwick, 2020). Russo-Netzer and Ameli (2021) further reinforced the notion that meaning mediates resilience, self-transcendence, and post-traumatic growth, factors related to the prevention of crises, as well as healing and protection following trauma. Thus, fostering basic trust and sense of meaning can protect from the potentially debilitating effects of trauma related to MI (Breitbart, 2020; Marshall & Marshall, 2021).

Logotherapy and Existential Analysis in the Management of Moral Injury

The following interventions for the management of MI were derived from the principles and practice of logotherapy and existential analysis (LTEA) (Marshall & Marshall, 2012):

- *Point out what is intact, areas of freedom, and what remains.* The therapist's tasks following the experience of morally injurious events are to: (1) Point out areas that have remained intact, such as values already lived, meaning already actualized in the past, meaning actualized in the present, and the dimension of an intact spirit, the inner core and essence of the person; (2) Look for areas of freedom that are still available despite limitations, obstacles, and challenges; Self-discovery, appreciation of the uniqueness of each person, the ability to choose, responsibility, self-distancing, and self-transcendence are spiritual capacities that can be used in the search for meaning to be actualized in the future (Fabry, 1968/2013, 1988/2021).
- *Modify maladaptive attitudes.* External factors such as morally injurious events can frustrate the possibility of actualizing values the same way as they were actualized in the past. Maladaptive attitudes can affect people who are: (1) too much intending to avoid existential struggles (hyperintention); (2) focusing too much on existential suffering (hyper-reflection); (3) paying exaggerated attention to themselves; and (4) hyper-intending the duty they want to fulfill. Maladaptive attitudes are counterproductive because they distract from the reason and the purpose of personal experience. They block spontaneity of action, since the person cannot see beyond what seems easily attainable, immediate, or instantaneous. The therapist using LTEA aims to correct these maladaptive attitudes by helping a person achieve a healthy balance between focus on the self and focus on the task to be fulfilled for the sake of a value, for the sake of another, for the sake of the world, in accordance with universal values, respecting the uniqueness and dignity of each person and the value of life. A change of perspective can take place in a series of steps: (1) acknowledging the reality of values violations; (2) exploring the extent to which violation of values is inevitable; (3) considering strengths and possibilities; (4) correcting any undesirable unhelpful attitudes, such as hyperintention or hyper-reflection; (5) openly discussing new discoveries about oneself; (6) guiding a person in the discovery of meaning and toward the capacity for personal growth and development (Lukas, 2014, 2015; Marshall & Marshall, 2015a, b, 2016).
- *Affirm the will to meaning.* Help to develop an appreciation of personal values that contributed to existential struggles. Although excessive emotions can cloud

appreciation of personal values, emotions point to personal values. Thus, existential suffering can prompt us to re-examine what is worth living for.
- *Recognize the areas of freedom.* Our freedom is not absolute, we are conditioned and shaped by our environment, but we have enough freedom to realize possibilities by actualizing values in a unique historical context.
- *Mobilize the resources of the human spirit.* The mobilization of spiritual resources such as the will to meaning, conscience, the ability to distance oneself, and self-transcendence bring forth the activation of hope, gratitude, humor, optimism, ideas, and ideals. Self-distancing—the ability to observe oneself from the outside—helps the individual to decide which values can be actualized according to our abilities and possibilities. It helps the person to re-engage with the world. Self-transcendence allows for the engagement with the world of values. Meaningful goals are motivating. When individuals have a strong reason to overcome obstacles, they are capable of offering a sacrifice, even a sacrifice of themselves, if necessary.
- *Explore the areas where meaning can be found.* Therapists do not ascribe meaning or give meaning, but they help to orient toward areas in which meaning can be found through the actualization of creative, experiential, and attitudinal values. The recognition of the unique meaning potentials of each person is matched to their abilities, capacities, potentials, and particular circumstances.

Tragic Optimism

The use of LTEA helps to complement the tragic triad of suffering, guilt, and death with the triad of meaning, comprised of creative, experiential, and attitudinal values, which gives the essence of Frankl's (2014) *tragic optimism*:

> An optimism in the face of tragedy… at its best always allows for (1) turning suffering into a human achievement and accomplishment; (2) deriving from guilt the opportunity to change oneself for the better; and (3) deriving from life's transitoriness an incentive to take responsible action. (pp. 129–130)

Applied to the management of MI, these concepts translate to the following guidelines: (1) Be aware of unavoidable suffering and when it makes sense to change one's attitude—one can live according to ethical values despite suffering; (2) In the face of guilt, it makes sense to change oneself—guilt is a personal phenomenon since it is through conscience and discernment that a dissonance between the person's behavior and the realization of universal values can be perceived; and (3) faced with vulnerability and finiteness, it makes sense to act.

Through this concept of tragic optimism, Frankl (2014) pointed out that meaning can be found in every life situation, even in inevitable suffering. The principles of LTEA can be used in collaboration with a person who experienced values transgressions to: (a) evaluate life as a gift received, (b) point out difficulties as opportunities for growth, (c) highlight the ability to respond with meaning to the call of life, and (d) support decision making and action.

The practitioner of LTEA promotes the activation of the will to meaning to recover the well-being of people affected by MI. An orientation to meaning contributes to increasing basic trust and alleviating existential struggles. People can find meaning by realizing values in their unique situations. Meaning is not relative but relational. An experience of the self in relation to values guides one's path of life. Meaning in life is a resiliency factor that helps a person to manage pain, guilt, and finiteness toward the heights of human accomplishment and fulfillment (Marshall & Marshall, 2021).

Case Example

The following example is an extended dialogue with Dr. Ferri, who used logotherapy in his own life to recover after being infected with coronavirus during his work with ill patients in Italy. The story is told by Gonçalves de Oliveira (2020, used with permission):

> A doctor from Italy contacted me. He was quarantined in the city of the Brescia, Italy, because of the COVID-19 pandemic. He worked in Germany at the time of the Cold War. Subsequently, he worked in Italy and he spent his vacation time to work in Africa for 18 years. Presently, he was nearing his retirement. The hospital where he is currently employed is at the center of the pandemic. His services were recruited not in the capacity of a surgeon but to care for those who are infected with the virus.
>
> He wrote to me during the night to help him discern what life was demanding of him and how to find meaning at this time. He had visited the Viktor Frankl Museum in Vienna the year before. He said that this visit had an enduring impact on his life. In our communication he wrote: "I am going to console those who are dying, and I am going to hold their hands and say a Hail Mary. When a doctor can not heal, he must offer relief and comfort."
>
> Subsequently, he went to this hospital and he became infected with the COVID-19 virus. Reportedly, he was at peace and remained calm. He was placed under medical observation and again in quarantine. He wrote to us later saying that he was feeling better. We are hopeful that he will manage to overcome the illness. Currently, he is reflecting on the value of sacrifice and finding meaning in life.

With his permission, I would like to share with you an excerpt from a recent conversation that I had with Dr. Eugenio Ferri on April 19, 2020:

VGO: Dr. Eugenio Ferri, you specialize in Rheumatology and General Surgery. From 1990 to 2000, you were Surgeon at St Elisabeth Hospital in Leipzig, Germany. In the years between 2003 and 2011 you carried out 15 missions in Cameroon and Congo, Africa. For two years between 2013 to 2015 you were responsible for the Surgery Departments of Fontem in Cameroon. Since 2015, you were Laparoscopic Surgeon at SMN Hospital in Reggio Emilia, Italy. Since 2007 to the present, you are Surgeon at the Hospital Guglielmo da Saliceto in Piacenza, Italy. You tested positive for the Corona Virus while working at the hospital during the pandemic. You are currently recovering in quarantine.

Having met you in Vienna in 2019 and knowing that you are an avid reader and connoisseur of Viktor Frankl's works, I would like to ask you to tell us a little bit about your experience, answering a few questions.

Viktor Frankl had these words from Hillel, a Jewish Rabbi, by the door of his home in Vienna:

"If I don't it; Who will do it?"

"If I don't do it now; When shall I do it?"

"If I do it for myself; Who am I?"

As a surgeon you lived through many experiences in Africa, Germany and Italy. How do you experience the above lines now at the time of the Corona virus in Italy?

Dr. EF: Africa opened my eyes to a reality that is hardly felt by us anymore. Death belongs to life. African thought cannot be compared to the Greek way of thinking that most of us are familiar with. The Cameroonian author, Martin Nkafu, speaks of "Vitalogy."

Yes, I learned this during one of my first experiences there. My patient was a girl who presented with acute abdominal pain. I did not yet know exactly the diagnosis, but I could determine that it was pathology and that it was necessary to operate. To my surprise, I find blood and neoformations in the abdomen which my local medical colleague immediately recognized as an endemic tumor. After the operation, I asked questions, emphasizing that it was necessary to begin chemotherapy! However, my colleague replied to me with great serenity: "Don't worry… we will have another little angel in heaven." To hear this was absolutely shocking to me. I found myself in a complete state of impotence when, in our world, through many technologies, we finally live in a continuous certainty of immortality and death is most of the time, someone's mistake.

VGO: Could this phrase from Frankl relate to your experiences; "Every situation is a call that first must be heard and then answered?"

Dr. EF: In this period of the Corona virus, we experienced a situation that reversed our role as doctors from being the "donors of life" to "accompanying death!" I found myself in an infirmary for terminally ill patients, where there were not only elderly people. The rooms were full of ill and unconscious people with no relatives who could see them. For someone who is familiar with Jesus' human and divine experience of the Abandonment, this could have been—making an analogy—an image of Him. I walked among those beds, praying for each one, thinking about the life they lived, thinking about their possible biographies and Jesus… waiting for them.

I filled out up to six death certificates per day—A lifetime! The dignity of a life!

I also had to call the relatives to announce the worsening of their condition and then to report their death…. I was now the "announcer of death," instead of "life and hope." But within me, there was a kind of empathy within which there was the serenity of a certainty that life goes on.

VGO: What does love mean to you? How could you transmit it in these moments of emergency?

Dr. EF: In this situation, I think it means closeness, respect, empathy, hope. The verse from St. Paul comes to my mind: "to give reason to hope."

VGO: In what ways do you think that suffering had a positive impact on you?

Dr. EF: Suffering can be good. I realized that I was more understanding of everyone—as if I lived a pardon of a general amnesty—even with myself. In particular, with my coworkers, I see them also as Jesus during his passion when it comes to deprivation in a cultural, moral sense or lack of trust. (pp. 31–35)

Result: Dr. Ferri continued his sessions with the therapists that focused on values-based living. Subsequently, he returned to Africa, where he continues to work as a surgeon offering his best knowledge paired with a human closeness to those who suffer.

Analysis: Dr. Ferri is a deeply religious man and highly competent doctor. Logotherapy is an open system, accepting religious experience. The principles of LTEA have helped him to deepen his faith and to respond according to his core beliefs. His example demonstrates that these principles can be easily learned and applied; they can be life-affirming in extreme situations in which the question of values and meaning arise. They can be used to deepen already existing trust or to restore trust that was broken. In other words, the principles of LTEA can be applied by both religious and secular individuals. This is because the common propeller of spirituality and authentic religion, religion that is based on deep spirituality, is the same: the dimension of the spirit that is a universal human phenomenon.

Conclusions

MI, originally described in the military field, has been identified in health workers during the COVID-19 pandemic. The management of MI in health workers and in civil society requires a context-specific approach.

MI caused by morally injurious events overlaps with, but is a different concept than, PTSD caused by traumatic situations. MI can coexist with PTSD and, if not well managed, can lead to PTSD. The search for meaning is a resiliency factor following trauma and morally injurious situations.

From an existential point of view, MI occurs when a transgression of values takes place that gives rise to existential struggles, manifested in a loss of meaning and existential suffering. The opposite of an existential struggle is basic trust that affirms meaning in life.

Application of the theoretical framework of LTEA helps to conceptualize the concept of MI in the context of existential dynamics. As a meaning-centered orientation to psychotherapy, LTEA provides interventions that aim to restore basic trust and kindle the will to meaning to aid recovery and promote well-being.

The use of LTEA can point to areas that are still intact and areas of freedom that are still available. Those who apply LTEA can help others (and themselves) to appreciate what remains, modify maladaptive attitudes, strengthen the will to meaning, mobilize inner spiritual resources, and illuminate areas where meaning can be found.

Practitioners of LTEA recognize suffering as an unavoidable part of life. Only a fallible person can get back on their feet, only a vulnerable person can feel pain, and only a finite person can strive for values that endure. The image of each person as valuable, regardless of their condition, is the starting point toward reconciliation with oneself and the renewal of a sense of meaning in life.

Some challenges in life are easier to master than others, just as reaching certain peaks in mountaineering is much more demanding than a leisurely walk through the valleys. Mastering the heights, as in the case of people affected by MI, requires courage, practice, patience, and determination. It also helps to have a well-trained, unconditionally life-affirming guide. The resources for this journey are the resources of the spirit and the guide is conscience through which the call can sound through: "Life awaits!"

References

American Medical Association. (2019). *Physicians' well-being: Why organizational change matters*. Retrieved from https://www.ama-assn.org/practice-management/sustainability/physician-well-being-why-organizational-change-matters

American Psychiatric Association. (2013). *Diagnostic and statistical manual of mental disorders: DSM-5* (5th ed.). American Psychiatric Association.

American Psychiatric Association Committee on the Psychiatric Dimensions of Disaster and COVID-19. (2020). *Moral injury during the COVID-19 pandemic* [Guidance document]. Retrieved from https://www.psychiatry.org/file%20library/psychiatrists/apa-guidance-covid-19-moral-injury.Pdf

Asken, M. J. (2020). Now it is moral injury: The COVID-19 pandemic and moral distress. *Medical Economics*. Retrieved from https://www.medicaleconomics.com/view/now-it-moral-injury-covid-19-pandemic-and-moral-distress

Asken, M. J., & Goldman, J. D. (2021). Moral distress, physician wellness and bioethics training: What the COVID-19 pandemic tells us about the future. *Medical Economics*. Retrieved from https://www.medicaleconomics.com/view/moral-distress-physician-wellness-and-bioethics-training-what-the-covid-19-pandemic-tells-us-about-the-future

Bélanger, S. A. H., Cramm, H., Fletcher, K., & Demers, J.-S. (2018). PTSD vs. moral injury: A scoping review. *Journal of Military, Veteran and Family Health, 4*(1), 2–4. https://doi.org/10.3138/jmvfh.4.1.002

Berger, J. T. (2014). Moral distress in medical education and training. *Journal of General Internal Medicine, 29*(2), 395–398. https://doi.org/10.1007/s11606-013-2665-0

Boyle, P. A., Buchman, A. S., Barnes, L. L., & Bennett, D. A. (2010). Effect of a purpose in life on risk of incident Alzheimer disease and mild cognitive impairment in community-dwelling older persons. *Archives of General Psychiatry, 67*(3), 304–310. https://doi.org/10.1001/archgenpsychiatry.2009.208

Breitbart, W. (Ed.). (2017). *Meaning-centered psychotherapy in the cancer setting*. Oxford University Press.

Breitbart, W. (2020). Trust in the age of COVID-19. *Palliative & Supportive Care, 18*(6), 634–635. https://doi.org/10.1017/S1478951520001364

Breitbart, W., & Masterson, M. (2016). Meaning-centered psychotherapy in the oncology and palliative care settings. In *Clinical perspectives on meaning* (pp. 245–260). Springer.

Breitbart, W., & Poppito, S. (2014). *Individual meaning-centered psychotherapy for patients with advanced cancer*. Oxford University Press.

Browne, K. C., Trim, R. S., Myers, U. S., & Norman, S. B. (2015). Trauma-related guilt: Conceptual development and relationship with posttraumatic stress and depressive symptoms. *Journal of Traumatic Stress, 28*(2), 134–141. https://doi.org/10.1002/jts.21999

Bryan, C. J., Bryan, A. O., Roberge, E., Leifker, F. R., & Rozek, D. C. (2018). Moral injury, posttraumatic stress disorder, and suicidal behavior among National Guard personnel. *Psychological Trauma Theory Research Practice and Policy, 10*(1), 36–45. https://doi.org/10.1037/tra0000290

Case, A., & Deaton, A. (2015). Rising morbidity and mortality in midlife among white non-Hispanic Americans in the 21st century. *Proceedings of the National Academy of Sciences of the United States of America, 112*(49), 15078–15083. https://doi.org/10.1073/pnas.1518393112

Chen, Y., Koh, H. K., Kawachi, I., Botticelli, M., & VanderWeele, T. J. (2020). Religious service attendance and deaths related to drugs, alcohol, and suicide among US health care professionals. *JAMA Psychiatry, 77*(7), 737–744. https://doi.org/10.1001/jamapsychiatry.2020.0175

Currier, J. M., Holland, J. M., Drescher, K., & Foy, D. (2013). Initial psychometric evaluation of the moral injury questionnaire—Military version. *Clinical Psychology & Psychotherapy, 22*(1), 54–63. https://doi.org/10.1002/cpp.1866

Currier, J. M., Farnsworth, J. K., Drescher, K. D., McDermott, R. C., Sims, B. M., & Albright, D. L. (2017). Development and evaluation of the expressions of moral injury scale-military version. *Clinical Psychology & Psychotherapy, 25*(3), 474–488. https://doi.org/10.1002/cpp.2170

Currier, J. M., McDermott, R. C., Farnsworth, J. K., & Borges, L. M. (2019). Temporal associations between moral injury and posttraumatic stress disorder symptom clusters in military veterans. *Journal of Traumatic Stress, 32*(3), 382–392. https://doi.org/10.1002/jts.22367

Dean, W., Talbot, S., & Dean, A. (2019). Reframing clinician distress: Moral injury not burnout. *Federal Practitioner, 36*(9), 3. Retrieved from https://www.ncbi.nlm.nih.gov/pmc/articles/PMC6752815/pdf/fp-36-09-400.pdf

Drescher, K. D., Foy, D. W., Kelly, C., Leshner, A., Schutz, K., & Litz, B. (2011). An exploration of the viability and usefulness of the construct of moral injury in war veterans. *Traumatology, 17*(1), 8–13. https://doi.org/10.1177/1534765610395615

Erikson, E. H. (1980). *Identity and the life cycle*. Norton.

Fabry, J. B. (2013). *The pursuit of meaning: Viktor Frankl, logotherapy, and life*. Purpose Research. (Original work published 1968)

Fabry, J. B. (2021). *Guideposts to meaning: Discovering what really matters* (2nd ed.). Purpose Research. (Original work published 1988)

Frankl, V. E. (2000). *Man's search for ultimate meaning*. Perseus. (Original work published *Der Unbewusste Gott*, 1948 and English translation, *The Unconscious God*, 1975)

Frankl, V. E. (2014). *Man's search for meaning* (3rd ed.). Beacon Press.

Gonçalves de Oliveira, V. (2020). The testimony of Dr. Ferri. In M. Marshall & E. Marshall (Eds.), *Carried by the Spirit: Our hearts sing: Discerning meaning during the COVID-19 pandemic* (pp. 31–36). Ottawa Institute of Logotherapy.

Greenberg, N., Docherty, M., Gnanapragasam, S., & Wessely, S. (2020). Managing mental health challenges faced by healthcare workers during covid-19 pandemic. *BMJ*, m1211. https://doi.org/10.1136/bmj.m1211

Hines, S. E., Chin, K. H., Levine, A. R., & Wickwire, E. M. (2020). Initiation of a survey of healthcare worker distress and moral injury at the onset of the COVID-19 surge. *American Journal of Industrial Medicine, 63*(9), 830–833. https://doi.org/10.1002/ajim.23157

Hines, S. E., Chin, K. H., Glick, D. R., & Wickwire, E. M. (2021). Trends in moral injury, distress, and resilience factors among healthcare workers at the beginning of the COVID-19 pandemic. *International Journal of Environmental Research and Public Health, 18*(2), 488. https://doi.org/10.3390/ijerph18020488

Hossain, F., & Clatty, A. (2021). Self-care strategies in response to nurses' moral injury during COVID-19 pandemic. *Nursing Ethics, 28*(1), 23–32. https://doi.org/10.1177/0969733020961825

Kaplin, A., & Anzaldi, L. (2015). *New movement in neuroscience: A purpose-driven life*. Paper presented at the Cerebrum: The Dana forum on brain science.

King's College London. (2020) *The history of moral injury*. Retrieved from https://youtu.be/QX8_QkNUoy8

Koenig, H. G., Ames, D., Youssef, N. A., Oliver, J. P., Volk, F., Teng, E. J., et al. (2018). The moral injury symptom scale—Military version. *Journal of Religion and Health, 57*(1), 249–265. https://doi.org/10.1007/s10943-017-0531-9

Koenig, H. G., Youssef, N. A., & Pearce, M. (2019). Assessment of moral injury in veterans and active duty military personnel with PTSD: A review. *Frontiers in Psychiatry, 10*, 443–443. https://doi.org/10.3389/fpsyt.2019.00443

Koenig, H. G., Youssef, N. A., Ames, D., Teng, E. J., & Hill, T. D. (2020). Examining the overlap between moral injury and PTSD in US veterans and active duty military. *Journal of Nervous and Mental Disease, 208*(1), 7–12.

Koizumi, M., Ito, H., Kaneko, Y., & Motohashi, Y. (2008). Effect of having a sense of purpose in life on the risk of death from cardiovascular diseases. *Journal of Epidemiology, 18*(5), 191–196. https://doi.org/10.2188/jea.je2007388

Kopacz, M. S., Ames, D., & Koenig, H. G. (2019). It's time to talk about physician burnout and moral injury. *The Lancet Psychiatry, 6*(11), e28. https://doi.org/10.1016/s2215-0366(19)30385-2

Litz, B. T., & Kerig, P. K. (2019). Introduction to the Special Issue on Moral Injury: Conceptual challenges, methodological issues, and clinical applications. *Journal of Traumatic Stress, 32*(3), 341–349. https://doi.org/10.1002/jts.22405

Litz, B. T., Berke, D. S., Kline, N. K., Grimm, K., Rusowicz-Orazem, L., Resick, P. A., et al. (2019). Patterns and predictors of change in trauma-focused treatments for war-related post-traumatic stress disorder. *Journal of Consulting and Clinical Psychology, 87*(11), 1019–1029. https://doi.org/10.1037/ccp0000426

Lukas, E. (2014). *Meaning in suffering: Comfort in crisis through logotherapy*. Purpose Research. (Original work published 1986)

Lukas, E. (2015). *The therapist and the soul: From fate to freedom*. Purpose Research.

Lukas, E. (2020). *Logotherapy principles and methods*. Elisabeth Lukas Archiv.

Lukas, E. (2022). *Trust, basic trust, self confidence, and trust in god/interviewer: S. Baier* (M. Marshall, Trans.). Grandios Magazine, Regensburg, Germany.

Maftei, A., & Holman, A.-C. (2021). The prevalence of exposure to potentially morally injurious events among physicians during the COVID-19 pandemic. *European Journal of Psychotraumatology, 12*(1), 1898791. https://doi.org/10.1080/20008198.2021.1898791

Mantri, S., Lawson, J. M., Wang, Z., & Koenig, H. G. (2020). Identifying moral injury in healthcare professionals: The Moral Injury Symptom Scale-HP. *Journal of Religion and Health, 59*(5), 2323–2340. https://doi.org/10.1007/s10943-020-01065-w

Mantri, S., Lawson, J. M., Wang, Z., & Koenig, H. G. (2021a). Prevalence and predictors of moral injury symptoms in health care professionals. *Journal of Nervous and Mental Disease, 209*(3), 174–180. https://doi.org/10.1097/nmd.0000000000001277

Mantri, S., Song, Y. K., Lawson, J. M., Berger, E. J., & Koenig, H. G. (2021b). Moral injury and burnout in health care professionals during the COVID-19 pandemic. *Journal of Nervous and Mental Disease, 209*(10), 720–726. https://doi.org/10.1097/nmd.0000000000001367

Marshall, M., & Marshall, E. (2012). *Logotherapy revisited: Review of the tenets of Viktor E. Frankl's logotherapy*. Ottawa Institute of Logotherapy.

Marshall, M., & Marshall, E. (2015a). *Perpetuum mobile: A personal global concern*. Ottawa Institute of Logotherapy.

Marshall, M., & Marshall, E. (2015b). *Spiritual psychotherapy: The search for lasting meaning*. Ottawa Institute of Logotherapy.

Marshall, M., & Marshall, E. (2016). *Attentive: A competence to discern meaning*. Ottawa Institute of Logotherapy.

Marshall, E., & Marshall, M. (2021). *Logotherapy and existential analysis for the management of moral injury*. Ottawa Institute of Logotherapy.

Norman, S., & Maguen, S. (2021). *Moral injury*. Retrieved from https://www.ptsd.va.gov/professional/treat/cooccurring/moral_injury.asp

Norman, S., Haller, M., Kim, H. M., Allard, C., Porter, K., Stein, M. B., et al. (2018). Trauma related guilt cognitions partially mediate the relationship between PTSD symptom severity and functioning among returning combat veterans. *Journal of Psychiatric Research, 100*, 56–62.

Pearce, M., Haynes, K., Rivera, N. R., & Koenig, H. G. (2018). Spiritually integrated cognitive processing therapy: A new treatment for post-traumatic stress disorder that targets moral injury. *Global Advances in Health and Medicine, 7*. https://doi.org/10.1177/2164956118759939

Phoenix Australia Centre for Posttraumatic Mental Health. (2020). *Moral stress amongst healthcare workers during COVID-19: A guide to moral injury*. Retrieved from https://www.phoenixaustralia.org/wp-content/uploads/2020/07/Moral-Stress-Healthcare-Workers-COVID-19-Guide-to-Moral-Injury.pdf

Russo-Netzer, P., & Ameli, M. (2021). Optimal sense-making and resilience in times of pandemic: Integrating rationality and meaning in psychotherapy. *Frontiers in Psychology, 12*, 645926–645926. https://doi.org/10.3389/fpsyg.2021.645926

Schechner, J., & Zürner, H. (2013). *Krisen bewältigen: Viktor E Frankls 10 thesen in der praxis*. Braumüller Verlag.

Shay, J. (1994). *Achilles in Vietnam: Combat trauma and the undoing of character*. Scribner.

Shay, J. (2003). *Odysseus in America: Combat trauma and the trials of homecoming*. Simon and Schuster.

Shay, J. (2014). Moral injury. *Psychoanalytic Psychology, 31*(2), 182–191. https://doi.org/10.1037/a0036090

Southwick, S., & Charney, D. (2018). *Resilience: The science of mastering life's greatest challenges*. Cambridge University Press.

Southwick, S., & Charney, D. (2021). Resilience for frontline health care workers: Evidence-based recommendations. *The American Journal of Medicine, 134*(7), 829–830. https://doi.org/10.1016/j.amjmed.2021.02.010

Southwick, S., & Southwick, F. S. (2020). The loss of social connectedness as a major contributor to physician burnout. *JAMA Psychiatry, 77*(5), 449. https://doi.org/10.1001/jamapsychiatry.2019.4800

Southwick, S., Lowthert, B., & Graber, A. (2016). Relevance and application of logotherapy to enhance resilience to stress and trauma. In *Logotherapy and existential analysis: Proceedings of the Viktor Frankl Institute Vienna* (pp. 131–149). Springer.

Talbot, S., & Dean, W. (2019). Beyond burnout: The real problem facing doctors is moral injury. *Medical Economics Journal, 96*(10).

Volk, F., & Koenig, H. G. (2018). Moral injury and religiosity in active duty U.S. military with PTSD symptoms. *Military Behavioral Health, 7*(1), 64–72. https://doi.org/10.1080/21635781.2018.1436102

Wang, Z., Koenig, H. G., Yan, T., Jing, W., Mu, S., Hongyu, L., & Guangtian, L. (2020). Psychometric properties of the moral injury symptom scale among Chinese health professionals during the COVID-19 pandemic. *BMC Psychiatry, 20*(1), 1–10. https://doi.org/10.1186/s12888-020-02954-w

Williamson, V., Murphy, D., & Greenberg, N. (2020). COVID-19 and experiences of moral injury in front-line key workers. *Occupational Medicine (Oxford, England), 70*(5), 317–319. https://doi.org/10.1093/occmed/kqaa052

Yeterian, J. D., Berke, D. S., Carney, J. R., McIntyre-Smith, A., St. Cyr, K., King, L., et al. (2019). Defining and measuring moral injury: Rationale, design, and preliminary findings from the Moral Injury Outcome Scale Consortium. *Journal of Traumatic Stress, 32*(3), 363–372. https://doi.org/10.1002/jts.22380

Edward Marshall, MD, PhD, Viktor E. Frankl Professor of Psychotherapy and Spirituality at the Graduate Theological Foundation (USA). Diplomate Clinician in Logotherapy (USA). Lifetime Member and Faculty of the Viktor Frankl Institute (USA). Accredited Member of the International Association of Logotherapy and Existential Analysis (Vienna, Austria). Registered Psychotherapist in Ontario and co-founder of the Ottawa Institute of Logotherapy, Canada.

Maria Marshall, Ph.D., Mignon G. Eisenberg Professor of Logotherapy at the Graduate Theological Foundation (USA). Diplomate Clinician in Logotherapy (USA) and Certified with Logotherapeutic Qualifications (Elisabeth Lukas, Germany). Lifetime Member and Faculty of the Viktor Frankl Institute (USA). Accredited Member of the International Association of Logotherapy and Existential Analysis (Vienna, Austria). Registered Psychotherapist in Ontario and co-founder of the Ottawa Institute of Logotherapy, Canada.

The Suffering Hypothesis: Viktor Frankl's Spiritual Remedies and Recent Developments

Paul T. P. Wong and Don Laird

Part 1: An Age of Existential Crises and the Suffering Hypothesis

The coronavirus pandemic (COVID-19) awakened us to the fragility and finitude of human existence (Cowden et al., 2021, p. 31; Van Tongeren & Showalter Van Tongeren, 2021; Wong et al., 2022). The recent Russia-Ukraine war and threats of China's invasion of Taiwan have made people keenly aware of the catastrophes of nuclear war. In addition to these existential crises, people are also troubled by pocketbook issues, random violence, runaway inflation, and the prospects of global economic recession. In these troubling circumstances, many people, including the young, may ask "What is the point of striving? How can one be happy in times like these?"

Positive psychology in North America, created in times of peace and prosperity (American Psychological Association, 1999; Seligman & Csikszentmihalyi, 2000), can no longer provide an adequate answer to such anxious questions from suffering people because it is principally focused on "understanding how people rise from zero to positive eight" (Gable & Haidt, 2005, p. 103). In contrast, existential positive psychology (EPP), which has its roots in existentialism and ancient wisdom, is fundamentally concerned with the pressing question of how to ameliorate suffering and how to flourish even in the darkest hours (Wong, 2020a, 2021d; Wong et al., 2022).

P. T. P. Wong (✉)
Trent University, Toronto, ON, Canada

D. Laird
Carlow University, Pittsburgh, PA, USA

C. L. McLafferty, Jr., J. I. Levinson (eds.), *Logotherapy and Existential Analysis*, Logotherapy and Existential Analysis: Proceedings of the Viktor Frankl Institute Vienna 2, https://doi.org/10.1007/978-3-031-48922-8_6

On the surface, EPP appears to be the mere synthesis of existentialism and positive psychology or the second wave of positive psychology (PP2.0). But at a deeper level, it is a new paradigm asking the toughest question of how to achieve ultimate happiness by transforming hell into heaven (Wong & Bowers, 2018). Psychologists have a moral obligation to end suffering and help individuals create a better future. The *suffering hypothesis* is designed to show people how to end unnecessary suffering and transform inescapable suffering to find and manifest strength, happiness, and flourishing.

Suffering Is a Fertile Ground for Existentialism and the Quest for Meaning

Human suffering has always been the main focus of existential philosophy and psychology. This isn't too difficult to understand. We emerged from the Great War and the Great Depression both physically and psychologically bruised. Then came the Holocaust committed by Nazi Germany and the atomic bombings of Hiroshima and Nagasaki. People began to wrestle with the horrors of life: the existential crises of human evils, the sorrows, chaos, and absurdities of Being as well as the existential anxieties of meaningless, loneliness, death, and the abuse of human freedom.

All human suffering—physical, emotional, mental, spiritual, social, and economic—and the apparent meaninglessness of human existence became fertile grounds for existentialism (e.g., Kierkegaard, Nietzsche, Camus, Satire, Hildegard, Frankl). Hamm (2015) summarized this idea:

> Just as existentialism took root in Europe much as a response to the meaninglessness the First World War drove into people's hearts, the Second World War only reinforced this sense of powerlessness, and the meaninglessness of existence. After all, what could one person do? (p. 9)

The pandemic has amplified our existential concerns. The global death tolls and hospitalization rates loudly declare that anyone could be infected and die of COVID-19. Even mandatory lockdown is behind us in most countries. The fear of being infected and testing positive remain a daily possibility. People are afraid to shake hands or hug each other, as if everyone could be a transmitter of COVID-19 or its variants.

No wonder we are witnessing unprecedented levels of anxiety, depression, anger, violence, social turmoil, discrimination, confusion, hate, and anxiety. We read and hear the phrase "existential crisis" so often now that it has become part of our common nomenclature. In the era of COVID-19, even young people begin to question the meaning of life, feeling that it is rather pointless to strive for good grades and good jobs, because in the end, we all die.

However, existential writings are far from the nihilistic despair they are accused of being. In effect, they reflect just the opposite. From the lens of existentialism, meaning offers us a heroic way to survive and experience a deeper kind of happiness. Hamm (2015) wrote:

> Joy is a fundamental part of the existential writings of several authors in the tradition.... It is in this sense that existentialism offers a possibility of joy not as a needle in a haystack, but rather as a diamond in the rough. (p. 7)

More recently, Roncero (2021) made a more explicit case that an existential crisis can be an opportunity for positive transformation:

> Existential crises are often be associated with a negative impact on one's life, but we forget the positive effect it [*sic*] can have. An existential crisis means we have the opportunity to get back in touch with our values, meaning and purpose, and with what we want to make of our lives. This can help us evaluate, plan and adapt our actions and direction in order to lead the life we want and will be happy with. (para 1)

As counterintuitive as it may seem, embracing inescapable suffering is far more adaptive than trying to avoid it. According to existentialism, paradoxically, we become an authentic version of ourselves and flourish only when we are aware of our mortality.

Jean-Paul Sartre (1943/1989) penned "Human life begins on the far side of despair" (p. 119). The answer to life's greatest questions is found within creative action and meaning. Similarly, Albert Camus (1952/1969) wrote: "In the midst of winter, I found there was, within me, an invincible summer" (para 10).

Viktor Frankl (1946/1985) was the first psychotherapist to fully articulate both the power of meaning and the obstacles of finding meaning. Although many of his fellow prisoners perished as a direct result of crimes committed by the Nazis, Frankl observed firsthand that others died by suicide or withered when they had lost their will to survive.

However, those who found meaning—or a purpose to remain alive—were far better equipped to withstand suffering and torment at the hands of their captors (Frankl, 1946/1985). Despite the heartbreak and horror of it all, Frankl noted that they persisted because they saw meaning and purpose in their suffering. It helps us recognize the importance of why finding meaning in the face of suffering is fundamental to our existence as a species:

> We must never forget that we may also find meaning in life even when confronted with hopeless situation, when facing a fate that cannot be changed. For what then matters is to bear witness to the uniquely human potential at its best, which is to transform a personal tragedy into a triumph, to turn one's predicament into a human achievement. (p. 116)

The Suffering Hypothesis and the Ultimate Happiness

According to the suffering hypothesis, life is full of suffering, and it is an inescapable part of human existence, as shown in Fig. 1. Whether we are confronted with natural disasters, pandemics, a soulless and heartless culture of brutal competitions, corrupt government, or tormented by our inner demons of greed, envy, anger, or

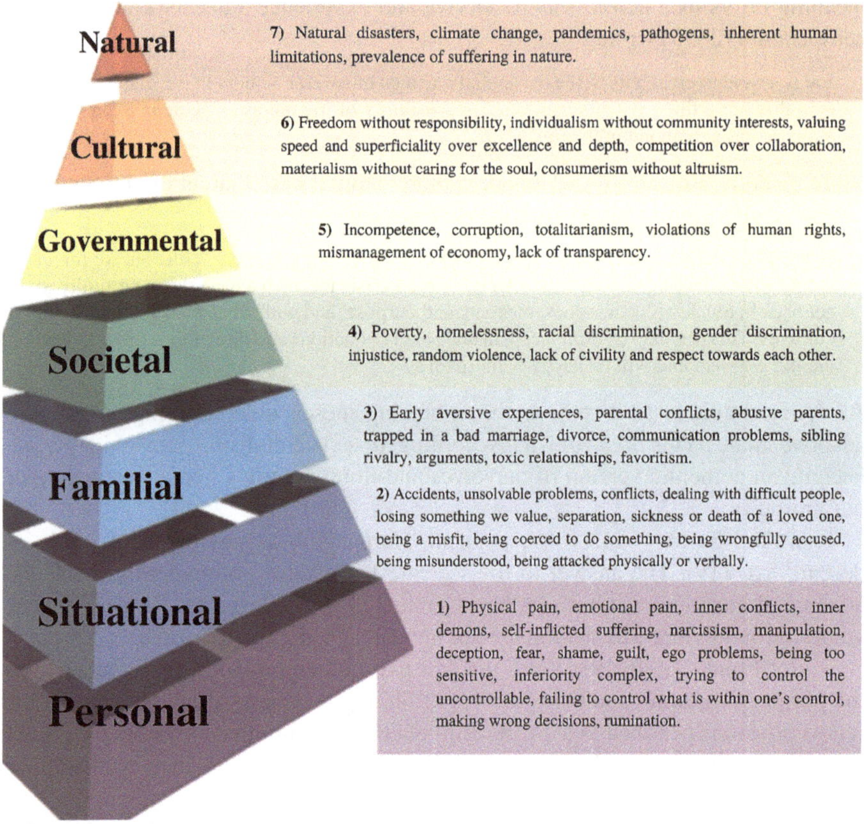

Fig. 1 A taxonomy of suffering

inferiority complex, we are carrying an enormous load of cares in our daily struggles for survival and happiness.

In Fig. 1, suffering caused by nature, culture, government, or society are mostly beyond personal control. Frankl suggested the use of attitudinal values to cope with these macro problems or to change oneself in order to accommodate these problems. The person can also exercise social responsibility to collaboratively improve our social ails. The last three levels (familial, situational, and personal) indicate that most of these problems are within the person's control. Therefore, individuals have the responsibility to resolve issue at these levels.

Barring any mishap, even an ordinary day can drain one's energy with its everyday hassles and frustrations of working with fake or unreasonable people. Suffering is everywhere, no matter what you do or where you go. One can be easily overwhelmed by the enormity and complexity of suffering, especially because most of our suffering is beyond human control. Thus, the brutal truth is that to live is to suffer and to suffer is to learn how to turn it into strength and flourishing.

The main attraction of our suffering hypothesis is that it is not suffering but how we respond to it that really matters. In other words, suffering can either destroy us or make us better and stronger. Inspired by Frankl's (1946/1985) testimony and teaching, we affirm that we have the capability to transform suffering into strength and add deeper meaning to our lives:

> The way in which a man accepts his fate and all the suffering it entails, the way in which he takes up his cross, gives him ample opportunity—even under the most difficult circumstances—to add a deeper meaning to his life. (p. 76)

It is important to note that Wong's (2003, 2021c) suffering hypothesis complements Jonathan Haidt's (2006) happiness hypothesis because the suffering hypothesis captures both functions of the soul, which is: (a) to satisfy the soul's spiritual yearning for happiness and (b) to satisfy the soul's ultimate need to come to terms with the dark side of human existence. These two functions need to work together to achieve healing and flourishing according to the dual-system model (Wong, 2012).

It is through integrating happiness and suffering that we can find the middle way—to be safely happy and to suffer joyfully (Soper, 2020; Wong, 2011, 2022b, c). It is through integration that we discover that ultimate happiness can be approximated by going through the gates of hell and moving upward toward heaven.

According to the suffering hypothesis, happiness is so intractable because life is always a mixture of happiness and suffering. No one is immune from pain, and we all live under the shadow of suffering and death. Furthermore, there is often a complex and dynamic relationship between happiness and suffering. There is a Chinese saying: "The extreme form of happiness produces sorrow." Just as happiness may lead to suffering, so does suffering may lead to happiness.

That is why the suffering hypothesis posits the following:

1. The pursuit of happiness can be a cause of suffering because of (a) frustration of unrealistic expectation and unexpected obstacles and (b) fear of losing what one values most.
2. The end of suffering is the beginning of true happiness because learning wisdom and virtues is needed for mature happiness.
3. We need wisdom and virtue because they lead to self-control, which helps us to avoid unnecessary suffering.
4. We need courage and virtue to endure, overcome, and transform inescapable suffering.
5. We rejoice in voluntary suffering for a worthy cause or someone we love more than ourselves.

> He who does not know of sorrows
> in this valley of sorrows,
> does not know of good things,
> nor has he tasted love,
> for sorrows is the garb of lovers. (De Jesús, 1955/1958)

Part 2: Frankl's Spiritual Remedies

Viktor Frankl occupies a unique place in the chronicles of psychology. While other psychologists do research on the behavior, cognition, or emotion of people through observation or self-report, Frankl studied real people in their struggles for survival and wholeness in a cruel world.

Frankl's (1946/1985) book *Man's Search for Meaning* remains a best seller because it touches people's hearts and souls and shows them how to find meaning whatever their circumstances. It is a shame that most research psychologists working on meaning are not familiar with the deep wisdom of his work on meaning.

The world seems to have gone wild, bent on self-destruction, with every person free to pursue their unbridled egotistic desires. What is the most promising solution to the perennial problem of human suffering? What is the best way to transform the hell of human evil, violence, and mental illness to the heaven of peace, love, and joy?

We propose that Frankl's cure (Wong, 2020b, 2021a, b) may show us the way. Frankl's logotherapy is both timeless and transcultural, because it speaks to the universal spiritual yearnings of human beings and discovers the universal human capacities to meet their spiritual needs for meaning: "Logotherapy's primary goal is to describe, phenomenologically, the essence of being via its different names, such as 'Dasein,' 'Tao,' 'self-realization,' 'Zen-consciousness,' and so on, and take this into consideration in the therapeutic encounter" (Ko, 1980).

Frankl's therapy is essentially a spiritual therapy in its assumptions and applications because of people's struggles with suffering and their inner "existential vacuum," even in the best of times.

Existential Vacuum as a Source of Human Suffering and Bad Behavior

Frankl (1946/1985) introduced the term *existential vacuum* to describe the condition of people who, for various reasons, do not have meaning in their lives and consequently experience boredom, emptiness, and loneliness. The lack of meaning and spiritual values, if unattended over a long time, may eventually result in an existential vacuum. People may resort to all kinds of distractions, even unethical and illegal activities, to fill that inner void. Frankl (1946/1986, 2004) considered it a noögenic (in the spiritual dimension) disorder, which called for a spiritual remedy. This existential vacuum accumulates and expands as people continue to reject what is meaningful in favor of what is expedient or meets the needs of their lower or baser instincts. As a result, weeds take over their soul in terms of bad habits, addictions, or indulgences in pleasures, pride, and egotism. Logotherapy is designed to help awaken a deep-seated need for meaning and spirituality in each person.

Frankl's Anthropology and the Spiritual (Noëtic) Dimension

Frankl (1946/1986) had a high view of the human being and opposed the prevailing view that we are "nothing but." His dimensional ontology recognized the somatic, psychological, and spiritual dimensions; he held a holistic view that these three dimensions were interrelated, with the spiritual dimension distinguishing us from the animal kingdom.

Against the dominant voices in the academia of Vienna (Freud's will to pleasure and Adler's will to power), Frankl (1969/1988) struggled to make his voice heard, to bring attention to the importance of the will to meaning as a spiritually rooted motivation. It is the spiritual yearning for meaning that enables us to transcend our physical and mental limitations. To ignore one's spiritual dimension, all kinds of problems may ensue, as we have already noted earlier.

There are three aspects of spirituality: (a) the will to meaning, which is one's spiritual motivation; (b) the meaning of life even in times of suffering, and (c) the capability to choose the spiritual orientation (Ryan, 2019).

The will to meaning is present in every person. In the *Unheard Cry for Meaning*, Frankl (1978) indicated that all human beings are crying out for meaning, but their cries are muffled by the voices of the secular world and egotistic desires. As Marseille (1997) noted, every person has the freedom and responsibility to reflect on one's own unhappy life and choose to re-orient toward a more meaningful and spiritual existence:

One cannot experience meaning in life without discovering the meaning of suffering:

> The meaning of suffering—unavoidable and inescapable suffering alone, of course—can be the deepest possible meaning. The art of being human is learning how to deal with those painful moments. These moments require an attitude of inner willingness to suffer, while remaining in touch spiritually with one's own extended dimensions.... When this inner struggle becomes calm, one can experience how the lower somatic and psychological dimensions influence the higher spiritual dimension but do not produce or cause it. One can discover despair despite success, and fulfillment despite failure. (Marseille, 1997, p. 6)
>
> It is one of the basic tenets of logotherapy that man's main concern is not to gain pleasure or to avoid pain but rather to see a meaning in his life. That is why man is even ready to suffer, on the condition, to be sure, that his suffering has a meaning. (Frankl, 1946/1985, p. 117)

The Spiritual Yearning for Ultimate Meaning

Frankl recognized three kinds of meaning—the meaning of the moment, one's meaning in life as a whole, and ultimate meaning (Wong, 2014). Belief in the ultimate meaning of life is necessary for logotherapy's basic tenet that life has intrinsic meaning up to the last breath. It reminds us of William James' (1895) affirmation of meaning: "Be not afraid of life. Believe that life *is* worth living and your belief will help create the fact" (p. 24).

Ultimate meaning makes the meaning of suffering possible. With a defiant attitude, we can still look at the shining stars in the darkest night and affirm one's faith in life's intrinsic and ultimate meaning: "The grandiose order, I believe, is what Frankl understands by logos, ultimate meaning. We can never hope to 'find' it in its totality, we can only pursue it to the best of our abilities" (Fabry, 1968/2013, p. 31).

Furthermore, Wong (2014) explained Frankl's idea in this way:

> In a sense, ultimate meaning belongs to the spiritual and transcendental realm. From time to time, we are given a glimpse of the glorious possibility that there is ultimate meaning and purpose in life. However, as we go through different stages of life and different experiences, our understanding evolves. This unending quest for ultimate meaning is simultaneously both uplifting and trying, and it has been at the centre of the human search for meaning since antiquity. (p. 163)

Joseph Fabry (1988/2021) added to this concept:

> If you are aware of ultimate meaning, in either a religious or a secular context, you will be able to respond meaningfully to the offerings of the moment because you have a built-in compass that points toward meaning. If you are not aware of ultimate meaning, you will respond to the meaning of the moment as best you can, and in the course of your life you will gradually approach understanding of ultimate meaning. (p. 3)

The Three Spiritual Values of Meaning

According to Frankl (1946/1986), there are three values or pathways to experience meaning:

1. *Creative values.* What I give the world with the value I create by doing what I do with all my heart, all my heart, and all my soul, and placing a stamp of my unique personality and imagination to the work, regardless of the occupation. Therefore, my work has meaning, because I do it as if unto God.
2. *Experiential values.* What I receive from the world with an attitude of gratitude and a humble attitude of learning some important lesson from God. This has spiritual value, because it takes one away from what makes me happy, but what stretches me and makes me become what I am meant to be.
3. *Attitudinal values.* What stance I take toward fate or suffering. "But most far-reaching are the attitude values which can be actualized to one's last breath" (Marseille, 1997, p. 6). Frankl (1946/1985) noted that "Man is that being who invented the gas chambers of Auschwitz; however, he is also that being who entered those gas chambers upright, with the Lord's Prayer or the *Shema Yisrael* on his lips" (p. 134).

The Human Capacities to Experience and Express the Spiritual Dimension

Frankl (1946/1985) held that there are three capabilities that enable us to express and experience our spiritual dimension:

Self-Determination The courage and freedom of the will to take personal responsibility for choosing to do what is right and what is meaningful rather than what gives us pleasure or power. This is a spiritual choice—to choose good rather than evil. As Solzhenitsyn (1973) noted:

> The line separating good and evil passes not through states, nor between classes, nor between political parties either—but right through every human heart—and through all human hearts. This line shifts. Inside us, it oscillates with the years. And even within hearts overwhelmed by evil, one small bridgehead of good is retained. And even in the best of all hearts, there remains… an unuprooted small corner of evil. (p. 168)

Self-Detachment The practice of pausing and keeping calm in order to get in touch with our conscience, and with God, allows us to do the right thing between stimulus and response. It is a very important skill to enable us to step back from our immediate concerns and the environment. We are not our problems. We are who decides how to best respond to all the events that happen to us. This little separation allows us to consult conscience and our forebrain before responding emotionally or habitually.

Self-Transcendence The essence of human existence. As Frankl (1946/1985) stated:

> By declaring that man is responsible and must actualize the potential meaning of his life, I wish to stress that the true meaning of life is to be discovered in the world rather than within man or his own psyche, as though it were a closed system. I have termed this constitutive characteristic "the self-transcendence of human existence." It denotes the fact that being human always points, and is directed, to something, or someone, other than oneself—be it a meaning to fulfill or another human being to encounter. The more one forgets himself—by giving himself to a cause to serve or another person to love—the more human he is and the more he actualizes himself. (p. 110–111)

Frankl (1946/1985) described in detail an experience of self-transcendence in the Nazi death camp:

> Another time we were at work in a trench. The dawn was grey around us, grey was the sky above, grey was the snow in the pale light of dawn, grey the rags in which my fellow prisoners were clad, and grey their faces…. I was struggling to find the *reason* for my sufferings, my slow dying. In a last violent protest against the hopelessness of imminent death, I sensed my spirit piercing through the enveloping gloom. I felt it transcend that hopeless, meaningless world, and from somewhere I heard a victorious "Yes" in answer to my question of the existence of an ultimate purpose. At that moment, a light was lit in a distant farmhouse, which stood on the horizon as if painted there, in the midst of the miserable gray of a dawning morning in Bavaria. "*Et lux in tenebris lucet*"—and the light shineth in the darkness. (pp. 40–41, italics in the original)

Elsewhere, Wong et al. (2021) fully described the different dimensions of self-transcendence and explained why it is important for us to become fully human by going beyond and above our physical and mental limitations and transcend all the negative forces that hold us back.

The Power of Meaning and Spirituality as an Antidote to Egotistic Desires and Human Suffering

What can we do about rampant human evil and widespread human suffering? Something needs to be done before more innocent people get killed and more people get addicted to drugs or commit suicide. Something needs to be done to help people with mental illness. Perhaps, we should at least give spirituality a chance. Perhaps most of the human and societal problems stem from the fact that we are like fish out of water in a secular and materialistic society. We have forgotten our spiritual roots and our need to be connected with our true selves, with people, and with God or Dao.

At a time when the world is full of disinformation and technological progress, we should expose all students to the spiritual power of meaning transformation. We need spiritual wisdom or moral transformation, one person as a time. We are not asking for a religious conversion to any particular faith tradition. We are proposing that Frankl's (1946/1985) view of a universal yearning for meaning, and his meaning interventions offer the possibility of awakening people's spiritual dimension and showing them the path to spiritual transformation through meaning.

Frankl took ethics very seriously. After the brutalities of Hitler, Frankl (1969/1988) wrestled with the question of how to prevent another Hitler and how to educate people to a more ethical or moral to treat each other (Wong & Reilly, 2017a, b). Frankl's spiritual remedies should result in loving our neighbors as ourselves rather than instruments to be used for our own gains.

Christian Miller (2017) made a compelling case that all of us are mixed bags of good and evil, and it is very important to become a better person and close the character gap. Of all the options to improve our character, Frankl's spiritual conception of meaning as self-detachment and self-transcendence is worth our serious consideration.

One cannot reason one's way to a virtuous life; nor can we find scientific guidance to live a moral life, because science is about the physical or natural world, not the moral realm. In the final analysis, one's moral mooring needs to be grounded in a transcendental reality, God, or Tao. To activate our spiritual dimension in order to get in touch with this ultimate meaning is a good start.

One moment of awareness can last a lifetime. One moment of responsible choice of will to meaning can change one's destination. Nothing can imbue life with more meaning and significance than such moments of encounter with God or the transcendental reality.

How to live a meaningful life is not just a matter of philosophical discussion or a matter of following the scientific findings of armchair psychology, but an urgent matter of how to become the best version of ourselves by becoming our true selves, guided by conscience, compelled by compassion, and consumed by the passion to pursue one's calling or what really matters.

It is a practical spirituality of walking on the narrow path of dirt but with our eyes toward an ideal that lifts up our spirit and fills our hearts and bellies with passion. It is the practical spirituality of making the best use of each day and the best use of every opportunity to turn hell into heaven. Frankl's spiritual remedies will not work if one treats logotherapy as intellectual knowledge rather than a blueprint or road signs for living a spiritually rooted meaningful life.

The universal spiritual hunger is evident not only in our own lives but in research. We can have spirituality without religion, and we can also have religion without belief in any set of dogmas (Borg, 1997; Goff, 2022, August 1). In his book *The God We Never Knew*, Borg (1997) affirmed the existence of God, but a God whose nature could not be expressed in human language, and hence who is not literally "all-knowing" or "all-powerful."

In the 2022 Gallup Survey:

> Gallup found 81% of Americans expressing belief when asked the simple question, "Do you believe in God?" This was down from 87% in 2017 and a record low for this question first asked in 1944, when 96% believed. It reached a high of 98% in the 1950s and 1960s. (Saad & Hrynowski, 2022, June 24, para 2)

In a recent article on spirituality's contribution to mental health, Sallcru (2022) defined spirituality as the transcendental ways of fulfilling human potential. After reviewing the extensive research evidence on the important role of spirituality in mental health and effective psychotherapy, Sallcru concluded: "From a personal perspective and professional capacity, I dare to say (without exaggeration) that spiritual practices could save anyone years of suffering and/or psychotherapy" ("Spiritual Practices…" para 1).

Therefore, there is enough empirical evidence and professional consensus that Frankl's spiritual remedies are aligned with human nature and contribute to mental health. However, Frankl's teaching is against the nihilism and narcissism supported by a secular, materialistic culture.

We have witnessed the devastations of developing only the brain power of intellect while starving the soul; and it is time for the wisdom of the soul and the virtues of living a purpose-driven and meaning-centered life (McLaughlin & McMinn, 2022; Wong, 2022b). In the eternal struggle between good and evil, a resurgence of spirituality and meaning may be our best hope of tipping the balance toward the good for individuals and society.

Part 3: Recent Developments

Logotherapy and the new science of suffering received increased attention during the pandemic (Chen et al., 2021; Van Tongeren & Showalter Van Tongeren, 2021; Wong, 2020b; Wong et al., 2022). These authors offered a glimpse of the progress made in extensions of logotherapy and the new science of suffering.

This section focuses on the research of Wong and others (Wong, 2009, 2010, 2015, 2016, 2019a, b, 2020b, 2022b; Wong & Bowers, 2018; Wong & Worth, 2017) in extending Frankl's work and providing a framework of existential intelligence and meaningful living. This framework covers five major sections, Acceptance, Belief, Commitment, Discovery, and Enjoyment (ABCDE): (a) *A*ccept life as it is—life is full of suffering and hardship; (b) *B*elieve in creating a preferred future through actualizing our potential, depending on others, and seeking help from God/Tao/Higher Power; (c) *C*ommit to personal growth and achieving one's life goal; (d) *D*iscover the resources available and the unexplored side of oneself; and (e) *E*njoy the intrinsic reward of living a meaningful life and the joy of turning hell into heaven.

A. *Accept life as it is—life is full of suffering and hardship.* Awareness of this reality better prepares us for the future and gives us the mindset that a good tomorrow depends on working hard today. This can be summed up as "don't pamper yourself!" If you are not hard on yourself, you will find life will be very hard and everyone is hard on you. Paradoxically, if you constantly endeavor to do your best and make continuous improvement, life will treat you better. The idea that a great person is hard on themselves but a small person is hard on others is widely attributed to Confucius. This principle also includes accepting ourselves fully, including our dark side and our mortality.
B. *Believe in creating a preferred future through actualizing our potential, depending on others, and seeking help from God/Tao/Higher Power.* Frankl (1946/1985) conceived of an ultimate meaning or supermeaning, as noted earlier:

> This ultimate meaning necessarily exceeds and surpasses the finite intellectual capacities of man; in logotherapy, we speak in this context of a super-meaning. What is demanded of man is not, as some existential philosophers teach, to endure the meaninglessness of life, but rather to bear his incapacity to grasp its unconditional meaningfulness in rational terms. Logos is deeper than logic. (p. 141)

Supporting this concept, Wong, (2019a) and Wong (2020b) articulated the power of faith in providing a sense of consolation, security, and guidance regardless of how horrible the circumstances. Elsewhere, Wong (2016) wrote about the responsibility of becoming the best version of ourselves through self-transcendence. To be mentally healthy, we need connections not just with our soul, but with others and with God (Rosmarin, 2021). These three connections represent the three pillars of positive mental health as the golden triangle in Fig. 2.

C. *Commitment to personal growth and achievement of one's life goal.* Belief needs to be followed by actions in order to narrow the belief-behavior gap or character gap (Miller, 2017). This involves making the best use of one's time to

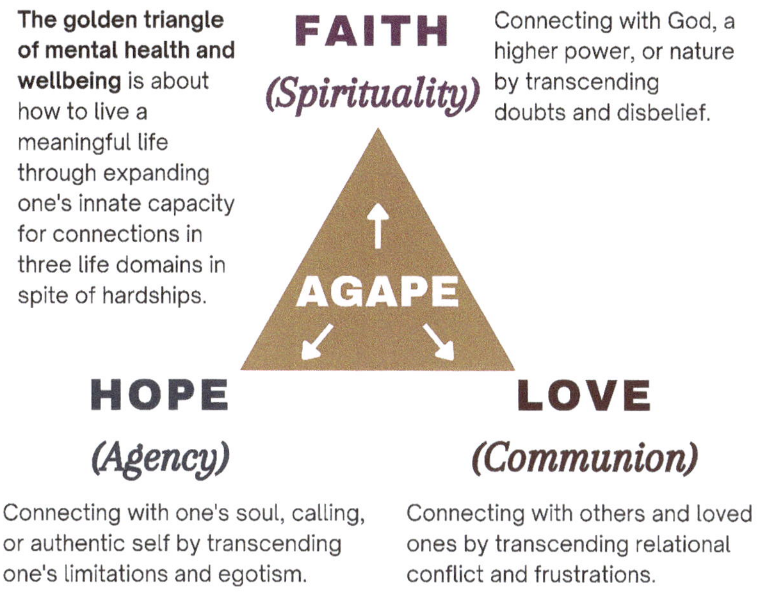

Fig. 2 The self-transcendence paradigm of global wellbeing and flourishing

become better, wiser, and stronger through the discipline of hard work (Wong, 2019a). This principle also involves the double-vision strategy of keeping one's feet on solid ground but keeping one's eyes on the highest ideals. What is personal is universal, and vice versa, in terms of human predicaments (Wong, 2015).

D. *Discover the resources available and the unexplored side of oneself.* According to Wong and Worth's (2017) deep-and-wide hypothesis, one does not know how strong or resourceful one is until one digs deeper and wider. Wong (2019b) also reported numerous studies demonstrating that both animals and humans can be trained to be extremely persistent and resourceful through increasing demand. Furthermore, we also discover the unexplored areas of oneself and the inexhaustible grace of, and resources in, God for the beliefs who pray to him for help.
E. *Enjoy the intrinsic reward of living a meaningful life and the joy of turning hell into heaven.* By practicing the above four principles of existential positive psychology and meaning therapy, one will reap the following benefits:

    1. Know how to suffer well and end unnecessary suffering. As Tolle (2010) noted:

        > Is suffering really necessary? Yes and no. If you had not suffered as you have, there would be no depth to you as a human being, no humility, no compassion. You would not be reading this now. Suffering cracks open the shell of ego, and then comes a point when it has served its purpose. Suffering is necessary until you realize it is unnecessary. (p. 39)

    2. Know how to maintain hope even in hopeless situations (Leung et al., 2021; Wong, 2009).
    3. Learn wisdom and virtue (Wong, 2022b).

4. Learn how to maintain inner peace, balance, and harmony regardless of the situation (Wong & Bowers, 2018).
5. Live the best possible life of depth and tranquility in a troubled world (Wong, 2022a). The ABCDE strategy is the main intervention for integrative meaning therapy (Wong, 2010) which incorporates the basic principles of logotherapy. Every step requires the exercise of the spiritual freedom and responsibility to pursue the core spiritual value of will to meaning.

Conclusion

Even though the world seems to be full of suffering and evil and we often wonder whom we can trust, there is hope. Miller (2017) provided a compelling case that we are all a mixed bag of good and evil, and no matter how bad a person may be, that person still has the image of God within and is capable of improvement.

As illustrated in this chapter, Frankl's (1946/1985) logotherapy and Wong's (2010) five principles for spiritual transformation (ABCDE) provide a promising way of positive education program to complement the existing Cs of youth development program (Lerner, 2009).

We offer an existentially oriented and spiritually rooted program based on the foundation of Frankl's logotherapy. It is holistic rather than one dimensional. It accepts the dark reality yet believes in the power of faith in God; it embraces suffering yet believes that one needs to experience hell in order to attain heaven. Instead of offering a fast and easy way to achieve positive transformation, it advocates the slow and difficult way of making the tough choices and the lifelong discipline of cultivating wisdom and virtue.

Wong (2021b) pointed out that our society often prefers instant gratification and quick fixes rather than taking the long view of learning how to live and how to endure hardships and resolve problems:

> For many people, concepts like responsibility, self-transcendence, and suffering are much more difficult to understand and accept than happiness, success, and flourishing. It is difficult because most people view life through the lens of hedonism, materialism, and egotism. They tend to react instinctively by rejecting and avoiding anything that makes them uncomfortable. They prefer distractions or instant relief to the bitter medicine provided by Frankl. (pp. v–vi)

My [Wong's] recent extensions of Frankl's work present a very different vision of positive youth development with its emphasis on meaning and spirituality as the two main pillars. We believe that this more realistic and spiritual worldview can better prepare our young people for a difficult present and an uncertain future. When we combine individual responsibility and effort with faith in God's spiritual resources and protection, we are undefeatable.

Guttmann (2008) highlighted the spiritual roots of Frankl's logotherapy:

> According to the theory of logotherapy, the struggle to achieve meaning in life is the most important struggle.... As long as one struggles, one is alive emotionally. One gets more mature. More seasoned, and richer spiritually by this struggle. Sisyphus found meaning in his suffering, and that meaning gave him the strength to carry on his suffering and find a few minutes of grace. (p. 61)

"Yes" to suffering, "Yes" to meaning, and "Yes" to the joy of living; thanks to the amazing grace of spiritual power. In the end, we are responsible for our wellbeing and our future, because we are the products of our choices. Successful execution of the ABCDE principles depends on spiritual activation of our faith and courage to say "Yes" to life, and "Yes" to doing the right thing no matter what.

Conflict of Interest We have no known conflict of interest to disclose.

References

American Psychological Association. (1999). The APA 1998 annual report. *American Psychologist, 54*(8), 537–568. https://doi.org/10.1037/0003-066x.54.8.537

Borg, M. J. (1997). *The God we never knew: Beyond dogmatic religion to a more authentic contemporary faith.* Harper Collins.

Camus, A. (1969). *Retour à Tipasa [Return to Tipasa]* (E. C. Kennedy, Trans.). Alfred A. Knopf. (Original work published 1952)

Chen, C.-H., Chang, S.-M., & Wu, H.-M. (2021). Discovering and approaching mature happiness: The implementation of the CasMac model in a university English class. *Frontiers in Education, 6*. https://doi.org/10.3389/feduc.2021.648311

Cowden, R. G., Rueger, S. Y., Davis, E. B., Counted, V., Kent, B. V., Chen, Y., et al. (2021). Resource loss, positive religious coping, and suffering during the COVID-19 pandemic: A prospective cohort study of US adults with chronic illness. *Mental Health, Religion and Culture, 25*(3), 288–304. https://doi.org/10.1080/13674676.2021.1948000

De Jesús, C. (1958). *The life of St. John of the Cross [Vida de San Juan de la Cruz]* (K. Pond, Trans.). Longmans and Harper & Brothers. (Original work published 1955)

Fabry, J. B. (2013). *The pursuit of meaning: Viktor Frankl, logotherapy, and life*. Purpose Research. (Original work published 1968)

Fabry, J. B. (2021). *Guideposts to meaning: Discovering what really matters* (2nd ed.). Purpose Research. (Original work published 1988)

Frankl, V. E. (1969/1988). *The will to meaning: Foundations and applications of logotherapy*. Meridian. (Original work published 1969)

Frankl, V. E. (1978). *The unheard cry for meaning: Psychotherapy and humanism*. Simon and Schuster.

Frankl, V. E. (1985). *Man's search for meaning* (3rd ed.). Washington Square Press/Pocket Books. (Original work published 1946)

Frankl, V. E. (1986). *The doctor and the soul* (R. Winston, & C. Winston, Trans.). Alfred A. Knopf. (Original work published in 1946 as *Ärztliche Seelsorge*)

Frankl, V. E. (2004). *On the theory and therapy of mental disorders: An introduction to logotherapy and existential analysis* (J. DuBois, Trans.). Brunner/Routledge. (Original work published *Theorie und Therapie der Neurosen Einfuhrung in die Logotherapie und Existenzanalys*)

Gable, S. L., & Haidt, J. (2005). What (and why) is positive psychology? *Review of General Psychology, 9*(2), 103–110. https://doi.org/10.1037/1089-2680.9.2.103

Goff, P. (2022, August 1). Why religion without belief can still make perfect sense. *Psyche*. Retrieved from https://psyche.co/ideas/why-religion-without-belief-can-still-make-perfect-sense
Guttmann, D. (2008). *Finding meaning in life, at midlife and beyond: Wisdom and spirit from logotherapy*. Praeger.
Haidt, J. (2006). *The happiness hypothesis: Finding modern truth in ancient wisdom*. Basic Books.
Hamm, R. F., III. (2015). *It's all uphill from here: Finding the concept of joy in existential philosophy and literature*. Doctoral dissertation, Purdue University. Retrieved from https://docs.lib.purdue.edu/dissertations/AAI3719195/
James, W. (1895). Is life worth living? *International Journal of Ethics, 6*(1), 1–24. Retrieved from https://www.jstor.org/stable/pdf/2375619.pdf
Ko, B.-H. (1980). Zen and the noetic dimension. In S. A. Wawrytko (Ed.), *Analecta Frankliana: The proceedings of the First World Congress of Logotherapy* (pp. 295–300). Institute of Logotherapy Press.
Lerner, R. M. (2009). The positive youth development perspective: Theoretical and empirical bases of a strengths-based approach to adolescent development. In S. J. Lopez & C. R. Snyder (Eds.), *The Oxford handbook of positive psychology* (pp. 148–164). Oxford University Press.
Leung, M. M., Arslan, G., & Wong, P. T. P. (2021). Tragic optimism as a buffer against COVID-19 suffering and the psychometric properties of a brief version of the life attitudes scale. *Frontiers in Psychology, 12*, 646843–646843. https://doi.org/10.3389/fpsyg.2021.646843
Marseille, J. (1997). The spiritual dimension in logotherapy: Viktor Frankl's contribution to transpersonal psychology. *The Journal of Transpersonal Psychology, 29*(1), 1–12. Retrieved from https://www.atpweb.org/jtparchive/trps-29-97-01-001.pdf
McLaughlin, P. T., & McMinn, M. R. (2022). *A time for wisdom: Knowledge, detachment, tranquility, transcendence*. Templeton Foundation Press.
Miller, C. (2017). *The character gap: How good are we?* Oxford University Press.
Roncero, A. (2021). What is an existential crisis, and how do you overcome it? *BetterUp*. Retrieved from https://www.betterup.com/blog/what-is-an-existential-crisis
Rosmarin, D. H. (2021). *The connections paradigm. Templeton Press.*
Ryan, W. F. (2019). The elements of ethics in Viktor Frankl. *Ultimate Reality and Meaning, 36*(1–2), 47–63. https://doi.org/10.3138/uram.36.1-2.47
Saad, L., & Hrynowski, Z. (2022, June 24). *How many americans believe in God?* Retrieved from https://news.gallup.com/poll/268205/americans-believe-god.aspx
Sallcru, S. (2022). Spirituality and its contribution to mental health. *Psychology Today*. Retrieved from https://www.psychologytoday.com/us/blog/psychology-insights-new-world/202208/spirituality-and-its-contribution-mental-health
Sartre, J.-P. (1989). *No exit and three other plays* (S. Gilbert, Trans.). Vintage. (Original work published 1943)
Seligman, M. E. P., & Csikszentmihalyi, M. (2000). Positive psychology: An introduction. *American Psychologist, 55*(1), 5–14. https://doi.org/10.1037/0003-066x.55.1.5
Solzhenitsyn, A. I. (1973). *The Gulag Archipelago, 1918–1956: An experiment in literary investigation* (T. P. Whitney, Trans.). Harper & Row.
Soper, C. A. (2020). *The evolution of life worth living: Why we choose to live*. C. A. Soper.
Tolle, E. (2010). *Stillness speaks*. New World Library.
Van Tongeren, D. R., & Showalter Van Tongeren, S. A. (2021). Finding meaning amidst COVID-19: An existential positive psychology model of suffering. *Frontiers in Psychology, 12*, 641747. https://doi.org/10.3389/fpsyg.2021.641747
Wong, P. T. P. (2003). Finding happiness through suffering [President's Column]. *Positive Living Newsletter.* Retrieved from https://www.meaning.ca/archives/presidents_columns/pres_col_aug_2003_happiness-through-suffering.htm
Wong, P. T. P. (2009). Viktor Frankl: Prophet of hope for the 21st century. In A. Batthyany & J. Levinson (Eds.), *Existential psychotherapy of meaning: Handbook of logotherapy and existential analysis*. Zeig, Tucker & Theisen.

Wong, P. T. P. (2010). Meaning therapy: An integrative and positive existential psychotherapy. *Journal of Contemporary Psychotherapy, 40*(2), 85–93. https://doi.org/10.1007/s10879-009-9132-6
Wong, P. T. P. (2011). Positive psychology 2.0: Towards a balanced interactive model of the good life. *Canadian Psychology/Psychologie Canadienne, 52*(2), 69–81. https://doi.org/10.1037/a0022511
Wong, P. T. P. (2012). Toward a dual-systems model of what makes life worth living. In *The human quest for meaning: Theories, research, and applications* (2nd ed., pp. 3–22). Routledge.
Wong, P. T. P. (2014). Viktor Frankl's meaning-seeking model and positive psychology. In A. Batthyany & P. Russo-Netzer (Eds.), *Meaning in positive and existential psychology* (pp. 149–184). Springer.
Wong, P. T. P. (2015). Meaning therapy: Assessments and interventions. *Existential Analysis, 26*(1), 154–167.
Wong, P. T. P. (2016). Self-transcendence: A paradoxical way to become your best. *International Journal of Existential Psychology and Psychotherapy, 6*(1), 9. Retrieved from http://journal.existentialpsychology.org/index.php/ExPsy/article/view/178
Wong, P. T. P. (2019a). *Inspirations for difficult times (L. C. J. Wong, Ed.). INPM Press.*
Wong, P. T. P. (2019b). *Learned helplessness or learned resourcefulness?* Retrieved from http://www.drpaulwong.com/learned-helplessness-or-learned-resourcefulness/
Wong, P. T. P. (2020a). Existential positive psychology and integrative meaning therapy. *International Review of Psychiatry, 32*(7–8), 565–578. https://doi.org/10.1080/09540261.2020.1814703
Wong, P. T. P. (2020b). *Made for resilience and happiness: Effective coping with COVID-19 according to Viktor E. Frankl and Paul TP Wong*. INPM Press.
Wong, P. T. P. (2021a). The Frankl cure for the 21st century: Why self-transcendence is the key to mental health and flourishing. *The International Forum for Logotherapy, 41*(2), 33–50.
Wong, P. T. P. (2021b). Preface: Frankl's cure for a soulless psychology and a sick society. In N. Krasovska & C.-H. Mayer (Eds.), *Psychobiography of Viktor Frankl* (pp. 1–8). Springer.
Wong, P. T. P. (2021c). The suffering hypothesis: How the new science supports the ancient wisdom of meaningful suffering [President's Column]. *Positive Living Newsletter.* Retrieved from https://www.meaning.ca/article/the-suffering-hypothesis-how-the-new-science-supports-the-ancient-wisdom-of-meaningful-suffering/
Wong, P. T. P. (2021d). What is existential positive psychology (PP 2.0)? Why it is necessary for mental health during the pandemic? *International Journal of Existential Positive Psychology, 10*(1), 1–16. Retrieved from http://www.drpaulwong.com/what-is-existential-positive-psychology-why-is-it-necessary-for-mental-health-during-the-pandemic/
Wong, P. T. P. (2022a). *The best possible life in a troubled world: The seven principles of self-transcendence.* Retrieved from http://www.drpaulwong.com/the-best-possible-life-in-a-troubled-world/
Wong, P. T. P. (2022b). The wisdom of the soul: The missing key to happiness and positive mental health? [Review of the book *A time for wisdom: Knowledge, detachment, tranquility, transcendence*, by P. T. McLaughlin & M. R. McMinn]. *International Journal of Existential Positive Psychology, 11*(2), 1–14.
Wong, P. T. P. (2022c). Towards a general theory of mental health and wellbeing [Review of the book The Evolution of Life Worth Living, by C. A. Soper]. *International Journal of Wellbeing*.
Wong, P. T. P., & Bowers, V. (2018). Mature happiness and global wellbeing in difficult times. In N. R. Stilton (Ed.), *Scientific concepts behind happiness, kindness, and empathy in contemporary society* (pp. 112–134). IGI Global
Wong, P. T. P., & Reilly, T. (2017a). *Frankl's self-transcendence model and virtue ethics—Part 1 of 2.* Retrieved from https://thevirtueblogdotcom.wordpress.com/2017/08/15/frankls-self-transcendence-model-and-virtue-ethics-part-1-of-2/

Wong, P. T. P., & Reilly, T. (2017b). *Frankl's self-transcendence model and virtue ethics—Part 2*. Retrieved from https://thevirtueblogdotcom.wordpress.com/2017/08/16/frankls-self-transcendence-model-and-virtue-ethics-part-2/

Wong, P. T. P., & Worth, P. (2017). The deep-and-wide hypothesis in giftedness and creativity. *Psychology and Education: An Interdisciplinary Journal, 54*(3–4), 11–23.

Wong, P. T. P., Arslan, G., Bowers, V. L., Peacock, E. J., Kjell, O. N. E., Ivtzan, I., & Lomas, T. (2021). Self-transcendence as a buffer against COVID-19 suffering: The development and validation of the self-transcendence measure-B. *Frontiers in Psychology, 12*, 648549–648549. https://doi.org/10.3389/fpsyg.2021.648549

Wong, P. T. P., Mayer, C.-H., & Arslan, G. (2022). COVID-19 and existential positive psychology (pp 2.0): The new science of self-transcendence [Editorial, Special issue]. *Frontiers in Psychology*. https://doi.org/10.3389/978-2-88974-153-3

Paul T. P. Wong, PhD, CPsych, is professor emeritus of Trent University and Trinity Western University. He is a Fellow of APA, APS, and CPA, and the founding president of the Internatonal Network on Personal Meaning and the Meaning-Centered Counseling Institute. He is editor-in-chief of the International Journal of Existential Positive Psychology and Consulting Editor of the Journal of Humanistic Psychology. As a research psychologist, he is well known as a leading authority on Viktor Frankl and logotherapy. As a pioneer of the positive psychology of suffering, he is responsible for a major paradigm shift from positive psychology to the existential positive psychology of flourishing through suffering. He has published 8 books and more than 300 articles and book chapters. He has been invited to give keynotes, webinars, workshops and lectures on all 7 continents.

His spiritual mission as a clinical psychologist is to spread the good news of self-transcendence—the hope of awakening people to their potential to see the light and to be the light in darkness through faith in God. The struggle of turning suffering into highest achievement will make people strong and whole with a sense of peace and harmony.

His brand of integrative meaning therapy aims at unlocking the transforming power of suffering. It incorporates various therapeutic modalities, such as cognitive behavior therapy, narrative therapy, and cross-cultural therapy, with meaning as the central integrating construct. Rather than focusing on symptom reduction, integrative meaning therapy emphasizes that both healing and flourishing can be achieved by meeting the basic human need for meaning, relationships, and faith.

Don Laird is a Licensed Professional Counselor and a National Certified Counselor who has invested over three decades helping those struggling with meaning and mental health issues. His specialties include anxiety, depression, death and existential anxiety, grief and loss, meaning and purpose, parenting, relationship issues, suffering, and life and career transitions.

In addition to providing professional therapy and clinical services, existential life coaching, and LPC supervision, Don serves as the clinical director at eTalkTherapy. Since 2012, he has been an adjunct professor at Carlow University where he teaches graduate courses in existential psychotherapy, psychology of film, and counseling theory. As a board member with the International Network of Personal Meaning, he is the chair of professional development and education and has coauthored several papers.

Writing Therapy and the Search for Meaning: A Case History

Daniele Bruzzone

Those in literature see psychology in fiction.
It's our turn to see the fiction in psychology. (Hillman, 1983, p. 18)

We are reminded by Irving Yalom (2015), a great teacher of existential psychotherapy, that the art of the psychotherapist is that of the storyteller and poet. For it is only when we tell the story of a life that the meaning sustaining it, or the lack of meaning afflicting it, can come to light. All therapeutic actions, if we analyze them closely, are no more than attempts to *weave a story* that is as healthy as possible to enable the person to keep on living and growing no matter what, even in the face of suffering.

Each therapy is a different story, and in all stories, something happens that does not perfectly coincide with the theories we use to explain it. Narrative language is much more appropriate to the human being than is scientific language, because it allows us to grasp *meaning*, which inevitably transcends the *facts* of the situation. Transformation increasingly depends more on the meaning individuals attribute to the facts that occur than on the facts themselves.

Thus, in this chapter, I do not present an empirically founded scientific report (although research in recent decades has largely confirmed the intuitive concepts of which I speak) but rely on a story to explain what can happen within the therapeutic encounter when it becomes a narrative laboratory with the capacity to produce change.

D. Bruzzone (✉)
Università Cattolica del Sacro Cuore, Milan, Italy

Italian Association for Logotherapy and Existential Analysis (ALÆF; www.alaef.com), Viktor Frankl Institut, Vienna, Austria
e-mail: daniele.bruzzone@unicatt.it

C. L. McLafferty, Jr., J. I. Levinson (eds.), *Logotherapy and Existential Analysis*, Logotherapy and Existential Analysis: Proceedings of the Viktor Frankl Institute Vienna 2, https://doi.org/10.1007/978-3-031-48922-8_7

Prisoners of a Tale

Each therapy is similar to a fairytale: Suddenly, something unexpected happens (whether thanks to or despite the techniques that we draw on to make it happen) that frees the individual—or rather, the *character* played by them—from the evil spell that had been keeping them in prison. Sometimes, this turning point is thanks to a "brainwave," which, as observed by Ludwig Binswanger (2007), is a creative act that nonetheless requires a level of experience that cannot be improvised. In psychotherapy, the best intuitions never arise by chance, but always come after a latent incubation period.

The clinical case that follows concerns one such insight and the way in which it contributed to enhancing my understanding of the therapeutic process.

Viktor Frankl (2009), in a 1949 paper entitled *Über die Lehrbarkheit und Lernbarkheit der Psychotherapie* (in English: *Is it possible to teach and learn psychotherapy?*), claimed that psychotherapy resembles an equation with two unknowns: on the one hand, the individuality of the patient; on the other, the personality of the therapist. This implies that therapy must be "reinvented from scratch" with each new patient. And indeed, it is impossible to reduce therapy to a precise formula revealing the secret of its own workings: Therapy *happens* and, in a certain sense, each instance of it represents *something new*. Therefore, Frankl argued, the only thing that is really worth teaching (and that must be learned in order to become a psychotherapist) is the ability to "personalize" and "improvise" therapy (p. 16).

The improvisation that I found myself putting into practice in the case study that follows was the use of *writing as a complementary therapeutic tool* in the context of an existential counseling relationship. Of course, I had read widely and heard much about the value and power of writing: I had learned from Jerome Bruner (1992) that human experience is always organized in the form of a narrative; I had understood, thanks to Paul Ricoeur (2011), that our very identity is structured as a story; and I had been struck by the claims of psychoanalysts, such as Schafer (1999) and Spence (1987), that narrative and symbolic truth play a far more decisive role in the life of a person than does historical truth. Despite this, I had no idea how to incorporate writing into the helping process; I had no precedents to guide me.

The practice of logotherapy, as we know, mainly draws on Socratic dialogue, a true instrument of "spiritual midwifery" (Frankl, 1974; see also Bruzzone, 2007, 2019), along with other conversational and argumentative strategies aimed at fostering the key spiritual dynamics of self-detachment and self-transcendence. As far as we know, Frankl did not use writing with his patients. Nevertheless, he himself wrote that man "reveals himself through his biography: it reveals… what this man really is, in terms of both the meanings he has actually lived out and his possibilities of meaning" (Frankl, 2005, p. 68; see also Bruzzone, 2021). This statement gave me much to consider: It was as though Frankl was saying that a person's life story contains not only their *past* but also their *future*.

Indeed, in the story that I am going to describe, the future was simultaneously present and denied: Constrained deterministically by the past (or rather: by the *story* of the past), it was waiting to be set free. To liberate the future and discover new possibilities, this story needed to be revisited, that is to say, it was necessary to transform the past, not in the *historical* sense (which would simply be impossible), but in the *narrative* sense. Let us see how.

Martha's Narrative Cage

The setting was a career guidance service set up by the local city council in collaboration with the university for people with occupational/career transition issues. Hence, my intervention was not clinical in nature but involved *existential counseling,* a kind of *existential coaching*, aimed at helping those availing of the service to redefine their professional selves and futures.

Martha (a pseudonym) was a 48-year-old woman with a complex history of abuse and hardship that stretched back to her disadvantaged childhood. Born in a marginalized area of a Southern Italian town, she had lost her father while still a child; from then on, she had lived in a family setting that was highly problematic, characterized by extreme poverty, emotional insecurity, criminality, and violence.

At the age of 18 years, Martha met a nun whom she came to see as a substitute for the mother she had lacked. Shortly afterward, she decided to join the religious life and entered a convent. However, she described the 30 years that she spent in this religious order as greatly troubled due to the extreme austerity, inflexible discipline, and even abuse and violence to which she and her fellow nuns were subjected. As a result of this difficult life, Martha suffered from a series of chronic health problems.

After a painful period of time outside of the convent, Martha now lived in a city in the north of the country, where she was provisionally a guest at another convent; she had resumed her studies and wished to find a job to support herself. However, she had no qualifications, no money, and no family behind her. Given that she knew nobody in the new town, she had turned to our service for help.

After the first couple of sessions, it was clear to me that Martha was afflicted by a deeper need than the mere requirement to find paid employment. Of course, she did have an immediate and concrete need (finding a job), but the real and crucial problem was another, and it was deeply rooted in her past.

Occasionally, Martha mentioned tragic fragments of her story, which I gradually began to perceive as generative themes around which her existence had come to be based. I began to realize that if she did not revisit the past that was holding her hostage, Martha would not be able to imagine or plan a different life for herself. Clearly, she was going through a period of profound *biographical change* in her life, but this implied an *existential transition* that was far more complex and required working at a deeper level and over a longer timeframe. Given that the setting we were in did not permit us to tackle this kind of work, I decided to resort to a parallel strategy that would allow Martha to begin working on herself outside of the space devoted to our discussions.

Some years beforehand, Martha had written a diary or, more precisely, an autobiographical memoir. She had been asked to do so by a psychiatrist she was seeing during a course of therapy that she had given up on after a few months. She expressed the desire to give it to me as a sign of trust and I agreed to read it on condition that we would continue to pursue our study and work objectives without wavering.

In this case, therefore, a body of writing was already available. This prompted me to look for a way to draw benefit from it. First, I carried out a narrative analysis of the text. Indeed, Martha's autobiography made me understand more clearly, not so much the *events* that had marked her life, but rather the *story* in which she framed them. It now became clear to me that she had converted the events of her life into a true narrative paradigm, which she used to interpret everything that was ever going to happen to her. For example, she told of several significant relationships with other people, but each one seemed to be variations on the same script; she even used the same words to describe them.

The narrative paradigm around which Martha had woven the tale of her existence was the negative paradigm of the victim: *Everything* had always gone wrong; in her life *everybody* had betrayed her in the end; *no one* had ever really loved her, etc. And the fact that this conviction was to some extent borne out by actual past events was relatively unimportant, because her story was so rigidly fixed that it excluded any other possibilities. Thus, if someone expressed concern for her or interest in her situation, her expectation was that sooner or later that person would abandon her. If not, she would drive the person away by making their life impossible. This shows how important (though painful) it was for her that her "script" should continue to be confirmed. It is not easy to take on the role of victim, but it is even more difficult to cast it off if an individual has never identified with any other role.

A Story Between the Lines

I was reminded of Binswanger's (1973) explanation of the origin of psychosis (see also Bruzzone, 2023). Existence, according to the Swiss psychiatrist, is always thematic: that is to say, it unfolds around a set of key themes. If, however, one particular theme takes over and becomes exclusive and recursive, it turns into a "fixed ideal," or idée *fixe*. In these cases, existence has "increasingly yielded to a particular view [of the world] by which it is gripped or overwhelmed" (p. 287).

Similarly, James Hillman (2006), in an account of a woman who had been in therapy with him, wrote that "the story needed to be doctored, not her: it needed reimagining.... She was indeed a victim, not of her history but of the story in which she had put her history" (pp. 20–21).

This was how Martha appeared to me: caged into a negative destiny. What she needed to do was to let go of her victim role and make space for a new story of herself. However, this was not a foregone conclusion because the idée fixe was still a way—albeit an extreme one—of attributing meaning to experience, or at least imposing a certain level of structure and predictability on it. It was therefore necessary to *interrupt this story in order to begin another.*

The opportunity to do so was provided, physically, by her writings. I realized that Martha's diary occasionally featured positive passages, words of gratitude, hints of self-esteem, hope, or faith. Though generally submerged by the rhetoric of pessimism and victimization, it seemed to me that these words could offer Martha a good start in reconstructing her story.

How? I took the liberty, in this case, of doing something a little unorthodox, that at first sight might even seem a little reckless. I photocopied the pages of her diary that contained these "healthy" words and I cut them out. We began to *recompose a new text* by pasting these small fragments onto a blank sheet of paper. As the new text took shape, a new Martha began to appear, who was more resilient, more confident, sometimes even more ironic, a Martha who had remained hidden "between the lines" for years.

In the beginning, it was almost like a game or a somewhat provocative experiment. In truth, Martha herself was not happy about it at all: This unusual collage was challenging her certainties and forcing her to become responsible for a story that, until that time, always resulted in her as the victim. But it was precisely this resistance that made me think we were on the right track. I believe that, for Martha, reflecting on this text was a crucial exercise in self-detachment: She was finally becoming aware that her narrative was not the only one possible and that, underneath the old Martha, perhaps there was another Martha who deserved to be given a hearing.

Her process of change began here. In 3 years, she did the things that she had not done in the previous 30: She completed her degree, found a job, began to live independently, learned to drive, and so on.

So the idea was confirmed, that changing the syntax of one's story can change the syntax of one's life.

New Words, New Worlds

When I felt that this new text had been consolidated, not only on the written page, but in Martha's life (she had stopped feeling sorry for herself and, when she remained focused on her objectives, was far less aggressive), I suggested that she go back to keeping a diary. However, at this stage, I did not give her permission to write about anything at all: I knew that it is one thing to bring about change and another thing to consolidate it. We were still at a delicate stage, in which writing could even lead Martha to regress should the voice of pessimism and discouragement again become dominant; what one writes is more indelible (including psychologically) than what one says, and this could have jeopardized all of our work to this point. Just as with any other *pharmakon*, writing has the potential to be toxic: In certain cases, it can even reinforce dysfunctional patterns or hyper-reflective tendencies. And this was not what we needed. Rather, my aim was to use writing to re-educate

Martha's gaze and reinforce her capacity for self-transcendence. This required a therapeutic prescription that set boundaries for her to respect. Martha was not yet ready to freely write her thoughts, but rather needed to free her thoughts through the exercise of writing. Thus, I did not initially ask her to write about herself, but about something positive that had brightened her day (such as a pleasant feeling, a scene of natural beauty, a personal satisfaction, a nice encounter, a funny thought).

The last act of this narrative work was suggested to me by Frankl (2000) himself, who in a 1938 article (the same one in which he spoke of "logotherapy" for the first time) described a method that he would later take up again in his *Ärztliche Seelsorge*:

> We guide the patient to imagine life as a novel in which he is the main character; the unfolding of events rests on him, as does determining what will happen in the following chapters.... Finally, and more powerfully, we can appeal for his active personal engagement by inviting him to imagine that he has reached the end of his life and must write his autobiography.... This image will lead him to live and act according to his sense of responsibility. (pp. 120–121)

Thus, following on the *reflective* writing and *expressive* writing, now we were introducing a sort of *fictional* writing. I invited Martha to start writing a new story (a hypothetical one, for the moment) about her future, about what the "new" Martha would have wished and what she would be able to achieve. This time there were no restrictions. I wanted Martha to have a space of her own in which she could feel free to dream and reimagine her future. In a word: where she could begin to hope again. I was surprised to discover that the imaginary scenario she came up with in reality had nothing unlikely about it. Martha's desires were quite "normal" and totally feasible: to have a job, a home of her own, to find new friends, etc., things that before seemed almost impossible—and now Martha was doing on a daily basis.

Sometimes, when the tension between us was running high, Martha would lash out at me, saying: "One day you will write a book about me and become famous!"

So, Martha, I have not written that book. *You* wrote it yourself with your new life. But in these pages, I have set out to tell how you succeeded in transforming a rigid script that was holding you prisoner into a tale of healing and freedom. You deserve a round of applause for that, as do all patients who teach us to be better therapists.

References

Binswanger, L. (1973). *Essere nel mondo* (G. Banti, Trans.). Astrolabio Ubaldini. (Original work published in English as *Being in the world*, 1963)

Binswanger, L. (2007). *Per un'antropologia fenomenologica* (E. Filippini, Trans.). Feltrinelli. (Original work published in German as *Ausgewählte Aufsätze und Vorträge*, 1955)

Bruner, J. (1992). *La ricerca del significato* (E. Prodon, Trans.). Bollati Boringhieri. (Original work published in English as *Acts of meaning*, 1990)

Bruzzone, D. (2007). Ricerca di senso e cura dell'esistenza. In *Il contributo di Viktor Frankl a una pedagogia fenomenologico-esistenziale*. Erickson.

Bruzzone, D. (2019). Vom Wissen zum Gewissen. Grundlagen einer sinnorientierten Erziehung. *Erziehung und Unterricht, 5-6*, 471–483.

Bruzzone, D. (2021). Meaning making and narrative in the illness experience: A phenomenological-existential perspective. *Encyclopaideia: Journal of Phenomenology and Education, 25*(59), 11–19.
Bruzzone, D. (2023). *Emotional life. Phenomenology, education, and care*. Springer.
Frankl, V. E. (1974). *Psicoterapia nella pratica medica* (B. Frick, Trans.). Giunti-Barbera. (Original work published in German as *Psychotherapie in der Praxis*, 1947)
Frankl, V. E. (2000). *Le radici della logoterapia* (E. Fizzotti, Trans. & Ed.,1st ed.). LAS.
Frankl, V. E. (2005). *Alla ricerca di un significato della vita* (E. Fizzotti, Trans.). Mursia. (Original work published in German as *Das Menschenbild der Seelenheilkunde*, 1974)
Frankl, V. E. (2009). *Si può insegnare e imparare la psicoterapia?* (E. Fizzotti, Trans.). Magi. (Original work published in German as "Über die Lehrbarkeit und Lernbarkeit der Psychotherapie," in J. U. Hubert (Ed.). *Festschrift zum 70. Geburtstag von Otto Pötzl*, 1949)
Hillman, J. (1983). *Healing fiction*. Station Hill.
Ricoeur, P. (2011). *Sé come un altro* (D. Iannotta, Trans.). Jaca Book. (Original work published in French as *Soi-même comme un autre*, 1990)
Schafer, R. (1999). *Rinarrare una vita* (E. Frattucci, Trans.). Giovanni Fioriti. (Original work published in English as *Retelling a life*, 1992)
Spence, D. P. (1987). *Verità narrativa e verità storica* (G. Noferi, Trans.). Martinelli. (Original work published in English as *Narrative truth and historical truth: Meaning and interpretation in psychoanalysis*, 1982)
Yalom, I. (2015). *Creature di un giorno: E altre storie di psicoanalisi*. Neri Pozza. (Original work published in English as *Creatures of a day*, 2015)

Daniele Bruzzone, PhD, is Full Professor of Education, Università Cattolica del Sacro Cuore, Milan (Italy). Director of the CARE Research Centre and editor-in-chief of *Encyclopaideia: Journal of Phenomenology and Education*. He is president of the Italian Association for Logotherapy and Existential Analysis (A.L.AE.F.) and board member of the Viktor Frankl Institute, Vienna. Research topics include: philosophy of education and care, emotions in helping relationships, and the search for meaning and existential wellbeing in life transitions. Among his recent books: *Emotional Life: Phenomenology, Education and Care* (Springer, 2023).

On Tragedy and Transformation: A Logotherapeutic Autoethnography

Benjamin D. Aiken

In this autoethnography, I share the story of my confrontation with an existential crisis of meaning following the untimely death of my best friend and life partner in the prime of our young adulthood. This confrontation with the greatest of all life contingencies—that is, the inevitability of my own death and the death of all whom I cherish—thrust myself into a realm of uncertainty that would take me across the world in search of meaning. Frankl (2000) asserted that:

> Man is not he who poses the question: "What is the meaning of life?" But he who is asked this question, for it is life itself that poses it to him… and man has to answer to life by answering for life; he has to respond by being responsible. (p. 29)

This is a story of my quest to answer the most unanswerable of all questions: "What is the meaning of life?" and "What is the meaning of suffering?"

Frankl's (1986) existential philosophy and theory of logotherapy has been profoundly instrumental in finding these answers. This autoethnography is neither a comprehensive account of logotherapy nor is it the story of my late partner's life and death. It is instead a story about coming to understand, in the most experiential way imaginable, that suffering and loss are fundamentally intricate features of the human condition. This autoethnography is also a story of transforming loss into a meaningful achievement—of rising meaningfully, as it were, above and beyond unavoidable and immeasurable suffering.

I have discovered a personally unique and singular answer to those questions, nearly 9 years after his death, in my new career as an academic and as a professional counselor. While my life journey has centrally informed my path toward newfound meaning in these roles, it is through these roles that I now advocate for

B. D. Aiken (✉)
Counselling Psychology Program, Adler University Vancouver, Vancouver, BC, Canada
e-mail: baiken2@uwyo.edu

C. L. McLafferty, Jr., J. I. Levinson (eds.), *Logotherapy and Existential Analysis*, Logotherapy and Existential Analysis: Proceedings of the Viktor Frankl Institute Vienna 2, https://doi.org/10.1007/978-3-031-48922-8_8

others—students and clients alike—to help them to discover their own unique and personal meaning in life. This autoethnography serves as an affirming testament to that possibility for all.

Relational Ethics: The Researcher's Aspirational Ethical Stance

We all live in communities connected to family members, friends, colleagues, and intimate others with whom we interact in our daily lives (Lapadat, 2017). This autoethnographic account of my experiences is, therefore, not my own; it implicates others in my life (Ellis, 2007). How to portray others in an autoethnographic account, particularly when the relational other is deceased, constitutes a significant ethical challenge that requires taking into account considerations beyond those of ethical theories and models of moral reasoning (Schwandt, 2014).

Relational Ethics

Carolyn Ellis (2007) informs my aspirational ethical stance. Slattery and Rapp (2003) described relational ethics as doing what is necessary to be "true to one's character and responsible for one's actions and their consequences on others" (p. 55). According to Ellis (2007), autoethnography starts with personal experiences and studies "us" in relationships and situations. Its process involves a back-and-forth movement between experiencing and examining a vulnerable self and observing and revealing the broader context of that experience.

As with the onset of death itself, my partner had no way of knowing I would one day share this story—*my story*—in which he is the central informant of my recorded accounts. I have vacillated between considering the constraints of telling and the possibility of healing, as well as a loyalty to him to create the best self I could become after his death. Given the context that 13 years of togetherness affords, I believe that if posthumously asked what to say or exclude, he would reply resoundingly—while playing out Eddie's character from the 1990's British sitcom *Absolutely Fabulous*, and with the roar of his memorably hearty laugh—"just make it fabulous!" In this manner, I trust he would have approved of my purposively selected contents.

In this autoethnography, I considered what I needed to tell for myself while honoring him the best I could. This included protecting us together and individually as well as protecting other people—including family members—in the story. I thus tried to tell a truthful account for readers, while I omitted things and occasionally changed details of a scene—all techniques commonly used in ethnographic storytelling and therapeutic memoir writing (Ellis, 2007). I endeavor to eulogize his positive characteristics, as well as the rituals, emotions, and experiences that followed his death. I also may, however, unavoidably divulge some personal details that show flaws, disappointments, and weaknesses in my character and his, as well as our strengths, achievements, and good judgment. As I know he would have wanted, this account of our experience in the world together—and the tremendous posthumous influence he continues to exert in my life—will, I trust, portray him in the most endearing light possible.

The Living Years: 1997–2010

On a balmy February afternoon in 1997, our paths serendipitously crossed at the Olin Library on the Rollins College campus in Winter Park, Florida. I was a 21-year-old undergraduate majoring in political science. He—then 23—had recently transferred from a college in New England, where he was majoring in history. While more than 25 years have since elapsed, that was the most pivotal and influential moment of my adult life.

Central Florida: The Formative Years

On a Saturday morning during the spring semester of 1997, while enrolled in a class called *The Politics of Feminism and Poverty in Rural Brazil,* I visited the library on my college campus in search of a particular book. Electronic search engines had yet to replace the card catalog system in those days. In my frantic scouring of the shelves, I happened upon a handsomely tall and dark-haired guy who was also looking for a particular book. There was a strikingly long and awkward pause as our glances caught one another's attention. Our banter continued for 20 minutes or so, as we each went back and forth from the shelves to the card catalog, until when, in passing, he said, "Hey I'm Dennis. So… do you go to school here?"

"I do," I said, "and you?"

What followed was a precarious chat, albeit brief, about much of nothing in particular. Both uncertain of ourselves and each other, we maintained a stance of *straightness*, as it were, as he shared about recently transferring from Boston, his majoring in history, and his love of the French language. After a few awkward minutes, he cautiously said, "Hey, I have a couple of tickets to Arabian Nights"—a central Florida–themed dinner venue—"that I got from one of my Uncle's clients. We should go sometime!"

We did not have cellphones in those days; I gave him my landline number, and he gave me his pager number. Also, back then I had a fax machine that was integrated into a dial-up modem. My computer at home just happened to be switched to fax mode, resulting in his incoming call being answered by the sound of a now-antiquated modem screech. A few days had lapsed when I returned home one afternoon to a message on my computer that a fax had been received. It was a note that he had faxed from his uncle's office: "I'm hoping you didn't give me the wrong number. If you get this, let's hang out this weekend." That evening we went to Arabian Nights!

The performance showcased the wedding between Princess Amirah and Prince Aswan, which brought together the two most powerful Bedouin kingdoms, aided by the magical abilities of the great Genie and the mysterious Sorcerer. The Stallions that pranced across the stage that evening added to the spectacle, and their speed was matched by the dissipation of the guarded demeanor that we had maintained at the library just a few days prior.

Over the two and a half years that followed, we grew closer, and our friendship grew stronger. We became a confidant to each other in our respective struggles to identify with our emerging individual and collective selves, though always at a certain distance that instilled a sense of social safety. I knew of his friends and family through the stories he shared, and the same was true of him and my friends and family. In almost every way, while often at arm's length, we supported each other in the coming of age as two young gay men. In that process, we grew in friendship and love.

A Momentous Decision

Fast forward to a thunderous and stormy evening on June 2, 1999. Until that day, our friendship had been kept a secret from our families. His mother and stepfather were on an extended trip out of state, and I was spending a lot of time with him at their home, where he kept watch of their cats. I had just graduated with my bachelor's degree, and he was beginning his last semester.

"You know, when I first saw you (two and a half years ago) at the library, I thought to myself, 'now if that guy were gay, I'd come out with it'…" he jokingly said, to which I laughed in retort, "I had a similar thought!" We laughed at the fate of our similar experiences—a glimpse into the inherent struggles of young gay men finding themselves in a heteronormative world, and a celebration of our togetherness, all at once. It was that evening that we committed ourselves to each other in a decision to never let what we had come to an end. We decided to forge a life together in a new place following his graduation. We decided that evening that we would figure out how and when to come out to our families and friends. We carefully chose Cape Town, Los Angeles, and Seattle—each for very different reasons—as our three contenders for a destination, and we selected December 26 as our day of departure. California won out in the end because of its progressive social and political values. Because of California's Same-Sex Domestic Partnership Bill, we were able to register our union soon following our arrival and enjoyed the benefits of marriage in our newly adopted home state.

During those two and a half years, in retrospect, we had individually and collectively found our place into heteronormative society as two young gay men; we embarked upon that journey together. Society's openness to gay culture was only beckoning in those years. Our mission was a beautifully sweet testament to the strength of our friendship and our love. Frankl (1967) said, "Man is not free from conditions, be they biological, or psychological, or sociological in nature. But he is—and always remains—free to take a stand toward these conditions; he always remains free to choose his attitude toward them" (p. 3). Those formative experiences shared with him established my understanding of this truth. It was not a comfortable journey for two young men in the 1990s. Contrary to all our fears, however, we were both accepted by our families and friends.

That December, I attended his graduation with his entire family. A few weeks later, on Christmas day—one day ahead of schedule—we departed from his now-late grandparents' driveway in Central Florida, with a U-Haul in tow and a cat in the backseat. We drove west into three sunsets and toward the rest of our natural lives together.

Southern California: Launching Ourselves into the World

We arrived in Los Angeles after three consecutive days of driving, with our Maine Coon cat screaming in the backseat all the while. We stopped only once to sleep, just west of Houston. On arrival, we checked into a cheap hotel in Van Nuys and remained there until after the millennium New Year. Before the end of the first week of the new millennium, we found a small apartment to rent just south of the 101 Freeway in Tarzana. Our life in the City of Angels had begun!

Goethe (1795/1824) may have foreseen the events that ensued from our decision to start a new life in Southern California, as he wrote about the power of Providence in the face of commitment in his seminal work, *Wilhelm Meister's Apprenticeship and Travels*. I found an entry-level job in the commercial investment real estate industry in February, and he found his dream job with an international publishing company in April. That August, I began business school, working toward my MBA. In November, we took our first vacation abroad to Paris, the first of many adventures that would take us around the globe to its far-reaching corners. The following spring, in 2001, we purchased our first home in Studio City. It would become my responsibility to manage the affairs of our household, and his never-abating mission to make our house a home.

Just a few months later, on December 23, 2001, Baby Ruth—our beloved teacup-sized Miniature Doberman Pinscher—entered the scene at 9 weeks old. We lost our beloved Pookie—the Maine Coon cat who came with us from Florida—a few years later. Then Rusty, an American shorthair we rescued from a feral colony along the Los Angeles River, entered our home.

In all the years that followed, our lives revolved around Baby Ruth. Our most relished past times included obedience classes at the Chateau Mar-Mutt in West Los Angeles, hikes at Runyon Canyon in the Hollywood Hills, walks through Woodbridge Park near our home, and Sunday drives to the beach in Santa Barbara, all with Baby Ruth. Just before completing this manuscript, I was once again reminded that life is temporal. Our beloved Baby Ruth suffered a stroke and passed away at 17 years old, and Rusty—our beautiful feline—died soon after of old age.

As the years carried on, I finished my MBA and began climbing the corporate ladder toward senior management. He settled into a position that he loved, frequently traveling to New York and elsewhere across the culinary world. He so enjoyed treating me, and our family and friends, to the most exceptional international culinary experiences. Though we had become accustomed to fine dining, our favorite regular spots were hole-in-the-wall establishments in Echo Park, North Hollywood, and downtown Los Angeles. We always sought out and enjoyed the full spectrum of every experience.

Spontaneity and loving companionship characterized our first decade of the twenty-first century. Charitable trust and mutual respect were the foundations of our relationship. We shared a great passion for our health and wellness and our explorations of the world—and we took trips that were not for the faint of heart. While the *W*-brand was his favorite hotel chain, our most cherished memories came from sleeping on the beach in Sri Lanka, trekking across the Saharan desert in Libya, and hiking the Drakensburg in South Africa, to name a few.

Ten years after our move to California, I was recruited by a real estate investment trust in Denver to fill a vice president position. That was the quintessential destination aspired to by young MBAs—a corner office with an executive title. It was an ideal opportunity for us to step further into the future we both envisioned for ourselves. We sold our home in Studio City and relocated to Denver, Colorado.

Colorado: A Future Lost

A few months after purchasing our new home in the Capitol Hill neighborhood of Denver, with many of our things still in boxes and I barely settled in my new job, Dennis experienced sudden death resulting from an illness that ran its full course at lightning speed. All at once, it seemed I had accumulated everything I could ever have wanted, on the one hand, though, on the other hand, I had just lost it all. Delirious and confused, I found myself on a flight from Denver to the East Coast the next morning—with Baby Ruth—to be with his family. He was interred at a cemetery near his mother's home. I spent 2 weeks there with his family before returning to Colorado, a place that was then as foreign to me as the new life I was about to embrace, forever void of his presence.

My Crisis of Meaning My earliest memory of being back in Denver, by myself and after his funeral, was the very moment I pulled my car into the garage after returning from the airport with Baby Ruth. That was also the very moment I first realized—or remember being aware of—the tremendous personal power that exists between stimulus and response. I was aware that remaining seated in the running car with the garage door closed was one of many options from which I could choose to alleviate my suffering. At that moment, I had a vivid awareness that nothing would ever be the same again, though it would be entirely up to me to figure things out, to choose my way forward into a catastrophically altered reality that I did not get to decide.

An Existential Crisis of Meaning The memory in my mind's eye kept returning to the precise moment the undertaker closed the casket before his internment. As if experienced in slow motion, that moment amplified ominous darkness that accompanied knowing, that for all time and eternity, I would never see him again. At that moment, his uncle—the same uncle who provided those tickets to Arabian Knights 13 years earlier—was standing next to me and gave me a robust sideways hug.

The sting of loss became too intoxicating to function during the day and too heavy to sleep at night. My doctor prescribed a medication to get through the day, another to sleep through the night. I also began weekly counseling with an existentially oriented psychotherapist, my first time working with a therapist, which continued for more than 4 years. Very early in our therapeutic relationship, my therapist suggested I read *Man's Search for Meaning*—Viktor Frankl's (2006) seminal work. It was on the existential principles outlined by Frankl that my compass shifted toward meaning and reconciliation of loss, and then later toward a new career as an academic and a professional counselor.

During the aftermath of his death, I searched feverishly outside of myself for an answer to the *why* and *how* of suffering. It was beyond measure that I grieved his absence. I visited a past-life regression hypnotherapist in New Mexico who claimed to unearth evidence that we knew each other in 1921 Salisbury, in then-Southern Rhodesia, where he was a tobacco farmer, and I was an accountant. A medium in Cape Town and another in Colorado both seemed to connect with him in remarkable ways that affirmed his presence. I frequently dreamt of him calling my cellphone and of seeing him hiding behind cement columns in parking garages.

In the following year, I was visiting with one of his best friends in Miami's Little Havana neighborhood. As we were enjoying a Cuban colada while sharing stories from the past, she, at one point, lifted her hands as if toward the heavens and exclaimed: "If you're with us, give us a sign!" In that moment, the lights went out alongside that sudden descending thud that accompanies the instantaneous switching off of the electrical and air conditioning systems. As the sound of people's voices began to replace the sudden sound of silence, she and I just looked at one another and shared in the serendipity of the moment. Evidence that his essence remained, in spite of death, was everywhere, though these events were painful reminders of loss. These external experiences, each unvalidated in the practical sense, did not reconcile or resolve anything; they only exacerbated the sting of suffering.

Logotherapy: A Philosophy of Counseling and Psychotherapy

As a theoretical approach to counseling and psychotherapy, logotherapy is premised on Frankl's (1969) notion that the will-to-meaning—or an intense desire to discover a unique meaning and purpose to one's life—is the primary motivation in human beings. This will-to-meaning acts on the circumstances of one's life, according to (Joshi et al., 2014), as was activated through my experiences. It pushes the individual to discover meaning, which is an ongoing, lifelong process. Steger et al. (2006) said that when meaning is experienced, it "pulls together people's ideas about who they are, the kind of world they live in, and how they relate to people and environments around them" (p. 83). According to Joshi et al., the presence of meaning in life may also be described as the experience of integrating life's many facets, thus allowing for a sense of direction and purpose.

Logotherapy may, therefore, be translated as therapy through meaning, or as "healing through meaning" (Frankl, 1978, p. 19). Through its tenets and principles, logotherapy is a meaning-centered approach to counseling and psychotherapy that seeks to assist one in orienting toward meaning in life. Change occurs when one becomes capable of accepting discomfort. Instead of trying to eliminate it or to change one's environment in an unhealthy way, maladaptive coping strategies are replaced with the use of existential resources (Frankl, 1986). According to Dezelic (2017), these include the uniquely human ability to self-distance from and to self-transcend beyond (Frankl, 1969) the unavoidable conditions of human existence.

Martinez and Florez (2015) said the ultimate goal of logotherapy is to facilitate psychological flexibility, malleability to situations, and an authentic personality open to the world and others. This, in turn, widens one's phenomenological field, enables one to perceive different alternatives and realities of existence, and allows one to engage in other options that bring about more meaning to life.

Logotherapy: A Philosophy of the Human Condition

Logotherapy is also a philosophy of the human condition (Marshall & Marshall, 2012). As a philosophy, logotherapy asserts that life has unconditional meaning, and that meaning in life cannot vanish under any circumstance (Lukas, 2000). This belief argues that the whole of the world has meaning and purpose to it, and every life experience, therefore, potentially contains meaning in and of itself. Accordingly, Frankl (1986) determined that human life rests upon three fundamental pillars of existence: (1) the freedom of will; (2) the will to meaning; and, (3) the meaning of life.

The Freedom of Will The first pillar, the freedom of will, contends that humans have the capacity of free choice (Frankl, 1986; Sartre, 2007; Yalom, 1980). Humans are finite beings, and existential circumstances restrict human freedom; the freedom with which logotherapy is concerned is not freedom *from* conditions, but rather the freedom *to* choose one's attitude in any given set of circumstances and toward whatever conditions may exist (Frankl, 1969). Within the often-overlooked space that exists between stimulus and response exists our freedom of will—that is, our freedom to choose a response. With this uniquely human freedom comes the responsibility to choose one's own way. In the absence of outward choices, this includes the capacity to choose one's attitude in the face of unavoidable suffering.

The Will to Meaning In describing the second pillar, the will to meaning, Frankl (1969) asserted that no other creature, except for human beings, has ever reached the point of being aware of and confronted with life's finiteness and mortality. Lukas (2000) added that the will to meaning corresponds to a striving and yearning for meaning, which inspires every human being. The *will to meaning* is precisely that which allowed me to accept loss and embrace life, in spite of suffering.

The Meaning of Life The third pillar—the meaning of life—holds that life has unconditional meaning, which cannot vanish under any circumstance (Lukas, 2000). According to Marshall and Marshall (2012), this infers that life holds meaning in any situation, even the most miserable of circumstances. The true meaning of each person's life is something that must be discovered by activity in the world or through interaction with others (Frankl, 1986; Graber, 2004). To this end, logotherapy is an action-oriented approach to counseling and psychotherapy. By taking action—that is, by moving in a direction that sought to transform suffering into an achievement—I transitioned myself from an established career in business to become a professional counselor and an academic in counselor education.

"A doctor cannot give meaning to his patients," said Frankl (2000), "nor can a professor give meaning to his students" (p. 119). Frankl (1978) also noted that:

> A professor cannot tell a student what the meaning is, but he at least can show that there is a meaning in life, that it is available to everyone and, even more, that life retains its meaning under any condition. It remains meaningful literally up to its last moment, up to one's last breath. (p. 41)

The meaning I have discovered in my new roles—from accompanying a client along their path toward self-actualization to observing a student grasp an empowering concept—is a unique meaning that exists strictly but for the tragedy of loss.

A Turn Inward Toward Healing

In addition to my intensive weekly psychotherapy, I was also fortunate to have had the time and resources to travel to many of the places we had planned to visit together, and I did plenty of that in solemn contemplation. I hiked Machu Picchu, spending a day at the ruins writing a letter to him, which I left folded tightly between two rocks in the Peruvian jungle. I traveled to the Himalayas and flew around Mt. Everest in a helicopter, a trip that he had long been planning. I visited the Taj Mahal in India. For my 40th birthday, I sailed the Drake Passage and across the Southern Ocean to Antarctica—a trip he had planned for our 40th milestone—and I did so with his photo in my cabin aboard the Russian-built ice-breaking vessel.

I trekked the Cape to Cairo route and hiked Mount Kilimanjaro in Tanzania along the way. It was on Mount Kilimanjaro, at the first of three base camps, that I decided to enroll in a class at the University of Colorado, which just happened to be in the counseling program. I had no idea that my decision to take a class would move me in an entirely new life direction. It was merely my intention to do something different and to embrace life differently.

By the end of 2012, I had completed three graduate courses at the University of Colorado while maintaining my professional responsibilities during the day. Still, I had no intention of pursuing a new profession as a professional counselor or an academic, though I was finding tremendous meaning in my new circle of friends and from the new body of knowledge that I was acquiring. My values and perspectives began to shift, too. Some in my former profession said, "You're making a mistake by focusing too much on other things," asserting that I should direct my energies toward capitalistic values. Meanwhile, others in my new academic circle said, "How amazing that you're exploring new things." One group understood my motives, while the other, more familiar group, lacked the existential insight to do so.

One year later, I was presented with another decision that would carry momentous consequences for the future. A perfect collision of corporate circumstances provided me with an opportunity to step away from the company where I worked, which I did to focus full-time on my master's degree in counseling. I still was not committed to changing professions, though I did view a prolonged hiatus for study and travel to provide a much-needed reprieve.

Tragic Optimism: Healing in Spite of Suffering

Frankl (1969) coined the phrase *tragic optimism*, which refers to the uniquely human ability to thrive in the face of adversity. Said differently, tragic optimism is that which allows one to say *yes* to life, in spite of unavoidable suffering that can otherwise stand in the way. My healing occurred alongside awareness that a meaningful existence and tremendous pain are inextricably linked. It became clear to me, even in spite of the limitations of human existence, that life is a series of decisions. As I reflected on this notion, I began to realize that my choices reflect my answers to life's questions.

I made a series of decisions at their respective moments of opportunity. For every decision to be made, there always exists the potential to decide in the direction of meaning. Emerging from the sum of these choices was awareness that suffering is commensurate with life meaning. Suffering is inextricably linked to the experience of being alive in the world. Saying "yes to life" in spite of the loss, however, is possible. "The acceptance of finiteness is the precondition to mental health and human progress," said Frankl (1967), "while the inability to accept it is characteristic of the neurotic personality" (p. 47). It became clear to me that acceptance of finitude—both Dennis's and my own, and all whom I love—was a precondition to my healing.

Constructivism: A Researcher's Philosophical Stance

Constructivism grounds my approach to learning, growth, and development and frames my philosophical worldview. Embracing the transitoriness of life, I have learned, means saying yes to life and to the many questions it poses. My reconciliation of loss continued to occur by happenstance alongside my journey toward a new profession as an academic and a professional counselor. It was the result of a series of decisions that moved the trajectory of my existence toward a personal meaning in life. Subjectivity plays a tremendous role in determining the most suitable choice, or response, to every question posed by life.

As a professional counselor with a clinical orientation toward humanistic and existential philosophies, and as an Assistant Professor of Counselling Psychology, my clinical interests are focused on the subjectivity of human experience. Existentialism asserts that *existence precedes essence* (Sartre, 2007). That is, we as human beings arrive on this landscape of Earth without an awareness of life's purpose or meaning, or even without an awareness of how we came to exist in the first place. It is through the lived experiences that follow, which are filtered through numerous lenses, that one's *essence* is discovered.

Whereas an acorn is determined to become an oak tree by virtue of its very existence, that is by doing nothing other than *being*, just as a caterpillar is determined to become a butterfly or a tadpole is determined to become a frog, Frankl (1986) explained that determinism—but for the unavoidable givens of existence—is foreign to the human experience. As human beings, we must construct what it is that we will *become*, through the choices we make on a moment-by-moment basis. These choices and their corresponding actions create one's lived reality and define the *essence* of one's own unique and unrepeatable existence. Frankl (1967) also noted that "life is but a chain of questions, which one has to answer by answering for life, to which one has to respond by being responsible, by making decisions, and by deciding which answers to give to each individual question" (p. 17).

This stance becomes apparent in my counseling and psychotherapy work through my guidance toward meaning making and essence discovery. My research interests, in part, are similarly focused on the existential process of discovering one's meaning in life, and thereby raising awareness to the essence of one's very existence. Constructivists reject the view that human knowledge is objective (von Glasersfeld, 1995). Instead, they hold that knowledge is constructed through subjective experiences and interpretations of the world. That is, humans are not determined to become an oak tree as is true for the acorn, but instead, one's interaction with the world creates truth and meaning. From this viewpoint, truth and meaning are navigated to become what existential theory describes as the essence of one's own unique and unrepeatable existence.

Conclusion

My journey through healing and reconciliation of loss following my partner's untimely death—which led me to a new career as both an academic and a professional counselor—taught me that through the right attitude, one could transform unavoidable suffering into a heroic and victorious achievement. When we can no longer change a situation, we are challenged to change ourselves (Frankl, 2006). Unavoidable suffering—viewed from this perspective—does contain meaning if and when it provides opportunity for change for the better (Frankl, 1978). This is not to suggest that meaning lessens the sting of suffering. Finding meaning in loss, however, does make unavoidable pain more bearable.

Frankl (2000) stated that "The answer to the question, 'what is the meaning of life?' can only be given out of one's whole being—one's life is itself the answer to the question of its meaning" (p. 119). There is no such thing as a universal meaning of life, but meaning that is unique to each individual situation and waiting to be discovered. "Each life situation confronting us places a demand on us—presents a question to us… a question to which we answer by doing something about the given situation" (p. 141). This is what Frankl (1967) referred to as the existential act—that is, to rise meaningfully "above one's own psychosocial condition" (p. 136), by taking action and saying "yes" to life, in spite of the suffering that is inherent to the unavoidable givens of human existence.[1]

References

Dezelic, M. (2017). Meaning constructs and meaning-oriented techniques: Clinical applications of meaning and existential exploration. *Journal of Constructivist Psychology, 30*(1), 32–41.

Ellis, C. (2007). Telling secrets, revealing lives: Relational ethics in research with intimate others. *Qualitative Inquiry, 13*(1), 3–29.

Frankl, V. E. (1967). *Psychotherapy and existentialism*. Washington Square Press.

Frankl, V. E. (1969). *The will to meaning*. World Publishing Company.

Frankl, V. E. (1978). *The unheard cry for meaning: Psychotherapy and humanism*. Simon and Schuster.

Frankl, V. E. (1986). *The doctor and the soul (Original work published 1946 as Ärztliche Seelsorge; Vienna: Franz Deuticke.)* (R. Winston, & C. Winston, Trans.). Alfred A. Knopf.

[1]This autoethnography was written in loving memory of Dennis, my late partner, and Baby Ruth and Rusty, our beloved four-legged children. May the sound of their names always be a blessing.

Frankl, V. E. (2000). *Man's search for ultimate meaning*. Perseus. (Original work published as *Der Unbewusste Gott, 1948 and English translation, The Unconscious God, 1975)*
Frankl, V. E. (2006). *Man's search for meaning*. Beacon Press. (Original work published 1946)
Goethe, J. W. (1795/1824). *Wilhelm Meister's Apprenticeship and Travels* (T. Carlyle, Trans.). Retrieved May 11, 2023, from https://www.gutenberg.org/files/36483/36483-h/36483-h.htm#BOOK_I
Graber, A. V. (2004). *Viktor Frankl's logotherapy: Method of choice in ecumenical pastoral psychology*. Wyndham Hall Press.
Joshi, C., Marszalek, J. M., Berkel, L. A., & Hinshaw, A. B. (2014). An empirical investigation of Viktor Frankl's logotherapeutic model. *Journal of Humanistic Psychology, 54*(2), 227–253.
Lapadat, J. C. (2017). Ethics in autoethnography and collaborative autoethnography. *Qualitative Inquiry, 23*(8), 589–603.
Lukas, E. (2000). *Logotherapy textbook: Meaning-centered psychotherapy* (T. Brugger, Trans.). Liberty Press. (Original work published *Lehrbuch der Logotherapie*)
Marshall, M., & Marshall, E. (2012). *Logotherapy revisited: Review of the tenets of Viktor E. Frankl's logotherapy*. Ottawa Institute of Logotherapy.
Martínez, E. Y., & Flórez, I. A. (2015). Meaning-centered psychotherapy: A Socratic clinical practice. *Journal of Contemporary Psychotherapy, 45*, 37–48.
Sartre, J.-P. (2007). *Existentialism is a humanism* (C. Macomber, Trans.). Yale University Press.
Schwandt, T. A. (2014). *The Sage dictionary of qualitative inquiry*. Sage.
Slattery, P., & Rapp, D. (2003). *Ethics and the foundations of education: Teaching convictions in a postmodern world*. Allyn & Bacon.
Steger, M. F., Frazier, P., Oishi, S., & Kaler, M. (2006). The meaning in life questionnaire: Assessing the presence of and search for meaning in life. *Journal of Counseling Psychology, 53*(1), 80.
von Glasersfeld, E. (1995). Introduction: Aspects of constructivism. In C. T. Fosnot (Ed.), *Constructivism: Theory perspectives, and practice* (pp. 3–7). Teacher College Press. Available at http://www.vonglasersfeld.com/180
Yalom, I. D. (1980). *Existential psychotherapy*. Basic Books.

Benjamin D. Aiken, Ph.D., LPC, RCC, is an Assistant Professor of Counselling Psychology at Adler University Vancouver in Canada. He is a Licensed Professional Counselor in Colorado and Wyoming, and a Registered Clinical Counselor in British Columbia. He is also an Academic Associate of Logotherapy and a diplomate candidate at the Viktor Frankl Institute of Logotherapy. This manuscript was written when he was a doctoral candidate at the University of Wyoming and updated shortly before publication.

Finding Meaning in Life in a Changing World

Rachel Bolaji Asagba

Finding meaning in life is an ongoing endeavor because it is a universal search. This concept was developed by Viktor Frankl (1995/2000), starting in his childhood and high-school days in the 1920s. Frankl had contact with the first great Viennese psychotherapist, Sigmund Freud, because of his interest in psychoanalysis; he even contributed to Freud's journal. Later, Frankl determined that humans do not merely search for pleasure as their primary motivation; he then became involved with Alfred Adler, the second great Viennese psychotherapist. Adler had also been a member of Freud's inner circle, but departed because of his own concept of the *power principle* as the primary motivation of human beings. This departure from Freud's *pleasure principle* caused Adler to develop his own school, known as *individual psychology*.

Editorial note: The following article was written by the late Rachel Asagba (1953–2021). We are grateful for permission to print this article from her daughter, Olatunde Asagba, and her son, Tundebola Asagba.

In the late 1980s, she became inspired by Viktor Frankl's writing and visited him in Vienna. She completed her logotherapy training with Elisabeth Lukas in 1992 and was mentored by Frankl.

In 1998, Rachel Bolaji Asagba joined the Department of Psychology at the University of Ibadan as an assistant lecturer, where she distinguished herself in the field of psychology. Her hard work and dedication over the years was finally rewarded in 2019 when she was promoted as Professor of Clinical Psychology.

Professor Rachel Asagba was the founder of the Nigerian Logotherapy Group at the University of Ibadan. She had a robust and vast archive of completed publications, journals, and research that cut across a wide range of fields in addition to her area of specialization. Asagba is undoubtedly one of the pioneers of logotherapy in Africa; this article demonstrates the manner in which she applied and adapted logotherapy to her environment and culture. It is difficult to convey the energy and positivity that she shared with everyone she met. Truly, she lived logotherapy.

R. B. Asagba (Deceased) (✉)
Ibadan, Oyo State, Nigeria

C. L. McLafferty, Jr., J. I. Levinson (eds.), *Logotherapy and Existential Analysis*, Logotherapy and Existential Analysis: Proceedings of the Viktor Frankl Institute Vienna 2, https://doi.org/10.1007/978-3-031-48922-8_9

After his time in the Freudian and Adlerian groups, Frankl (1995/2000) developed the idea that neither pleasure nor power was the primary human motive in life; rather it was *finding meaning in life* (Asagba, 1993, 2002, 2006; Fabry, 1968/2013; Frankl, 1969/1988; Graber, 2004; Kalmar, 1982; Lukas, 2020). Frankl stated: "I suspended what I had learned from my great teachers and began listening to what my patients were telling me, trying to learn from them" (as cited in Fabry, 1968/2013, p. 7). He spent his life lecturing worldwide and demonstrating this meaning principle.

The Search for Meaning as the Primary Human Motivation

According to Frankl (1969/1988), the search for meaning is the primary motivation of the individual. Recent findings by contemporary scholars have confirmed that finding meaning is a primary human motivation (Evans, 2012; Kleftaras & Psarra, 2012; Maddi, 1970; Reker & Wong, 1988; Steger et al., 2011). Frankl believed that the human ability to search for meaning makes us unique and different from lower animals and plants. This is due to the nature of the complete, whole human being as existing in three, interlacing dimensions, each interacting with the environment: body (*soma*), emotions and intellect (*psyche*), and spirit (*noös*). If humans seek completeness, they must therefore be able to function well in all these aspects from the holistic point of view. It is in the noös, also known as the noëtic dimension, that the individual searches for meaning. The complete human being uses the *freedom of will* and the ability to choose to discern the most meaningful choice from the many available alternatives (Lukas, 2015).

Frankl (1946/1985) noted:

> Mental health is based on a certain degree of tension, the tension between what one has already achieved and what he still ought to accomplish, or the gap between what one is and what one should become. Such a tension is inherent in the human being and therefore is indispensable to mental well-being. We should not, then, be hesitant about challenging man with a potential meaning for him to fulfill. It is only thus that we evoke his will to meaning from its state of latency. I consider it a dangerous misconception of mental hygiene to assume that what man needs in the first place is equilibrium or, as it is called in biology, "homeostasis," i.e., a tensionless state. What man actually needs is not a tensionless state but rather the striving and struggling for a worthwhile goal, a freely chosen task. What he needs is not the discharge of tension at any cost but the call of a potential meaning waiting to be fulfilled by him. What man needs is not homeostasis but what I call "noödynamics," i.e., the existential dynamics in a polar field of tension where one pole is represented by a meaning that is to be fulfilled and the other pole by the man who has to fulfill it. (pp. 104–105)

Frankl (1969/1988) contrasted Freud's materialism (which is known as depth psychology) with human ideals and values (which he called "height psychology"):

> Contrary to the homeostasis theory, tension is not something to avoid unconditionally, and peace of mind, or peace of soul, is not anything to avow unconditionally. A sound amount of tension, such as that tension which is aroused by a meaning to fulfill, is inherent in being human and is indispensable for mental well-being. (pp. 47–48)

According to Asagba (1993, 2002, 2006), a complete, healthy human being comprises the biological (somatic), psychological (psychic), and spiritual (noëtic) dimensions. An example is someone who takes good care of the three dimensions by maintaining good harmony. Such individuals maintain a healthy lifestyle as much as possible. For instance, they eat balanced meals daily and practice good hygiene, both personal and environmental. From the psychological point of view, they maintain and balance emotions. At the same time, their spiritual needs are also well taken care of, both in times of health and during illness. This is why there is an absolute need to refer patients to the right specialists and the need for a multidisciplinary approach in treating them. In this way, a holistic approach is maintained, as advocated in logotherapy.

Frankl (1969/1988) argued that meaning is available to everyone via the three tenets that make up the building blocks of logotherapy. These are labeled: the *meaning of life*, the *will to meaning*, and the *freedom of will*. These tenets suggest that the meaning potential of a situation can be assessed by a person. At an individual level, a person can be seen as having a "life battery" that contains meaning potentials that can be charged by actualizing meanings of the moments of life.

The following demonstrates that everyone has choices to make in life: Imagine we are all stranded in a desert with no means of sustenance except for a train that can take anyone to their ultimate meaning. The decision to get on board the train must be voluntary, because we are free to make choices. Therefore, everyone in the desert has the freedom to stay behind—by doing nothing in life—or to board the train and stop at station one, station two, or station three, etc., or even to stay on the train and refuse to get off. It is worth noting that when a person does not make a choice, they have made one by not making the choice. Therefore, everyone always has a choice to make because we all have that freedom, even if we choose to not choose.

Change in the World Is Part of the Normal Phenomenon

The world is changing and this change is not new to us—it has been so from the beginning of humanity. However, the changes of today cannot be compared with those of the Stone Age or the World War era. The rate of change during the Stone Age or the World War era was much slower than that between Frankl's time to the present. Frankl (1969/1988) realized this when he commented on the changes in traditional values:

> Today we live in an age of crumbling and vanishing traditions. Thus, instead of new values being created by finding unique meanings, the reverse happens. Universal values are on the vane. That is why ever more people are caught in a feeling of aimlessness and emptiness or, as I am used to calling it, in the existential vacuum. However, even if all universal values disappeared, life would remain meaningful, since the unique meanings remain untouched by the loss of traditions. To be sure, if man is to find meanings even in an era without values, he has to be equipped with the full capacity of conscience. It therefore stands to reason that

> in an age such as ours, that is to say, in an age of the existential vacuum, the foremost task of education, instead of being satisfied with transmitting traditions and knowledge, is to refine that capacity which allows man to find unique meanings. (p. 64)

We are in the computer age with webcasts, social networks, blogs, and other social media. Developing countries such as those in Africa are rapidly emerging, but not everyone is carried along. As a result, there is a large gap between the rich and the poor. Unfortunately, the young, who make up the bulk of the population, share more of that burden because the majority of them are unemployed. This might help explain unpredictable events experienced worldwide. Terrorist attacks, uprisings in the Middle East and Africa (e.g., Alshaba in East Africa and Boko Haram in Nigeria), and world events such as the economic meltdown have an effect all around the world. These factors should help us realize that we are now in a world that may appear to be meaningless. We need to promote the principles of logotherapy worldwide. Although we cannot give meaning to people, we can try to live out our meaning by example to our families, friends, coworkers, and governmental officials. The use of the principles of logotherapy could be a starting point.

Utilization of the Concept and Principles of Logotherapy

Our changing world poses many of life's questions to us, which all of us must answer. It is now that we must act—it is the current *meaning of the moment* that Frankl (1969/1988) talked about. I am quite sure that some may wonder: "How do I start now with all those challenges facing me?" The answer is simple: We must use ourselves as our starting point. We must start with ourselves through a *Socratic dialogue* (Fabry, 1988/2021; Frankl, 1978) to first discover ourselves and to look inward objectively. Then we ask ourselves questions such as the following: "What are we giving to the world?" "Who are we encountering in our daily lives?" or "What kind of attitude would life expect me to show to the distressed around me?"

Frankl (1969/1988) recommended that individuals act on the meaning of the current moment. In the same vein, Burdman (2008) remembered Frankl advising her to "listen to the person on the street, he or she will be your teacher" (p. 72). Burdman extended the thought:

> Who is that person on your street? In the market? On the subway? Or seated with you at the conference table? Or anywhere you find yourself?
>
> Are we listening? What are we hearing? If we can stay awake when our lives are changing, secrets will be revealed to us about ourselves, about the nature of life, and about the eternal source of meaning that is always available and that is renewable day by day. (p. 72)

Asagba (1993) described how to find meaning in developing countries:

> Logotherapy distinguishes situations of fate (which we cannot change) and those of freedom (which we can change). We must accept our genetic "fate" that we are Africans or Nigerians, but also we must use our areas of freedom, tempered by responsibility, and develop self-reliance with our capabilities. Instead of searching for white-collar jobs—not everyone can be a doctor or manager—we can go back to the land and plant crops or make use of our raw materials to produce something that is needed. (p. 32)

Few people think of what they can do for their country; instead, they complain about the situation. We cannot change our fate of being Nigerians, but we can work together and see to it that our country develops like Germany or Austria did after the first and second World Wars. We can transform Africa into a better place to live.

The Need to Promote the Act of Finding Meaning, Starting from the Care Providers

In promoting the act of finding meaning, we need to practice the concept and principles of logotherapy. For instance, Graber (2004) found the use of her Reflections on the Meaning Triangle as a tool to increase awareness of personal strengths which could not only help our clients—but also the care providers or professionals—to find meaning. Graber noted:

> Reflecting upon the following questions will help you to discover meaning experienced at some time in your life. Answer the following questions with the first impression that comes to mind:

1. What creative gifts have I offered to others through my talents, my work, deeds done, goals achieved that held meaning for me?
2. What experiences have I received from encountering others in relationships of all kinds, from nature, culture, or religion that were deeply meaningful?
3. What attitudinal values have I realized by taking a stance toward situations or blows of fate that was courageous or self-transcending? (p. 94)

The activities found in the *Meaningful and purposeful goals workbook* (Hutzell & Jerkins, 2009) provide another way of exposing ourselves to awareness of meaning in our daily activities. A variety of exercises can also be found in *Guideposts to meaning: Discovering what really matters* (Fabry, 1988/2021). Other relevant literature also can be found at http://www.viktorfrankl.org, the official website of the Viktor Frankl Institute in Vienna.

Conclusion

The search for meaning in life by human beings in a changing world is an ongoing challenge. This search is a part of human existence and is a primary motivation. Finding meaning involves the *how*, the *when,* and the *where*, and each person is responsible to find it uniquely. While ultimate meaning is unattainable because individuals must continue in their search until the last breath, the meaning of moment is available to us and can be reached. This meaning of moment varies from one situation to the other, due to the uniqueness of each person and the uniqueness of each situation.

Change is a normal phenomenon: Although it affects our traditional values, it does not affect our unique meaning, as long as we make responsible choices with commitments and sensitivity to other people around. The utilization of the concept and principles of logotherapy must start from us. It is necessary for all of us to be role models to our family, neighbors, colleagues, and others.

References

Asagba, R. B. (1993). Logotherapy's knowledge and wisdom. *International Forum for Logotherapy, 16*(1), 31–34.

Asagba, R. B. (2002). *Logotherapy and cultural development*. Spectrum NG Press Ltd.

Asagba, R. B. (2006). *Logotherapy from an African perspective*. University Press Nigeria Ltd.

Burdman, G. M. (2008). *Search for significance: Finding meaning in times of change, challenge, and chaos*. Bellevue Press.

Evans, W. F. (2012). *The world still cries for meaning: Are we still listening?* Paper presented at the The Future of Logotherapy World Congress, Viktor Frankl Institut, Vienna, Austria.

Fabry, J. B. (2013). *The pursuit of meaning: Viktor Frankl, logotherapy, and life*. Purpose Research. (Original work published 1968)

Fabry, J. B. (2021). *Guideposts to meaning: Discovering what really matters* (2nd ed.). Purpose Research. (Original work published 1988)

Frankl, V. E. (1978). *The unheard cry for meaning: Psychotherapy and humanism*. Simon and Schuster.

Frankl, V. E. (1985). *Man's search for meaning* (3rd ed.). Washington Square Press/Pocket Books. (Original work published 1946)

Frankl, V. E. (1988). *The will to meaning: Foundations and applications of logotherapy*. Meridian.

Frankl, V. E. (2000). *Recollections: An autobiography* (J. B. Fabry & J. Fabry, Trans.). Basic Books. (Original work published 1995 as *Was nicht in meinen Büchem steht*)

Graber, A. V. (2004). *Viktor Frankl's logotherapy: Method of choice in ecumenical pastoral psychology*. Wyndham Hall Press.

Hutzell, R. R., & Jerkins, M. E. (2009). *A workbook to increase your meaningful and purposeful goals (MPGs)* (2nd ed.). Viktor Frankl Institute of Logotherapy Press. Retrieved from: http://www.viktorfrankl.org/assets/pdf/hutzell_workbook_2009.pdf

Kalmar, S. (1982). A brief history of logotherapy. In S. A. Wawrytko (Ed.), *Analecta Frankliana: The proceedings of the first World Congress of Logotherapy, 1980*. Institute of Logotherapy Press.

Kleftaras, G., & Psarra, E. (2012). Meaning in life, psychological well-being and depressive symptomatology: A comparative study. *Psychology, 3*(04), 337. https://doi.org/10.4236/psych.2012.34048

Lukas, E. (2015). *The therapist and the soul: From fate to freedom*. Purpose Research.

Lukas, E. (2020). *Meaningful living: Introduction to logotherapy theory and practice* (J. B. Fabry, Trans.; 2nd ed.). Purpose Research.

Maddi, S. R. (1970). *The search for meaning: An introduction*. Washington Square Press.

Reker, G. T., & Wong, P. T. P. (1988). Aging as an individual process: Toward a theory of personal meaning. In V. L. Bengtson & J. E. Birren (Eds.), *Emergent theories of aging*. Springer.

Steger, M. F., Oishi, S., & Kesebir, S. (2011). Is a life without meaning satisfying? The moderating role of the search for meaning in satisfaction with life judgments. *The Journal of Positive Psychology, 6*(3), 173–180.

The late Rachel Bolaji Asagba (1953–2021), obtained a diploma in Nutrition and Dietetics from the University of Vienna, where she studied between 1973–76. In the US, she earned a bachelor's degree from the College of Mount St. Vincent in 1985, then a master's degree in psychology and nutrition from Clayton University in 1986.

She received her logotherapy training from the Viktor Frankl Institute, Vienna from 1989–1992 and was mentored by Viktor Frankl. She remained a strong advocate for logotherapy over her personal and professional life. In 1998, she was appointed as an assistant lecturer in the Department of Psychology, University of Ibadan, Oyo State. Her hard work and dedication were rewarded in 2019, when she was promoted to professor of clinical psychology.

Rachel Asagba was the founder of the Nigerian Logotherapy Group at the University of Ibadan. She has a robust and vast archive of completed publications, journals, and research that span a wide range of fields in addition to her area of specialization.

International Negotiation and Conflict Resolution: Hope, Optimism, and Meaning Through Logotherapy-Enhanced Rational-Emotive Behavior Therapy

Matti Ameli, Pninit Russo-Netzer, and Clara Benacerraf

International Negotiation and Conflict Resolution: Hope, Optimism, and Meaning Through Logotherapy-Enhanced Rational-Emotive Behavior Therapy

Conflict negotiation largely refers to a process of resolving a disagreement or a conflict through the care for each side's needs and addressing their interests to allow satisfactory outcomes. Granted, this is a dynamic, complex, and challenging process that has been explored in depth through various perspectives, from a problem-solving, third-party approach to international and intercommunal conflicts resolution (Burton, 1984; Kelman, 2005), to coordination strategies and resources (see Nan & Strimling, 2006, p. for a review) and peacemaking, peacebuilding, and peacekeeping (Handelman, 2019), to name a few. Other approaches, such as nonviolent communication (Rosenberg, 1999), involve communication tools applied to resolve conflicts in various contexts (e.g., in educational, therapeutic, and organizational settings). In their pioneering work, Aquilar and Galluccio (2008, 2011) offered a comprehensive analysis of cognitive, emotional, and communicative aspects involved in international negotiation, highlighting the beneficial input of cognitive behavioral therapy in the negotiation process. More particularly, they highlighted three macro categories involved in such process: prevention (identification and

M. Ameli (✉)
Private Practice, Valencia, Spain

P. Russo-Netzer
Achva Academic College, Arugot, Israel

Department of Counseling and Human Development, University of Haifa, Haifa, Israel

C. Benacerraf
International College Spain, Madrid, Spain

C. L. McLafferty, Jr., J. I. Levinson (eds.), *Logotherapy and Existential Analysis*, Logotherapy and Existential Analysis: Proceedings of the Viktor Frankl Institute Vienna 2, https://doi.org/10.1007/978-3-031-48922-8_10

modification of dysfunctional beliefs), managing (focusing on interpersonal and metacognitive processes), and reparation (offering psychotherapeutic help to the victims) (Aquilar & Galluccio, 2008). These broad macro categories inform our proposed model discussed in this chapter.

In an attempt to outline a holistic approach that integrates broad philosophies of life, psychotherapy, and tools into the multilayered process of conflict resolution, this chapter focuses on two such perspectives, in order to integrate viewpoints of both rational emotive behavioral therapy (REBT) and logotherapy (a meaning-oriented approach). The authors of this chapter come from different cultural backgrounds, with experience in the clinical and educational field, aiming to translate these ideas, rooted in REBT and logotherapy, into international negotiation and conflict resolution processes. At the clinical level, the integration between REBT and logotherapy has provided promising directions for the cultivation of optimal sense making (Russo-Netzer & Ameli, 2021), suggesting that such an integrative model may also promote an optimal negotiation mindset for hopeful and meaningful conflict resolution.

What Facilitates Conflict Resolution?

Results from a study project involving 120 negotiators from 15 EU countries show that communication, creativity, and empathy are among the central characteristics that positively contribute to the negotiation process, whereas suspicion of deceit, aggressiveness, and rigidity are considered dangerous and detrimental for negotiation. The importance of hope is also highlighted as it deeply relates to emotions, meaning, and morality in international negotiation, facilitation, and mediation (Aquilar & Galluccio, 2008). Various experts in the field have also shared interesting ideas regarding the inclusion of psychological concepts in the frame of conflict resolution and peace negotiation.

Howard Gardner (2011) proposed a ninth form of intelligence, *existential intelligence*, which he considered to be one of the most important types of intelligence for negotiators. Paul Gilbert (2011) introduced the concept of *cooperative social mentality*, which draws on caring and compassion, in contrast to *competitive social mentality*, where self-promotion is the primary motive. Carolyn Saarni (2011) focused on the concept of *emotional competence*, highlighting that negotiators are better prepared if they are knowledgeable about the emotional cultural customs, based on the values and beliefs of their counterpart's culture. Finally, Aimée Karam (2011) reported that resilience and wisdom are important elements in successful negotiation and reconciliation. She highlighted the importance of familiarity with procedures that could increase resilience in the face of adversity and severe conflict management.

What may underlie all of these aforementioned facilitators of conflict resolution are sense-making processes that allow for the cultivation of such structures. In this context, logotherapy (Frankl, 1984b), a values-based meaning-centered approach, emphasizes self-transcendence, compassion, wisdom, and resilience and goes beyond the strict clinical domain to bring its support to all areas of human activity where the question of meaning arises in a significant way. According to Frankl, if voluntary commitment to a common meaningful task has the potential to overcome aggressiveness and violence for individuals and groups, then it could also be applied for humankind as a whole for the establishment of peace. Marshall and Marshall (2012) suggested that logotherapy has been used as a vehicle of dialogue and reconciliation, to help find meaningful ways to resolve inner conflict as well as conflicts among people. From clinical therapy to counseling, from pedagogy to education, from the field of law to that of the economy—particularly the world of work—logotherapy offers insights into various decision-making practices and offers a potential contribution to negotiation, conflict resolution, and arbitration.

Following a brief overview of both REBT and logotherapy, an integrative model for negotiation will be presented along with ideas on how to include logotherapy within the training program proposed by Aquilar and Galluccio (2008).

Overview of Rational Emotive Behavioral Therapy

Rational Emotive Behavioral Therapy was founded by the American psychologist Albert Ellis in 1955. Ellis (1962) believed that a dogmatic and rigid philosophy of demandingness based on absolutistic beliefs expressed in terms of "musts," "shoulds," "oughts," and "have tos"—toward self, others, and life or the world—lies at the heart of psychological disturbances. This may lead to three other types of irrational beliefs: *awfulizing* (an extreme exaggeration of the negative consequences of a situation), *frustration intolerance* (demanding comfort and ease at all times and not tolerating discomfort), and *global evaluation of worth of self or others* (the idea that human beings are ratable and some are worthless or less valuable than others) (DiGiuseppe et al., 2014). While rigid and dogmatic beliefs are at the core of psychological disturbance, psychological flexibility based on relativism, non-dogmatic preferences, and unconditional acceptance is a key feature of psychological health (DiGiuseppe et al., 2014; Ellis & MacLaren, 2005). The REBT model of psychotherapy promotes a rational life philosophy which emphasizes unconditional self-acceptance, unconditional acceptance toward others, and unconditional life acceptance (Ellis & Ellis, 2011). Practitioners of REBT distinguish between unhealthy/maladaptive and healthy/adaptive negative emotions. Healthy negative emotions such as concern, annoyance, sadness, disappointment, and regret or remorse are based on rational beliefs, whereas unhealthy negative emotions such as anxiety, depression, clinical anger, shame, and guilt are based on irrational beliefs. The target is unhealthy and maladaptive negative emotions (DiGiuseppe et al., 2014; Dryden, 2012).

The main goal of REBT is to identify, dispute, and modify: (a) rigid, irrational, and unhealthy philosophies based on absolutistic demands; and (b) a lack of unconditional acceptance of self, others, and life/world into a flexible and healthy philosophy based on preferences and unconditional acceptance (Ellis & Ellis, 2011). *Disputing* is the best-known method of REBT. It aims at helping clients to identify their irrational beliefs and substitute them with adaptive and healthy beliefs. This method has been found effective for a large spectrum of population and clinical psychiatric disorders (David et al., 2018).

As one of the charter members of the APA Division of Peace Psychology, Ellis (1992) was interested in the use of psychotherapeutic principles to promote peace; "Rational-Emotive Approaches to Peace" reflected his ideas and thoughts on that topic. He highlighted that REBT had the potential to promote a more peaceful relationship with oneself, toward families and neighbors, and ultimately toward foreign ethnic and political groups. He suggested the following peace-enhancing attitudes and actions: negotiation and compromise, altruism and social interest, encouraging empathy, enhancing hope for the future, and promoting nonviolence and internationalism. Those attitudes are largely rooted in acceptance (self, others, and world) and would fit mostly in the macro category of *prevention* proposed by Aquilar and Galluccio (2008). Ellis also pointed out the value of REBT for overcoming the following: depression and despair, prejudice and arrogance, labeling and semantic errors, vulnerability and defensiveness, rage and hostility, rigid and absolutistic thinking, low frustration tolerance, and communication difficulties. Those would largely fit in the categories of *managing* and *reparation* as proposed by Aquilar and Galluccio.

Ellis (2008) highlighted the element of choice, pointing out that peace negotiators can choose peaceful negotiation strategies or combative methods for solving national and international conflicts. Analyzing the roots and causes of fighting, conflicts, and disagreements, Ellis (1992) pointed out that demandingness was involved in most cases. Demandingness—expressed in absolutistic musts, should, and oughts—constitutes the essence of anger, fury, rage, and combat and could lead to the three derivatives, *awfulizing* ("Not getting what I want is terrible"), *frustration intolerance* ("I can't stand losing, being wrong," etc.), and *global evaluation of another's worth* ("You are a rotten or damnable person"). Ellis (2004) called for trying our best to stop damning ourselves, others, and life while remaining strongly motivated to encourage and work for our own and others' improvement.

Research has demonstrated that cognitions related to revenge are the best predictors of the state of anger, followed by demands that the event should not have happened. Demands of others is another significant variable. (DiGiuseppe & Froh, 2002) found a positive correlation between items related to others' unfairness, condemnation, lack of respect, and others behaving immorally with the intensity of state anger. Several meta-analyses also suggest that there is substantial evidence for anger management and aggression interventions based on cognitive-behavioral approaches (DiGiuseppe & Tafrate, 2003; Lee & DiGiuseppe, 2018).

DiGiuseppe and Tafrate (2007) differentiated between two forms of anger. One type is defined as a functional or "healthy anger" that promotes constructive change and leads to long-term positive outcomes; it is based on rationality (flexible, healthy beliefs), planning, and strategic thinking and has a long-term purpose. The other type is dysfunctional or "unhealthy anger" and is based on impulsivity and short-term gain; its main goal seems to influence the impression of others by demanding respect or fairness and is based on dogmatic and rigid beliefs that could lead to aggression and revengeful actions.

Referring to the Black Lives Matter movement, DiGiuseppe (2021) pointed to the term "righteous indignation" as a possible way to express that healthy anger held by its followers. As an example of healthy anger, he referred to Nelson Mandela who was able to implement a revenge-less strategy in South Africa by choosing to use anger to build a better future instead of focusing on the past and on seeking revenge. Empirical research on conflict resolution has suggested that anger in the absence of hatred could be constructive to move toward compromise (Halperin et al., 2011). In line with this, Handelman (2019) highlighted the importance of an innovative multidimensional approach for a revolutionary peace process which includes peacemaking, peacebuilding, and peacekeeping. Tafrate and Kassinove (2009) concluded that forgiveness is a process that involves letting go of anger and resentment and choosing a perspective of understanding, compassion, and goodwill toward the offender. They proposed a five-stage model of forgiving: (1) uncovering anger, (2) deciding to forgive, (3) defining forgiveness, (4) understanding why others behave badly, and (5) giving something of value to the wrongdoer (p. 112). As an example, they made reference to Viktor Frankl and his experiences in the Nazi concentration camp, along with his meaning-based theory of logotherapy as an example for overcoming anger and life adversities by strengthening trust in life's meaningfulness and people's dignity.

Overview of Logotherapy

The Austrian neurologist, psychiatrist, and Holocaust survivor Viktor Frankl (1988/1969) pioneered logotherapy during the 1930s. It is generally defined as an empirically based meaning-centered approach to psychotherapy. Frankl envisioned logotherapy, the "third Viennese School of Psychotherapy," as an undogmatic system of therapy that is open to collaboration with other psychotherapeutic orientations. Frankl portrayed the human person as existing in three overlapping dimensions: somatic (physical body), psychological (emotions and intellect), and noëtic (uniquely human dimension). The noëtic dimension is considered the site of authentically human phenomena and includes qualities such as self-distancing, self-transcendence, humor, values, imagination, love, and gratitude. In contrast with the first two dimensions where our reactions are often automatic, in the noëtic dimension we can choose how to behave (Lukas, 2000). The physiological, psychological, and noëtic (or spiritual) dimensions constitute a human person and hence cannot be rejected or overlooked (Marshall & Marshall, 2022; Russo-Netzer et al., 2016). Each of these dimensions reflects a layer of qualities and functions that interact with each other but is nonetheless ontologically independent from one another (Frankl, 1986). The fundamental tenets of logotherapy are freedom of will, will to meaning, and meaning in life (Frankl, 1988/1969). *Freedom of will* asserts that human beings have the freedom to choose their response within the limits of given possibilities, under all life circumstances. *Will to meaning* points out that the main motivation of human beings is to search for the meaning and purpose in their lives. *Meaning in life* highlights that life has meaning under all circumstances, even in unavoidable suffering and misery. According to Frankl (1984a), we can discover meaning in life in three different ways, known as the categorical values: *Creative values* consist of what we give to the world, such as accomplishing a task, creating a work, or doing a good deed; *experiential values* are what we take from the world, such as the experience of truth, beauty, and love toward another human being; and *attitudinal values* reflect the stand we take toward an unchangeable situation or unavoidable suffering. Frankl (1984a) used the term *tragic optimism* to refer to remaining optimistic through hope, faith, and love in spite of the tragic triad of pain, guilt, and death. Frankl based this concept on the principle that life is meaningful under all circumstances and that human beings have the capacity to make responsible choices in any given situation by creatively turning the negative aspects into constructive ones (Frankl, 1984a; Lukas, 2000). Logotherapists focus both on the client's "current positives" (assets and strengths) and "future potentials" or possibilities for expansion (Lukas, 2000). The goal of the logotherapist, thus, is to tap into the client's unique human capacities such as intentionality, responsibility, and freedom of choice and to broaden their visual scope to discover and actualize the meaning potentials in their lives (Ameli, 2016a, 2016b). The logotherapist is active during the therapy session, pointing out inconsistencies, sharing ideas, and disagreeing with clients when their values are not adjusted to reality (Lukas, 2000). In clinical practice, logotherapy has been found to be useful in various interventions and contexts such as depression, anxiety, alcohol/drug abuse, psychosis, grief, and despair associated with incurable disease (Marshall & Marshall, 2017; Schulenberg et al., 2008). Furthermore, the importance of meaning in life as a resource for both coping and thriving has been emphasized across populations and diverse cultural subgroups (e.g., Abu-Raiya et al., 2021; Pavlacic et al., 2021; Russo-Netzer & Bergman, 2020; Steger et al., 2008), among immigrants/ non-immigrants (Russo-Netzer et al., 2021) and throughout the lifespan, from childhood (Shoshani & Russo-Netzer, 2017) and adolescence (Russo-Netzer & Shoshani, 2020) to late adulthood (Russo-Netzer & Littman-Ovadia, 2019).

Although logotherapy did not offer an explicit framework for conflict resolution, Frankl's own personal life story as well as his disciples have offered some insightful ideas and insights that may contribute to further develop current models of conflict resolution. Frankl's (1984a) idea of collective guilt suggests that it is "unjustified to hold one person responsible for the behavior of another person or a collective of persons" (p. 149). In other words, the collective (e.g., a country) cannot be held accountable for the deeds of a group of individuals. Along these lines, Elisabeth Lukas (2020b) proposed the concept of "*dissonance of conscience*" (p. 84). According to this idea, if we send a positive signal to our opponents, it would make it difficult to answer with a negative, since something positive has been received. The positive received would help them decide on something positive to send and to move toward meaning, which means the "good *for all concerned*" (p. 84). Further suggestions derive from logotherapeutic applications and techniques in an international educational setting. These include a focus on international-mindedness, enabling students to reflect on their own perspective, culture, and identities and on those of others. By learning to appreciate different beliefs, values, and experiences and to collaborate across cultures and disciplines, students are equipped with the necessary skills to move toward a more peaceful and sustainable world (International Baccalaureate Organization, 2023). From a logotherapeutic perspective, conflict resolution involves teaching children to be self-determined, non-judgmental, and focused on hope for the future.

The following key techniques for conflict resolution are a good fit with logotherapeutic principles and have been incorporated at an international school in Madrid:

- *The peace bridge* is a kinesthetic conflict-resolution tool for children, consisting of a series of steps that lead to a mutually beneficial and peaceful solution.
- *The wheel of choice*, a conflict resolution tool inspired by "positive discipline" (Nelsen, 1996), offers children the opportunity to learn how to manage conflict by making responsible choices without using violence.
- *The calming sequence* (Buron & Curtis, 2012) is a self-regulation tool for children, which helps them manage their thoughts, feelings, and actions in situations of stress, anger, or anxiety.
- *Creative compassion*, for which Swindler (2012) identified four basic principles, which are (a) knowing ourselves and our personal values; (b) knowing other people's values, avoiding stereotypes and prejudices; (c) learning about the interconnectedness between our values and the values of others; and (d) practicing the ability to imagine being born or raised in another religious and cultural context.

Proposal of an Integrative Model for Conflict Resolution and International Negotiation

We propose an adaptation of the "optimal sense-making" concept, proposed by Russo-Netzer and Ameli (2021) and based on the integration of rationality and meaning in the clinical field, along with logotherapeutic concepts in the educational setting applied in an international school with over 70 nationalities, to the conflict resolution field. The integrative model envisions a dynamic model for negotiation based on the four macro categories: prevention, managing, and reparation proposed by Aquilar and Galluccio (2008) in which REBT and logotherapy are integrated, along with an additional new category, *holistic transformation*, which reflects the exclusive input from logotherapy. We suggest the importance of an *optimal negotiation mindset* that would facilitate rational and meaningful agreements and steps toward prevention, managing, recovery, and resilience (see Fig. 1). Referring to the ideas of Albert Ellis (1992) on how to implement REBT for conflict resolution and peace negotiation, we propose the following ideas on how to integrate REBT and

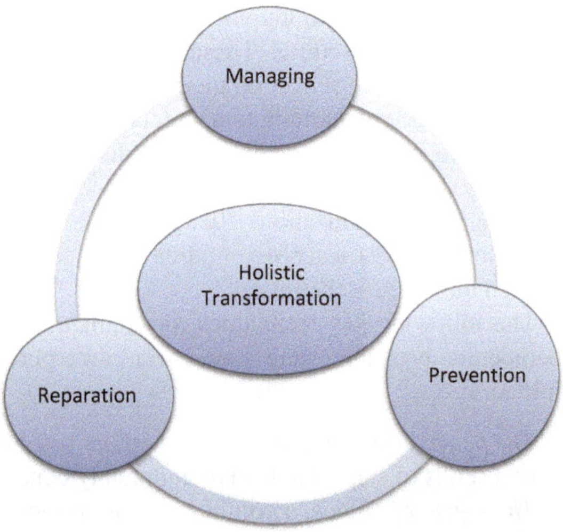

Fig. 1 Suggested integrative model for conflict resolution

logotherapy in each of the macro categories and provide ideas on a fourth possible category based on logotherapeutic concepts.

Prevention

The *prevention* category is mostly focused on overcoming dysfunctional beliefs and includes actions related to social communication with the goal of discouraging terrorist organizations and followers (Aquilar & Galluccio, 2008). Albert Ellis (1992) referred to areas such as negotiation and compromise, altruism and social interest, encouraging empathy, enhancing hope for the future, and promoting non-violence and internationalism. Those elements would largely fit in that category. We propose to enhance REBT by adding key concepts and strategies from logotherapy that are used in the frame of educational counseling within an international setting, such as the international school in Madrid (Benacerraf, 2016, 2020). Strategies could be implemented with children at an early age and adapted to adults within the frame of international conflict resolution and negotiation, which include:

- *Negotiation and compromise.* The peace bridge entails the use of Socratic dialogue, a child-friendly method rooted in logotherapy as defined by Benacerraf (2020). It is a process that opens up children's way of thinking, including the exploration of complex ideas, and guides them toward self-transcendence and meaningful solutions.
- *Altruism and social interest.* Creative compassion is used in international settings to teach children how to identify each other's values and preferences, so they are able to empathize with each other without being judgmental. This reinforces two basic concepts in logotherapy: the uniqueness of every human being

and their ability to make decisions freely and responsibly. In turn, these two concepts are deeply connected to altruism and self-transcendence (Benacerraf, 2016).

- *Encouraging empathy.* Creative compassion and the wheel of choice require that all parties have a shared responsibility to move from a conflictive place to a more promising, peaceful one. Through role-playing and storytelling, children model how to make meaningful choices and discover new meanings through self-transcendence and compassion.
- *Enhancing hope for the future.* Through play therapy, art therapy, and drama, children have the opportunity to be freethinkers and envision a more tolerant, peaceful, and hopeful future.
- *Promoting nonviolence and internationalism.* In an international setting, as children interact with each other, they realize that people think and act differently. Sometimes, this may lead to lack of tolerance and aggression. The calming sequence technique helps children to regulate their emotions, prevent impulsiveness, and promote peaceful dialogue. Through projects and celebrations of the multicultural diversity present in over 70 nationalities, children learn the values of respect, tolerance, and internationalism.

Managing

The *managing* category includes interpersonal and metacognitive processes; the objective is to promote dissuasive actions directed to active followers (Aquilar & Galluccio, 2008). Within the frame of REBT, Ellis (1992) referred to overcoming issues such as prejudices and arrogance, labeling, rage and hostility, rigid absolutistic thinking, frustration intolerance, and communication problems, which largely fit in this category.

In the beginning of a conflict or in a moderate conflictive situation, a first step could be helping the parties identify each of their most valuable cultural, social, and religious values that would fit in the creative values, according to logotherapy. The objective would be to identify the common values and turn them into potentially meaningful opportunities for collaboration. The values awareness technique proposed by Hutzell and Jerkins (2009) is a valuable tool in clinical practice to help clients identify their values and define goals aligned with those values. It would be interesting to adapt that technique or create a similar logotherapeutic tool in the frame of international negotiations.

As for contrasting values in the category of creative values (for example, religious-based rituals or cultural customs), the objective could be to negotiate ways to lead to constructive compromise. As a first step, we propose for negotiators to implement REBT strategies and techniques to identify and substitute irrational beliefs with healthy and adaptive beliefs. The second step would be to add logotherapeutic concepts and strategies based on the freedom of choice and dereflection that helps to counteract metacognitive processes, such as secondary disturbance or rumination, to promote meaningful beliefs. Some of the approaches to the stage of managing are:

- *Overcoming prejudices and arrogance.* The application of REBT could promote the concept of unconditional acceptance of others as human beings. Frankl's (1988/1969) logotherapeutic concept of shared humanity or *monanthropism* (p. 98) complements REBT along with the "creative compassion" of Swindler (2012): We all belong to the human race and we all matter; we have the option to understand our opponents' contrasting values by imagining being born and raised in their country and culture.
- *Overcoming labeling.* Overgeneralizing the actions of another and labeling them as bad or evil could be addressed by REBT's philosophy of imperfection and fallibility, as well as our inherent self-worth. The concepts in logotherapy related to the uniqueness of human beings, self-transcendence, and focus through dereflection on the others' strengths could complement REBT: Each culture is unique and we have the option to focus on the positive aspects of an opponents' culture in order to move toward agreement and action.
- *Overcoming rage and hostility.* It would be important for negotiators to help express the feelings of the parties involved in a healthy way that could lead to constructive compromises and actions. Teaching the differences between "unhealthy" and "healthy" anger (or righteous indignation) that would lead to long-term planning and strategizing of constructive actions would be key. Applications of logotherapy could complement the use of REBT by transforming anger into responsible and meaningful action through dereflection: We can choose to focus on agreeing on meaningful actions that would lead to peace and forgiveness.
- *Overcoming rigid absolutistic thinking.* Using the strategies of REBT, it would be important to identify the "shoulds" and "musts" and promote a flexible way of managing the conflict by turning them into preferences and desires. The dereflection technique of logotherapy would be complementary in transforming the preferences into meaningful actions. The technique of the wheel of choice could be adapted to promote responsible collaboration in a nonblaming manner.
- *Overcoming frustration intolerance.* It would be important during the negotiation process to teach methods that would help to counteract the tendency to react violently against unfair practices, political issues, etc. by demanding that they absolutely must not exist and seeking immediate gratification at any cost. Application of the meaningful philosophy of logotherapy, based on self-transcendence, would complement REBT in finding powerful reasons to help tolerate frustration and discomfort: for the sake of peace, nonviolence, children's future, etc. The peace-bridge technique could be adapted to take steps toward meaningful agreements.
- *Overcoming communication problems.* The strategies of REBT could be used to teach an assertive communication style to minimize violence and awfulizing. Although each party could perceive events such as bombing or killing as awful,

repeating these incidents in retaliation would lead to violent exchange. The logotherapeutic concept of "dissonance of conscience" (Lukas, 2020b, p. 84) would be valuable in order to promote initiative in reciprocal positivity.

Reparation

The *reparation* category involves offering psychotherapeutic help to the victims and survivors of war and psychological support for repentant terrorists as well (Aquilar & Galluccio, 2008). Within the frame of REBT, Ellis (1992) referred to issues such as overcoming depression and despair, rage, hostility, and low frustration tolerance, which fit in this category. We propose to add issues related to trauma, post-traumatic stress disorder (PTSD), and guilt. Southwick et al. (2006) have cited examples of the use of logotherapy as an adjunctive treatment for war-related PTSD. Russo-Netzer and Ameli (2021) have provided ideas on the integration of REBT and logotherapy based on "optimal sense-making" at the clinical level, which has the potential to promote acceptance, frustration tolerance, self-transcendence, perseverance, resilience, and post-traumatic growth. We propose the following ideas for integration, emphasizing attitudinal values:

- *Overcoming depression and despair.* The techniques of REBT could be used to modify the unhealthy beliefs and dysfunctional behavioral patterns as well as to promote unconditional acceptance of self and life. Activating the will to meaning through attitude modulation (Lukas, 2020a, pp. 47–76) would help overcome despair and discover meaning in suffering, leading to resilience.
- *Overcoming trauma.* The cognitive, behavioral, and emotive techniques of REBT could be implemented to process the trauma and move toward unconditional acceptance of life/world, The use of the concept of tragic optimism from logotherapy would be a good complement to address meaning in adversity in order to promote post-traumatic growth.
- *Overcoming rage.* The disputing techniques and psychoeducation of REBT could be used to transform rage and unhealthy anger into indignation, along with unconditional other acceptance, and move toward the process of forgiveness as described by Tafrate and Kassinove (2009). By orienting the person toward the meaningful attitudinal choices and actions available and implementing forgiveness, the application of logotherapy could be used (Pattakos & Dundon, 2014).
- *Overcoming frustration intolerance.* The disputing techniques of REBT could also be used to facilitate frustration tolerance; the concept of self-transcendence of logotherapy could be implemented to find a worthwhile reason to tolerate the discomfort and the pain: for the sake of a loved one, a meaningful mission, a task, etc.
- *Overcoming guilt.* This would be relevant mostly in the case of repentant terrorists. As a first step, the disputing techniques of REBT could be helpful to transform guilt into remorse and emphasize unconditional self-acceptance. As a

second step, logotherapy's concepts of tragic optimism and redemption (Frankl, 1986) could be valuable in order to turn remorse into an opportunity to compensate the wrong done. For example, the repentant terrorist could help to rebuild something valuable that he has destroyed or damaged like a school or hospital. Lukas (2015, p. 168) addresses guilt highlighting three types of reparations: (a) to the same person, (b) to another person, and (c) on a moral level. The last type would lead to repentance, a change in inner attitude that would potentiate knowledge, meaning, and growth.

Beyond the three meta-categories suggested by Aquilar and Galluccio (2008) of prevention, managing, and repairing, we propose a fourth macro-category which transcends rational resolution and allows a more holistic approach toward transformation and growth.

Holistic Transformation

When we examine the etymology of the word *health*, we find that the Latin source of the word is *hal*, which means "whole"; capturing this etymological connection, one of the dictionary definitions found in the *Cambridge dictionary* (online, n.d.) of *to heal* is *to make whole*. In this sense, it may be suggested that wholeness involves healing of the divided and fragmented parts of an individual, a system or society at large (Russo-Netzer, 2018, p. 2). In the context of negotiation and conflict resolution, aiming at wholeness as a guiding principle requires a more complex, holistic, and nuanced view of human experience. In order to gain a holistic view, we also need to keep in mind that our current conceptualizations and insights may only reflect a limited and specific perspective on the infinite and complex processes to which we have only partial access.

Although challenging, becoming aware of our own set of theoretical and ideological conceptualizations and consciously suspending, or "bracketing," judgment, presumptions, and expectations derived from such previous knowledge is no less important than accumulating new information. Adopting a sense of humility enables us to remain self-conscious and not take for granted previously held paradigms with regard to human nature and experience. As Frankl (1984a) stated:

> Man is not fully conditioned and determined but rather he determines himself whether he gives in to conditions or stands up to them.... Man does not simply exist but always decides what his existence will be, what he will become in the next moment. (p. 131)

When we are willing to move beyond zero-sum structures and narrowing frameworks to the reality of human beings, we are more capable of exploring the full and rich range of colors and experiences in a holistic manner. This may allow us to capture a somewhat "in-between" phase of the change experience between the dissolution of current contextuality and the construction of new frameworks and core beliefs, as a glimpse to potentiality and situational freedom which facilitate the possibility for shift of intentionality and recalibrating lived experience. Such a stance may facilitate a new awareness of situational freedom, as was found as essential characteristics in transformative life experiences (Russo-Netzer & Davidov, 2020). In the context of conflict resolution, this may be reflected in a negotiation process that is managed to allow more focus on shared humane values, such as compassion and self-transcendence which move beyond each party's focus on current situation and fragmented view. The logotherapeutic idea of tragic optimism may enable a shift toward meaningful options, hope, growth, and resilience, as well as redeeming and compensation through meaning. This may include help rebuilding something valuable that was destroyed or damaged (e.g., school, hospital etc.), collaborate toward a mutually beneficial meaningful project (e.g., share resources, design new guidelines, etc.).

Logotherapy as an Integral Part of the Training Program for Negotiators

Aquilar and Galluccio (2008) described the features of a 15-day training program for negotiators that not only includes teaching based on REBT and cognitive-behavioral therapy but also concepts and strategies from art therapies (music, theater, poetry, etc.) and evolutionary psychology including attachment theory. The concept of compassion as proposed by Paul Gilbert (2011) has also been integrated. We propose to include logotherapy to enhance the training program. Concepts of logotherapy such as meaning, freedom of choice, self-transcendence, values, and tragic optimism would be valuable in preparing meaning-oriented negotiators. The training could be focused on three parts: (1) *Man's Search for Meaning*, Viktor Frankl's (1984a) life story and experiences during World War II, could be valuable; (2) a theoretical part, reflecting the main tenets and the philosophical basis of logotherapy, research, and applications to the negotiation process; and (3) a practical part, in which the main logotherapeutic techniques and tools are taught in combination with REBT and cognitive-behavioral therapy techniques as proposed in this paper and role played in potential negotiation settings, with a focus on resilience, post-traumatic growth, and holistic transformation.

Conclusion

Ellis (2008) placed an emphasis on the choice that negotiators have to choose peaceful negotiation strategies or combative methods. Frankl's (1984a) focus on self-transcendence facilitates reaching and maintaining peaceful choices by finding powerful reasons to do so that focus on meaning. Integrating logotherapeutic strategies and tools from both educational and clinical fields with the REBT framework could be beneficial in training both rational and meaning-oriented negotiators. A rational existential-philosophy of negotiation, as presented in this chapter, has the potential to lead to an optimal negotiation mindset that would facilitate the conflict resolution and peace negotiation process.

References

Abu-Raiya, H., Sasson, T., & Russo-Netzer, P. (2021). Presence of meaning, search for meaning, religiousness, satisfaction with life and depressive symptoms among a diverse Israeli sample. *International Journal of Psychology, 56*(2), 276–285. https://doi.org/10.1002/ijop.12709

Ameli, M. (2016a). Integrating logotherapy with cognitive behavior therapy: A worthy challenge. In *Logotherapy and existential analysis: Proceedings of the Viktor Frankl Institute Vienna* (pp. 197–217). Springer International Publishing.

Ameli, M. (2016b). Reason, meaning, and resilience in the treatment of depression: Logotherapy as a bridge between cognitive-behavior therapy and positive psychology. In P. Russo-Netzer, S. E. Schulenberg, & A. Batthyany (Eds.), *Clinical perspectives on meaning* (pp. 223–244). Springer International Publishing.

Aquilar, F., & Galluccio, M. (2008). *Psychological processes in international negotiations: Theoretical and practical perspectives*. Springer.

Aquilar, F., & Galluccio, M. (2011). *Psychological and political strategies for peace negotiation: A cognitive approach*. Springer.

Benacerraf, C. (2016). *Counselling the IB learner profile: A logotherapeutic approach*. Paper presented at the NAE Regional Conference, Bratislava, Slovakia.

Benacerraf, C. (2020). *Using Socratic Dialogue in logotherapy with children and adolescents: Developmental considerations to facilitate self-discovery, attitudinal change and meaning fulfilment.* (Diplomate paper). Viktor Frankl Institute of Logotherapy,

Buron, K. D., & Curtis, M. (2012). *The incredible 5-point scale: Assisting students in understanding social interactions and controlling their emotional responses* (2nd ed.). AAPC Publishing.

Burton, J. W. (1984). *Global conflict: The domestic sources of international crisis.* Wheatsheaf Books.

David, D., Cotet, C., Matu, S., Mogoase, C., & Stefan, S. (2018). 50 years of rational-emotive and cognitive-behavioral therapy: A systematic review and meta-analysis. *Journal of Clinical Psychology, 74*(3), 304–318.

DiGiuseppe, R. A. (2021). *Understanding and overcoming anger* [Video]. Retrieved from https://www.youtube.com/watch?v=Mehk5MorKXY

DiGiuseppe, R. A., & Froh, J. J. (2002). What cognitions predict state anger? *Journal of Rational-Emotive and Cognitive-Behavior Therapy, 20*, 133–150.

DiGiuseppe, R. A., & Tafrate, R. C. (2003). Anger treatment for adults: A meta-analytic review. *Clinical Psychology: Science and Practice, 10*(1), 70.

DiGiuseppe, R. A., & Tafrate, R. C. (2007). *Understanding anger disorders.* Oxford University Press.

DiGiuseppe, R. A., DiGiuseppe, R., Doyle, K. A., Dryden, W., & Backx, W. (2014). *A practitioner's guide to rational-emotive behavior therapy*. Oxford University Press.

Dryden, W. (2012). *Dealing with emotional problems using rational-emotive cognitive behaviour therapy: A practitioner's guide*. Routledge.

Ellis, A. (1962). Reason and emotion in psychotherapy. L. Stuart.

Ellis, A. (1992). Rational-emotive approaches to peace. *Journal of Cognitive Psychotherapy, 6*(2), 79–104.

Ellis, A. (2004). *The road to tolerance: The philosophy of rational emotive behavior therapy.* Prometheus Books.

Ellis, A. (2008). Foreword. In F. Aquilar & M. Galluccio (Eds.), *Psychological processes in international negotiations: Theoretical and practical perspectives*. Springer Science & Business Media.

Ellis, A., & Ellis, D. J. (2011). *Rational emotive behavior therapy*. American Psychological Association.

Ellis, A., & MacLaren, C. (2005). *Rational emotive behavior therapy: A therapist's guide*. Impact Publishers.

Frankl, V. E. (1984a). *Man's search for meaning* (3rd ed.). Pocket Books. (Original work published 1946)

Frankl, V. E. (1984b). The meaning crisis in the first world and hunger in the third world. *International Forum for Logotherapy, 7*(1), 5–7.

Frankl, V. E. (1986). *The doctor and the soul* (R. Winston & C. Winston, Trans.). Alfred A. Knopf. (Original work published 1946 as *Ärztliche Seelsorge*)

Frankl, V. E. (1988/1969). *The will to meaning: Foundations and applications of logotherapy*. Meridian.

Gardner, H. (2011). Changing minds: How the application of the multiple intelligences (MI) framework could positively contribute to the theory and practice of international negotiation. In F. Aquilar & M. Galluccio (Eds.), *Psychological and political strategies for peace negotiation: A cognitive approach* (pp. 1–14). Springer.

Gilbert, P. (2011). International negotiations, evolution, and the value of compassion. In F. Aquilar & M. Galluccio (Eds.), *Psychological and political strategies for peace negotiation: A cognitive approach* (pp. 15–35). Springer.

Halperin, E., Russell, A. G., Dweck, C. S., & Gross, J. J. (2011). Anger, hatred, and the quest for peace: Anger can be constructive in the absence of hatred. *Journal of Conflict Resolution, 55*(2), 274–291.

Handelman, S. (2019). Peace revolution as a three-dimensional process: The Israeli-Palestinian case. In M. Nugmanova, H. Mikkola, A. Rozanov, & V. Komleva (Eds.), *Education, human rights and peace in sustainable development* (p. 279). IntechOpen.

Heal. (n.d.). *Cambridge dictionary* (4th ed.) Retrieved from https://dictionary.cambridge.org/dictionary/english/heal

Hutzell, R. R., & Jerkins, M. E. (2009). *A workbook to increase your meaningful and purposeful goals (MPGs)* (2nd ed.). Viktor Frankl Institute of Logotherapy Press. A PDF version is available at: https://www.viktorfrankl.org/assets/pdf/hutzell_workbook_2009.pdf

International Baccalaureate Organization. (2023). *What is an IB education?* (PDF). Retrieved from https://www.ibo.org/globalassets/new-structure/about-the-ib/pdfs/what-is-an-ib-education-en.pdf

Karam, A. (2011). Cognitive therapy in national conflict resolution: An opportunity. The Lebanese experience. In F. Aquilar & M. Galluccio (Eds.), *Psychological and political strategies for peace negotiation: A cognitive approach* (pp. 197–210). Springer.

Kelman, H. C. (2005). Building trust among enemies: The central challenge for international conflict resolution. *International Journal of Intercultural Relations, 29*(6), 639–650.

Lee, A. H., & DiGiuseppe, R. (2018). Anger and aggression treatments: A review of meta-analyses. *Current Opinion in Psychology, 19*, 65–74.

Lukas, E. (2000). *Logotherapy textbook: Meaning-centered psychotherapy* (T. Brugger, Trans.). Liberty Press. (Original work published in German as *Lehrbuch der Logotherapie*)

Lukas, E. (2015). *The therapist and the soul: From fate to freedom*. Purpose Research.

Lukas, E. (2020a). *Meaningful living: Introduction to logotherapy theory and practice* (J. B. Fabry, Trans.; 2nd ed.). Purpose Research.

Lukas, E. (2020b). *A unique approach to family counseling: Logotherapy, crisis, and youth* (C. L. McLafferty, Jr., Ed.). Purpose Research.

Marshall, M., & Marshall, E. (2012). *Logotherapy revisited: Review of the tenets of Viktor E. Frankl's logotherapy*. Ottawa Institute of Logotherapy.

Marshall, E., & Marshall, M. (2017). *Anthropological basis of meaning centered psychotherapy*. Ottawa Institute of Logotherapy.

Marshall, M., & Marshall, E. (2022). *Viktor E. Frankl's logotherapy and existential analysis: Theory and practice*. Ottawa Institute of Logotherapy.

Nan, S. A., & Strimling, A. (2006). Coordination in conflict prevention, conflict resolution and peacebuilding. *International Negotiation, 11*(1), 1–6.

Nelsen, J. (1996). *Positive discipline* (Revised ed.). Ballantine Books.

Pattakos, A., & Dundon, E. (2014). *The OPA! Way: Finding joy & meaning in everyday life & work*. BenBella Books.

Pavlacic, J. M., Schulenberg, S. E., & Buchanan, E. M. (2021). Experiential avoidance and meaning in life as predictors of valued living: A daily diary study. *Journal of Prevention and Health Promotion, 2*(1), 135–159. https://doi.org/10.1177/2632077021998261

Rosenberg, M. B. (1999). *Nonviolent communication: A language of life*. PuddleDancer Press.

Russo-Netzer, P. (2018). Healing the divide through wholeness: Holding on to what makes us human. *International Journal of Existential Psychology and Psychotherapy, 7*, 1–17.

Russo-Netzer, P., & Ameli, M. (2021). Optimal sense-making and resilience in times of pandemic: Integrating rationality and meaning in psychotherapy. *Frontiers in Psychology, 772*. https://doi.org/10.3389/fpsyg.2021.645926

Russo-Netzer, P., & Bergman, Y. S. (2020). Prioritizing patterns and life satisfaction among ultra-orthodox Jews: The moderating role of the sense of community. *The Journal of Psychology, 154*(3), 233–248. https://doi.org/10.1080/00223980.2019.1704392

Russo-Netzer, P., & Davidov, J. (2020). Transformative life experience as a glimpse into potentiality. *Journal of Humanistic Psychology*, 1–28. https://doi.org/10.1177/0022167820937487

Russo-Netzer, P., & Littman-Ovadia, H. (2019). "Something to live for": Experiences, resources, and personal strengths in late adulthood. *Frontiers in Psychology, 10*, 2452. https://doi.org/10.3389/fpsyg.2019.02452

Russo-Netzer, P., & Shoshani, A. (2020). Authentic inner compass, well-being, and prioritization of positivity and meaning among adolescents. *Personality and Individual Differences, 167*, 110248. https://doi.org/10.1016/j.paid.2020.110248

Russo-Netzer, P., Schulenberg, S. E., & Batthyany, A. (Eds.). (2016). *Clinical perspectives on meaning: Positive and existential psychotherapy*. Springer.

Russo-Netzer, P., Horenczyk, G., & Bergman, Y. S. (2021). Affect, meaning in life, and life satisfaction among immigrants and non-immigrants: A moderated mediation model. *Current Psychology, 40*, 3450–3458. https://doi.org/10.1007/s12144-019-00284-z

Saarni, C. (2011). Emotional competence and effective negotiation: The integration of emotion understanding, regulation, and communication. In F. Aquilar & M. Galluccio (Eds.), *Psychological and political strategies for peace negotiation: A cognitive approach* (pp. 55–74). Springer.

Schulenberg, S. E., Hutzell, R. R., Nassif, C., & Rogina, J. M. (2008). Logotherapy for clinical practice. *Psychotherapy: Theory, Research, Practice, Training, 45*(4), 447. https://doi.org/10.1037/a0014331

Shoshani, A., & Russo-Netzer, P. (2017). Exploring and assessing meaning in life in elementary school children: Development and validation of the meaning in life in children questionnaire (MIL-CQ). *Personality and Individual Differences, 104*, 460–465. https://doi.org/10.1016/j.paid.2016.09.014

Southwick, S. M., Gilmartin, R., McDonough, P., & Morrissey, P. (2006). Logotherapy as an adjunctive treatment for chronic combat-related PTSD: A meaning-based intervention. *American Journal of Psychotherapy, 60*(2), 161–174. https://doi.org/10.1176/appi.psychotherapy.2006.60.2.161

Steger, M. F., Kawabata, Y., Shimai, S., & Otake, K. (2008). The meaningful life in Japan and the United States: Levels and correlates of meaning in life. *Journal of Research in Personality, 42*(3), 660–678. https://doi.org/10.1016/j.jrp.2007.09.003

Swindler, L. (2012). *An online course in critical thinking and creative compassion to create deep dialogue. Section two: Creative compassion*. Retrieved from https://dialogueinstitute.org/creative-compassion

Tafrate, R. C., & Kassinove, H. (2009). *Anger management for everyone: Seven proven ways to control anger and live a happier life*. Impact Publishers.

Matti Ameli, MS, is a registered psychologist and certified professional coach with over twenty years of international experience. She has both studied and worked in France, the United Sates, and Spain. She practices with passion both rational emotive behavior therapy and logotherapy. She has published several innovative papers on the integration of cognitive behavior therapy, rational emotive behavior therapy, and logotherapy in international journals, and has presented at international congresses. She works in private practice in Valencia, Spain.

Pninit Russo-Netzer, PhD, is a senior lecturer and researcher and the head of both the Education Department and the Resilience and Optimal Development Lab at Achva Academic College. She is also the head of the Compass Institute for the Study and Application of Meaning and the founder and head of the Academic Training Program for Logotherapy at Tel-Aviv University. She has published numerous academic articles and chapters and is the coauthor of five books and coeditor of four books on the topics of meaning in life, positive psychology, existential psychology, as well as positive change and growth. Russo-Netzer serves as academic advisor and consultant to both academic and nonacademic institutions worldwide, including the World Trade Center (WTCHR). She is the recipient of the International Positive Psychology Association (IPPA) Spirituality and Meaning Researcher Award, recognizing exemplary professionals who have had—and continue to have—a substantially positive impact on research in spirituality/meaning.

Clara Benacerraf, MSc, is an educational psychologist and logotherapist. She serves as the Head of Counseling and the Designated Safeguarding Lead at the International School Spain in Madrid. As part of her commitment to fostering a strong school-parent partnership, she regularly contributes insightful articles to the school newsletter, sharing practical tips, research-backed strategies, and thoughtful reflections to support parents in navigating the challenges and joys of raising well-rounded individuals. She has shared her insights and knowledge at various Nord Anglia Education regional conferences and delivered lectures at the Viktor Frankl Institute of Logotherapy in Israel. Beyond the academic realm, Benacerraf has extended her reach to a wider audience through television appearances that address challenges and opportunities in the educational system as well as the importance of mental health in well-being.

Part III
Research in Logotherapy: Case Studies

Examples of Applications of Logotherapy

Robert R. Hutzell

How do you apply logotherapy? Viktor Frankl kept the application simple: You apply logotherapy by bringing an individual's value system forward from their spiritual dimension to let it exert its direction-giving effect. Such is my paraphrase of the explanation I heard Frankl give on more than one occasion.

Other persons have provided additional and helpful formulas. For example, Elisabeth Lukas outlined a four-step process (1977) and a five-step process (1984). Jim Crumbaugh (1973/1988) offered *logoanalysis*, which involved mental and paper-and-pencil exercises to help individuals consider their values and then pursue goals to fit those values.

This paper discusses a few of the ways I have applied logotherapy to myself and in clinical practice over almost 50 years. Included are examples of some simple applications as well as more complicated ones.

Applying Logotherapy to Yourself

You apply logotherapy on yourself whenever you tap into your value system to decide what to do, or what to experience, or what to stand for despite your circumstances. Often, this happens without intentional contemplation about it.

However, without contemplation or consideration, you might respond to opportunities in ways that are not in accordance with your true values or ideals; instead, you react from your emotions or your prior psychological conditioning. Or you react from physical drives. The everyday world tempts you to choose

R. R. Hutzell (✉)
Retired, Knoxville, IA, USA
e-mail: hutzells@iowatelecom.net

C. L. McLafferty, Jr., J. I. Levinson (eds.), *Logotherapy and Existential Analysis*, Logotherapy and Existential Analysis: Proceedings of the Viktor Frankl Institute Vienna 2, https://doi.org/10.1007/978-3-031-48922-8_11

psychologically conditioned behaviors and physical pleasures over your higher values. Advertisement industries and peer pressure excel at tempting you.

Your physical and psychological dimensions focus inward on yourself and your drives, wants, and pleasures. When you fail to attend to your spiritual aspect, you might not actualize your value ideals: You may make decisions that go against your true self and you don't perceive your life as fulfilled. This can leave a sensation of being less than you could be. It leaves you feeling dissatisfied, incomplete, and that you've wasted the day.

In contrast, your spiritual dimension leads you beyond yourself: *self-transcendence*, which leads you to loves, morality, principles, and personal sacrifices for entities or causes bigger than yourself.

Occasions exist when you access your value system to guide your actions despite the conflict between your psychophysiological and spiritual dimensions. Joe Fabry listed five circumstances in which you tap into your value system. He reported these as circumstances in which individuals experience meaning in their lives, and he discussed them in detail in two of his books: *The Pursuit of Meaning* (1968/1987) and *Guideposts to Meaning* (1988). The occasions Fabry noted as value-illuminating are when you:

- discover an idea about your true self.
- make pondered and well-considered choices.
- take responsible action.
- detect your personal uniqueness in the world.
- respond for the sake of someone or something beyond yourself.

One way I've found useful is to conduct logotherapy on myself daily: I keep a to-do list of meaningful goals. I contemplate my values hierarchy in conjunction with my available opportunities when I develop this list, using Fabry's five guides to help decide what goals to include on my list.

Each morning, I review my list and decide what fulfills the meaning of the moment. I choose the most meaningful goal-opportunity to tackle first. As my day continues, I check off completed goals and add new ones that come to mind. Sometimes these meaningful goals are small parts of what will add up to larger goals over time.

At the day's end, I review what I have marked off. When I have completed several items on my list, I sense the day has been meaningful. Before I end the day, I anticipate the next day by considering which items on my list might receive the highest attention when I wake up.

In the end, application of logotherapy seems simple, and you can do it for yourself. At the same time, many physical and psychological realities influence you to do otherwise. When you do not act in consonance with your values, and you thus experience frustration and lack of fulfillment, then outside help to apply logotherapy can be beneficial.

Experiences Applying Short-Term Logotherapy to Individuals

In my experience, logotherapy often takes only a few sessions; sometimes a single session is enough when problems come on fast and have existed a short time. Problems that have come on more slowly and existed for a longer time often require more sessions. This relationship between problem duration and therapy duration is a general guideline, not a concrete rule, which I noticed whether the problem started with a physical, psychological, or spiritual issue.

Example: Locked Ward Confinement

In my career as a clinical psychologist, the staff on locked psychiatric wards called me many times to see patients who displayed anger about their confinement behind locked doors. These patients initiated hostile disruptions on the ward, and staff could not discharge them to open wards until their uncontrollable activities decreased. My conversations with many patients went along these lines:

RH: Thanks for seeing me. I want to talk with you about what you think of this ward. I hear it upsets you.

Patient: I don't like it here.

RH: Staff tells me you show a lot of anger and cause problems on the ward.

P: I hate them. They keep me locked up. I want out.

RH: Yes, I wouldn't like being locked up either.

P: This stinks.

RH: What makes it bad for you? Tell me why you don't like it here.

P: I don't want to stay here. They tell you what to do. They control all of us. There's no freedom. I want out.

RH: You mentioned freedom. So, you're saying you value your freedom… it's important to you.

P: Yes… of course… highly important to me! I want out of this place. I want my freedom back.

RH: What if I told you they sent me here to talk about how to get you out of this locked ward and gain more freedom? Would it be worth any effort, any work, to have more freedom?

P: What do you mean? What work?

RH: Well, maybe we could develop a plan to get you out of here to a less restrictive ward. I've done that with a lot of other people.

P: And you will get me out?

RH: I can't discharge you myself.... Staff on the unit makes that decision when they think it's safe for you to leave. But I will tell you they called me over here to work with you, if you decide to, so they can let you go somewhere less confining for treatment. What do you think.... Is freedom worth some effort on your part?

P: I want my freedom. I want out.

RH: OK. They told me they keep you here because of unpredictable, disruptive behavior. So, it seems to me, getting out will require you to choose to become less unpredictable to them... less disruptive... which keeps you here and doesn't accomplish your goal of more freedom. Of course, you might instead continue as you have.... You can make that choice... but it hasn't worked thus far. Would it be worth the effort of us discussing a plan to get out of here to gain more freedom?

P: Well, I might consider it. I want out of here. I want my freedom.

RH: OK. Let's think of a plan together.

Conversations like this one refocused patients away from their emotional reactions to confinement in a locked ward onto their underlying values. In this example, the value was freedom. The patients became motivated to participate more in treatment plans and less on demonstrations of anger and disruption.

In logotherapy terms, I employed the *self-distancing* component of the patients' *defiant power of the human spirit* to let their value system provide its direction-giving effect. I first acknowledged the patients' emotional reaction of anger. Then I helped them step back and look at the situation as a problem involving more than their emotional reaction, more than their anger. The problem included their responsibility for their behavior and its impact on staff decisions. Once they stepped back from their hyper-focused anger, they could recognize a bigger picture of their situation and of their self. That broader view included their value for freedom.

We can gain a broader perspective when we step back from our immediate reactions. In terms of Fabry's (1968/1987, 1988) five circumstances in which we tap into our value systems, the guide I enlisted with the locked ward patients was to make pondered and well-considered choices.

Frankl (1946/2006, p. 104) time and again paraphrased Nietzsche: He who has a reason *why* can put up with almost any *how*. The locked ward patients' value for freedom helped them decide to take *response-ability* for, and control of, their angry feelings and choose to pursue a value more important to them: freedom. The decision led to participation in a plan of treatment, which, in turn, could lead to transfer. In other words, they put up with their inclination for anger and managed it and participated in treatment planning (the "how") in order to actualize their value for freedom (the "why").

Example: Terminal Medical Condition

Another situation in which the application of logotherapy helps is in the despair experienced by terminally ill patients. The practitioner of logotherapy recognizes that people disdain suffering, of course; and despair on top of the suffering makes it even worse.

Frankl (1985) developed a formula: Despair = Suffering – Meaning (p. 273). That is, despair is suffering without meaning. It is a consequence of meaningless suffering. When suffering cannot be eliminated, reduction of the sense of meaninglessness can at least help. The suffering may remain, but finding meaning to counteract the sense of meaninglessness reduces the added despair. Practitioners of logotherapy bring the individual's value system into awareness with ways to actualize one or more values, which increases meaning and thus reduces the despair.

Throughout many years of my career, physicians called me to the hospital beds of terminally ill patients. Within introductions, relationship building, and informed consent, my conversation included the fact that their doctor had consulted me to help them deal with their situation. I inquired about what had been important in their life. Here I sought glimpses into their values. Then I inquired what they could do now—despite their situation—to actualize those same values. Many conversations went along these lines:

RH: So your doctor asked me to talk with you regarding your circumstance. It's bad, I know. But I can discuss with you some things you might do even now… some things perhaps important to you. Tell me: What has been important to you in the past and remains important to you now and in the future regardless of your situation?

Patient: My family has always been important to me.

RH: Tell me about your family and what you did with them or for them.

The patient and I then discussed their relationships, interactions, and related accomplishments.

RH: Were there times when you put them ahead of yourself? Maybe there were times when you sacrificed what you preferred because of your love for them?

We proceeded to discuss situations where they put their loved ones ahead of their own preferences.

RH: Is there something to do for them even now, like you did so many times in the past?

P: I don't see how.

RH: Well, you've always loved them. That's clear. What might you do to love them even now? Maybe some words to say to them. Maybe some information you want them to know.

With this, and sometimes additional Socratic questions on my part, the patient could determine a way to show the family they still loved them, would always love them. At times, they brought up unfinished business. Other times, they brought up information they wanted loved ones to know. Often, they just wanted to tell the others what they meant to them.

RH: Now is the time to do that. Your situation calls for you to do it now. It might not be easy, but it's important. It fits an important value of yours, and you will feel positive about it even if it takes courage and energy on your part. In a way, it constitutes another sacrifice to make for their sake, just as you have sacrificed for them in the past.

The patient and I then developed a plan together to accomplish their new goal, emphasizing the actualization of the value of love. At times, these plans included rehearsal and role-play with the patient. Sometimes the plans included my presence with the patient and the family members together, but more often, the patient had the motivation to fulfill the plan without me present.

In logotherapeutic terms, I employed the other component of the defiant power of the human spirit: self-transcendence. This allowed the patient's value system to have its direction-giving effect.

In this scenario, I first acknowledged the patient's situation. Then I helped the individual focus on a value beyond the self. Next, we explored opportunities where it remained possible to respond in accord with their long-held value.

After the patient had a purpose consonant with their values—to fill the next moment, the next hour, the next day with a meaningful task regardless of their condition—they recognized a goal they could accomplish. Their suffering remained, but they focused on meaning despite their circumstances. Meaninglessness decreased, and thus the despair lessened.

Physicians told me their patients became less depressed, less despairing, after these interventions; and the physicians continued to consult me when they had similar cases. Sometimes, family members contacted me and thanked me for helping their loved ones find peace. More than one family even took out ads in the local newspaper to express their appreciation.

In the situations represented above, the application of logotherapy surfaced the individual's value system to let it provide its direction-giving effect. These situations were acute, with an abrupt onset, and needed immediate intervention. Only one, or a few, logotherapy sessions were required most times.

Experiences Applying Longer-Term Logotherapy in Groups

Sometimes the onset of problems in which logotherapy can help is not rapid or recent, such as with individuals who have addictions, prolonged depression, or pervasive dissatisfaction with life. The application of logotherapy proves useful in these situations in conjunction with other treatments and follows the same process:

surface the underlying value system to let it offer a meaningful direction in the individual's life. These longer-developed issues usually require more than one or two treatment sessions.

Although I employed logotherapy with numerous chronic conditions, three predominated: addiction, depression, and post-traumatic stress disorder (PTSD).

The use of logotherapy always involved helping people recognize their core value system and pay attention to it. After this increased awareness, many individuals identified healthy changes to make in their behaviors, relationships, and attitudes. Because the changes resonated with their innermost values, participants often established strong motivation to make the changes. Such is the intended outcome of logotherapy.

However, I learned that many people have to sharpen their goal-setting and planning skills in order to carry through to where their values pointed. They recognized what was important to them and could help them past their problems, but they needed to improve their ability to make this happen. They required new skills to keep moment-to-moment desires, emotional reactions, or outside pressures from derailing their progress.

For this, I adapted and expanded what my teacher, Jim Crumbaugh (1973/1988), termed "logoanalysis." Crumbaugh's logoanalysis guided individuals through values clarification and into the establishment of goals. The process involved structured mental exercises to help persons think about their values. Then the logoanalysis went on to emphasize the importance of pursuing goals to fit those values.

In Viktor Frankl's published cases, his patients set goals or changed their attitudes after they recognized their personally meaningful values. Crumbaugh found his clients often required further guidance about how to set specific goals to fit their values.

In my experiences, I noticed a lot of persons needed even further work. They needed not only to work on setting goals commensurate with their values, but also to gain skill in how to plan to accomplish the goals.

The process I developed, and employed over the years, incorporated four steps. First came focus on the individual's personal values: values clarification. Step two established goals that fit with their values: goal setting. The third step developed a plan to achieve the goals to actualize the individual's values: planning. The last step incorporated the individual's strengths and weaknesses into the plan in order to maximize the impact of individual strengths and minimize derailment by personal weak points: optimizing prospects for success. Thus, the fourth step magnified the possibility for success of the plan to achieve goals to actualize the individual's values. A motivational pull for the individual to follow through with the whole process flowed from the focus on their personal values.

Over the years, I conducted this course of mental exercises in groups for persons with addictions and other long-term problems. Ten group sessions (plus homework assignments) comprised the course, which, over time, several thousand individuals completed.

On occasions later, individuals came to me, and we held conversations along these lines:

Patient: Remember me? I was in your logo group a couple of years ago.

RH: Oh, hi. Good to see you again.

P: Remember in the group when you said… [here the individual stated a phrase or idea they had found significant].

RH: [I thought to myself: That sounds close to something I would have said.] And you recall it after all this time.

P: Yes. And I wanted to catch you to say the group turned my life around. I've been on track ever since. I want to thank you.

I then thanked the patient for letting me know of their success and assured them their accomplishments resulted from what they did with what they learned anywhere in the treatment program. Thus, they were responsible for their progress and could take pride in it. We shook hands, and I wished them continued success.

While I used group sessions for most of my logotherapy work in addictions, my application of logotherapy for depressed persons occurred more often in individual sessions. Persons with PTSD came in between. The steps, however, remained the same: surface the values, set goals to actualize the values, establish workable plans to reach the goals, and then incorporate the individual's unique assets and deficits into the plan to maximize the probability of success.

I have published papers in which I described the procedure in detail: one in *The International Forum for Logotherapy* (Hutzell, 1983), and the other in the *Joernaal/ Journal: Viktor Frankl Foundation of South Africa* (Hutzell, 2002). In addition, my colleague, Mary Eggert, and I adapted the first two steps to develop our *Workbook to Increase Your Meaningful and Purposeful Goals–MPGs* (Hutzell & Eggert, 1989). The workbook had many reprints. I have copies of 10 different printings in my files, so I know it was reprinted at least 10 times. Most recently, it has been available as a free PDF on the website of the Viktor Frankl Institute Vienna (Hutzell & Eggert, 2018), and it has been translated into a Spanish edition (Hutzell & Eggert, 1989/2021).

Other Logotherapy Approaches

I developed a variety of other logotherapeutic approaches for short-term and long-term therapy over the course of almost 50 years. However, those presented in the present paper were some of the most frequent I used. Among the other issues for which I commonly applied logotherapy were treatment adherence, diminution of institutionalization, and productive decision making despite current psychiatric and life situations. Often, these applications were offered via group formats, though at other times the sessions were individual. The application of logotherapy always involved helping individuals recognize their core value system and employ it as a guide for healthy decisions and choices to make.

There are many additional ways to employ logotherapy. A number of publications describe logotherapy's application in short- and long-term therapy, including recent reprints of books by two of my teachers, Joe Fabry (1968/2013) and Elisabeth Lukas (1984/2014). In each case though, the primary goal remains the same: to help individuals focus on their values and utilize those values for healthy decisions in their lives.

References

Crumbaugh, J. C. (1988). *Everything to gain: A guide to self-fulfillment through logoanalysis*. Institute of Logotherapy Press. (Original work published 1973)

Fabry, J. B. (1987). *The pursuit of meaning: Viktor Frankl, logotherapy, and life*. Institute of Logotherapy Press. (Original work published 1968)

Fabry, J. B. (1988). *Guideposts to meaning: Discovering what really matters*. New Harbinger Publications.

Fabry, J. B. (2013). *The pursuit of meaning: Viktor Frankl, logotherapy, and life*. Purpose Research. (Original work published 1968)

Frankl, V. E. (1985). Logos, paradox, and the search for meaning. In M. J. Mahoney & A. Freeman (Eds.), *Cognition and psychotherapy* (pp. 259–275). Springer.

Frankl, V. E. (2006). *Man's search for meaning*. Beacon Press. (Original work published 1946)

Hutzell, R. R. (1983). Practical steps in logoanalysis. *International Forum for Logotherapy, 6*, 74–83.

Hutzell, R. R. (2002). A general course of group analysis. *Joernaal/Journal: Viktor Frankl Foundation of South Africa, 7*, 15–26.

Hutzell, R. R., & Eggert, M. A. (1989). *A workbook to increase your meaningful and purposeful goals (MPGs)*. Institute of Logotherapy Press.

Hutzell, R. R., & Eggert, M. A. (2018). *A workbook to increase your meaningful and purposeful goals (MPGs)* (PDF ed.). Viktor Frankl Institute Vienna. Retrieved from http://www.viktor-frankl.org/assets/pdf/hutzell_workbook_2009.pdf

Hutzell, R. R., & Eggert, M. A. (2021). *Hacia una vida con sentido: Manual para incrementar tus metas significativas y con proposito* (*MSP*) (M. Ameli & M. Ortiz, Trans.) [Toward a meaningful life: A guide to increasing your purpose and meaningful goals (MSP)]. Independently published by the translators. (Original work published 1989)

Lukas, E. (1977). The four steps of logotherapy. *Uniquest: Festival of Meaning, 7*, 24–25.

Lukas, E. (1984). Human dignity and psychotherapy. *The International Forum for Logotherapy, 7*, 67–84.

Lukas, E. (2014). *Meaning in suffering: Comfort in crisis through logotherapy*. Purpose Research. (Original work published 1984)

Robert R. Hutzell (PhD, Clinical Psychology, Florida State University, 1975) was Editor of *The International Forum for Logotherapy* for many years. He is a Fellow of the American Psychological Association, a nationally certified Health Service Provider in Psychology, and a Logotherapy Diplomate. Prior to retirement, he served as a Clinical Psychologist in the Veterans Affairs Health Care System, and as an independent practitioner and department head at a community hospital. Bob has held professional organization leadership positions (including President of the National Organization of VA Psychologists, President of the Iowa Psychological Association). He has served as a review editor for psychological journals, has published widely, and has received several national and international recognitions.

Suicide Prevention in the Work of Viktor Frankl

Élison Silva Santos and Andrés Eduardo Aguirre Antúnez

The work of an author is marked by its theoretical construction. Science invites us to impartially analyze the methods and results of research. In the field of clinical psychiatry, the historical context, environment, and attitudes of Viktor Frankl and his theories about clinical interventions are relevant. Also, his perceptions, words, and attitudes were intertwined with the way his theories were applied to the disorders of patients in the field of clinical psychiatry.

Analysis of the phenomenon of suicide and the search for effective forms of prevention represent a great challenge to psychologists. Although it is widely recognized that environment and circumstances influence the development of suicidal thoughts (Cutler et al., 2001; Loureiro et al., 2013), the attitude of each person in their subjectivity is the primary object of study for clinical intervention.

Few theorists who were also clinicians experienced so many critical situations related to suicide as the Viennese psychiatrist Viktor Emil Frankl. Even as a young medical student, he was advocating for the creation of youth counseling centers. Shortly after graduating, he became head of the female suicide ward at the Steinhof Psychiatric Hospital in Vienna, seeing approximately 12,000 cases during the years he was there (Frankl, 2007, p. 211). He experienced the extremes of war as a prisoner of four concentration camps (Frankl, 1991), wrote approximately 40 books,

É. S. Santos (✉)
Sapiens Institute of Applied Sciences–IPSapiens, Chrysalis Center for Mental Health and Wellness, Washington, DC, USA

Lab of Mental Health Multi-Methods–LabSamm, University of São Paulo, São Paulo, Brazil
e-mail: elison@buscasentido.com

A. E. A. Antúnez
Department of Clinical Psychology, Institute of Psychology – University of São Paulo, Lab of Mental Health Multi-Methods – LabSamm, University of São Paulo, São Paulo, Brazil
e-mail: antunez@usp.br

C. L. McLafferty, Jr., J. I. Levinson (eds.), *Logotherapy and Existential Analysis*, Logotherapy and Existential Analysis: Proceedings of the Viktor Frankl Institute Vienna 2, https://doi.org/10.1007/978-3-031-48922-8_12

was a professor at several American universities, including Harvard, the University of Pittsburgh, the University of Texas at Dallas, and the United States University in San Diego. He received an honorary doctorate from 29 universities around the world, including the University of Brasília and the University of Rio Grande do Sul (Viktor Frankl Institute). There are documented records of his work from 1923 to 1997 when he died (Frankl, 2000, 2007).

The fundamental principle of his work is the search by human beings for meaning in life. After working with Freud and Adler, and with strong scientific, empirical, and philosophical foundations, Frankl (1978, 1986, 2003, 2016, 2020) founded logotherapy and existential analysis, the third Viennese school of psychotherapy. Concepts such as self-distancing, self-transcendence, the tragic triad, the will to meaning, finding meaning in life, and paradoxical intention added to the human capacity to find meaning in the face of suffering. Freedom and responsibility took on a prominent role in enabling individuals to face the greatest challenges of life, including suicidal ideation.

Frankl's Vienna

In the history of humankind, we will certainly find many instances in which a persistently high suicide rate was recorded, but perhaps circumstances similar to what happened in the city of Vienna, Austria, between the First and Second World Wars are rare. Sonneck, Hirnsperger, and Mundschütz (2010) noted that, at that time, the rate of suicide was recorded at 73 cases per 100,000 inhabitants: "In comparison, there were 189 suicides in Vienna in 2008, which was a suicide rate of only 11.2 per 100,000" (p. 115). Suicide rates rose sharply in the period between 1919 and 1939, with peaks in the first year of the Second World War in 1939, and at the end in 1945. Early twentieth-century Vienna was awash with reports of suicide in the newspapers. Many linked the high rate of suicide to the collapse of cultural or social norms as well as problems in families, work, or religious communities (Bowman, 2008, p.142).

As early as 1926, Frankl (2007) publicly advocated for the creation of Youth Advice Centers in the city of Vienna: "We clearly realize that few and rare are the occasions that nowadays offer young people the opportunity to ask questions that seem important to them" (p. 87). This highlighted the need for healthy environments in which young people could talk, for example, about the very meaning of life. He noted:

> A journalistic report recently reported that, during the first three months of 1926, 20 suicides or attempted suicides took place in Vienna solely due to fear of punishment, a reason which can only be assumed in the case of young people. How many cases will be added under the heading of "unknown reasons," until we come to understand the real consequences of [the existential vacuum]? (pp. 87–88)

Frankl highlighted the importance of psychology and the need for public institutions and society to understand the psychology of youth:

> One way or another, it's time to learn enough about the psychology of young people so that we don't respond to a young person's suicide by simply taking note of it or just making a gesture of compassion, so that we can immediately proceed with our everyday tasks. (p. 88)

In the 1920s and 1930s, it was common for anyone who tried to commit suicide to be taken to city hospitals for psychological evaluation. Those who were considered more serious were taken to Steinhof, the hospital where Viktor Frankl worked (Bowman, 2009, p. 142). About 12,000 cases were reported during the period that Frankl was in charge of the department; this number seems very high, about 3000 per year; truly, the data on suicide in the city at that time were alarming (Sonneck et al., 2012; Frankl, 2007). In comparison, a study of the rate of suicides in the city of São Paulo by Bando (2008) and Bando et al. (2012) showed that, between the years 1976 and 2005, there was an average suicide rate of 4.1 per 100,000 inhabitants. Between 1979 and 2003, there were 11,434 deaths by suicide in the city. In the following years, the rate increased, rising to 4.6 deaths per 100,000 inhabitants in 2007–2008 and 5.6 in 2013–2014.

The "Ethical Congregation," headed by educator and philanthropist Wilhelm Börner, working with Viktor Frankl, was active in suicide prevention through the Vienna Rescue Society in the Viennese Third District from 1928 to 1937 (Sonneck et al., 2012).

Biller et al. (2002) noted that Viktor Frankl was a consultant and professor of neurology and psychiatry at the University of Vienna. As a Jew, he had to close his private practice and give up his professorship in 1939, and was forced to take the position offered to him as head of the neurological section of the Rothschild-Spital in Vienna, where between 1939 and 1942 he worked with patients who had attempted suicide, including those that other doctors could not help. During this time, his wife lost their first child to an illegal abortion due to fear of deportation. Between 1942 and 1945, he survived four concentration camps, but lost his parents, brother, and wife in them. Despite all his sufferings, after the war he spoke out in favor of reconciliation and against the notion of collective guilt.

The Historical Context of Suicide in Psychology

In classical antiquity, suicide was seen as an act of freedom and was even honorable in some situations. Seneca took his own life before Nero did. If life was not worth living, it was acceptable to decide not to live anymore. Socrates, who was accused of corrupting the youth of Athens, committed suicide with hemlock and accepted death instead of denying his principles and teachings.

In the Middle Ages, Saint Augustine (1950) highlighted the prohibition of suicide by the Church, which increased with the passage of time. "No one ought to inflict on himself voluntary death, for this is to escape the ills of time by plunging into those of eternity" (Book I, Chapter 27). Thomas Aquinas (2011) stated that "someone's killing himself is contrary to a natural inclination and contrary to charity, by which everyone ought to love himself. And so killing oneself is always a mortal sin as being contrary to natural law and contrary to charity" (II-II, Q. 64, Art. 5). Suicide was seen as a sin against God, against life itself, and against the community. However, it was allowed if it were the result of obedience to a divine order; as Augustine (1996) stated:

> If allowed by the authority of a general, how much more accepted would it be with the authority of the Creator! Therefore, whoever already knows that it is not lawful to commit suicide… if he receives an order from one whose precepts it is not lawful to despise, let him take a good look if there is absolute certainty of the divine origin of such an order. (p. 172)

The idea that life does not belong to the person, but to God, is still very present today. Suicide is still seen by many religions as a sin.

The term *desperatio,* Latin for despair, was used to refer to a demonic influence; anyone who listened to the devil was sinning against God and the Church. The bodies of those who committed suicide were punished in various ways such as by dismemberment or hanging upside down. The family was penalized by not inheriting any property of the deceased; it was a dishonor against the family.

Robert Burton (1621/1857) published *The Anatomy of Melancholy,* in which he highlighted human suffering: "If there be a hell upon earth, it is to be found in a melancholy man's heart" (p. 261). [green = checked and verified against English edition]. At that time, the topic of suicide was no longer treated only as a taboo but took on connotations related to the mind, the idea that there is human suffering and it was not related solely to human will, relationships with the divine, or with the morality of honor and freedom.

It was also in that century that the works of Shakespeare (1564–1616) emerged in the world of the arts; suicide was present in his works 76 times. For example, as Hamlet faced the possibility of suicide his suffering was portrayed in the famous phrase: "To be or not to be, that is the question" (*Hamlet*, Act 3, Scene 1). Thus, suicide became a human dilemma during that period.

Goethe (1774/1987), in the 1774 book *The Sorrows of Young Werther,* told the story of a teenager who committed suicide by shooting himself in the head when he learned that his beloved was engaged to another boy. A wave of suicides took place around that time with individuals dressing up as Werther and shooting themselves in the head. This effect became known as the Werther effect.

Frankl (1986) quoted Goethe in what he noted should be the fundamental principle of every psychotherapist: "If we take people as they are, we make them worse. If we treat them as if they were what they ought to be, we help them to become what they are capable of becoming" (p. 8). According to Frankl, we need to overestimate people so that they become what they can be, a vision that established foundations not only for logotherapy but for what later became positive psychology.

In the 1897 publication of *Suicide*, Durkheim (1897/2011) inaugurated a sociological view of suicide. By observing the suicide rate in different European countries, at different times, and adjusting for professions, social classes, and marital status, he perceived suicide as a social phenomenon, going so far as to say that the family, the state, and the church would cease to function as factors of social integration after the Industrial Revolution. Durkheim's vision could be compared with Frankl's idea of the existential vacuum, in which the loss of traditions is one of the factors that causes the vacuum. Durkheim summarized his findings:

> Just as suicide does not result from the difficulties with which man may have to live, the way to stop this progress is not to make the fight less hard and life easier. If today people kill themselves more than in the past, it is not because we must make more painful efforts nor because our legitimate needs are less satisfied; it is because we no longer know how far our legitimate needs go and we no longer perceive the meaning of our efforts. (p. 506)

In his conclusions, Durkheim highlighted another aspect that is in line with Frankl's thinking: Meaninglessness plays a key role in suicide.

In the twentieth century, understanding suicide was expanded through advances in psychology. Freud (1917) presented aspects of the unconscious and psychic mechanisms that interfered in the person to the extent that suicide is considered. Melancholy was an object of his study:

> We perceive, as the primordial state from which instinctual life departs, such a formidable love of the ego for itself, that we see a release, in the anguish generated by the threat to life. Such an amount of narcissistic libido that we do not understand can lead to its own destruction. (p. 136)

Suicide was now seen with a magnifying glass and its cause was beyond biology; it was in the human psyche that it needed to be understood. It became possible to speak of an "I" and of the relationship with oneself and with the other. This self can also become an object. Freud (1917) stated:

> We have long known, it is true, that no neurotic harbours thoughts of suicide which he has not turned back upon himself from murderous impulses against others, but we have never been able to explain what interplay of forces can carry such a purpose through to execution. The analysis of melancholia now shows that the ego can kill itself only if, owing to the return of the object-cathexis, it can treat itself as an object—if it is able to direct against itself the hostility which relates to an object and which represents the ego's original reaction to objects in the external world. Thus in regression from narcissistic object-choice the object has, it is true, been got rid of, but it has nevertheless proved more powerful than the ego itself. (p. 252)

According to Freud (1917), melancholy highlighted the unique possibility of the ego killing itself when it treats itself as an object, being able to direct against itself the "hostility that concerns an object" (p. 252). There was recognition that in this dynamic, the object is more powerful than the self and that is why suicide is possible. Although Frankl viewed human beings from a different perspective than that of Freud, he was familiar with psychoanalysis, and it is possible to say that such explanations can be accepted, except for the assertion that the "Ego is subjugated by the object." Frankl would probably state that the "Ego subjugates itself to the object" because there is an intrinsic freedom to the Ego, both in what Freud refers to as "falling in love" and in "suicide."

Frankl (2003), unlike Freud, saw love as a phenomenon and not as an epiphenomenon. Therefore, if for Freud suicide was related to falling in love and the subjugation of the self, for Frankl the relationship was one of freedom of the self, both to love and to commit suicide:

> In the case of something like sublimation, it is always love that precedes this same sublimation as a condition of possibility; and that, for this reason, the ability to love—the presupposition of sublimation—could not by itself be the result of a process of sublimation… In short: only the Ego (Ich) that tends towards the Thou can integrate the Id (Es) true and proper. (p. 19)

In this way, the ability to love is found in human beings in a *primary and original* way. For Frankl, love was a specifically human capacity and was related to self-transcendence; love was a sublime way of finding the meaning of life. He went so far as to say that "the entry into the superhuman dimension, made effective in faith, is based on love" (p. 64).

In Frankl's critique of psychoanalysis, there was the question of will. Frankl (2003) cited the American psychologist Rollo May when he noted that "psychoanalysis becomes an accomplice of the patient's tendency towards passivity, leading him to consider himself deprived of the power to decide, without feeling responsible for their difficulties" (p. 101). He also cited the research of Crumbaugh and Maholik, who provided evidence to support the hypothesis that there is indeed a will to meaning in human beings.

In this way, Frankl (2003) continued to defend that love, faith, and hope are not controlled by the will. "I cannot want to believe, I cannot want to love, I cannot want to wait. Hence, it is useless to demand that a man 'wants meaning'" (p. 101). It was therefore necessary to "appeal to the will to meaning," (p. 101) which can mean a therapeutic path for suicide prevention. Frankl opened the way to think about the possibility that the therapist "can make the brightness of meaning emerge, putting at the disposal of the will whether to want it or not" (p. 101).

This is the potential appeal of the logotherapeutic process of suicide prevention, but for this appeal to occur, the therapist needs to at least believe that there is a meaning to be found and that it is possible for his patient to find it. Otherwise, this therapeutic path is unlikely.

The Meaning of Life and Psychology

According to Ewalds-Kvist and Lützén (2015), Frankl was the first existentialist to emphasize positive existential data for his theory, although he himself was deported to four Nazi camps between 1942 and 1945, including Auschwitz, where Josef Mengele directed him to the gas chamber. Against all odds, Frankl managed to get in line with people who were forced to live and work in the camps. During his imprisonment, Frankl was faced with many questions about his own meaning in life.

The option of preserving life was nevertheless clear and well documented (Frankl, 2007, 2019b). As he could not be considered a doctor, according to Nazi laws, with the beginning of the war, "Viktor Frankl worked from 1939 to 1942 as a

'Jewish therapist' and then as a 'Jewish specialist' at the Rothschild Hospital in Vienna, where he also witnessed cases of poisoning by sleeping pills, for those who were considered lost" (Sonneck et al., 2012, p. 117).

Frankl (2010) revealed a problem of the suicide of someone close to him when his assistant, Dr. Rappaport, protested that he was trying to save people who had attempted suicide. "Then came the day that Dr. Rappaport herself was ordered to appear for deportation; she then attempted suicide, was admitted to my department and brought back to life by me—and was later deported" (p. 95). He added: "I respect a person's decision to end their own life. But I would like my principles to be respected as well" (p. 95).

Frankl developed "a kind of suicide news service among the prisoners that immediately reported to him any hint of suicidal thoughts or intentions. He would then contact the potential suicide and try to dissuade him" (Sonneck et al., 2012, p. 118).

Pacciolla (2015) highlighted that Frankl's humanistic existentialism was present throughout his training process, in his performance before, during, and after the Second World War, "until the most complete organization of his thought in the 1950s, before the beginning of the DSM (1952) and before the phenomenological turn of the 1960s" (p. 20).

Regarding Frankl's orientation to phenomenology, Kühn (2015) stated:

> The contributions… around Viktor Frankl's thoughts are at the crossroads of phenomenology and psychotherapy. They arise from a double challenge around meaning as logos and therapy as a particular relational praxis. It is about showing, on one hand, that the therapy envisaged here does not only obey scientific and psychotherapeutic techniques or methods, but that it involves a radical phenomenological anthropology based on the affective and noëtic appearance of meaning for each individual. (p. 7)

Even in the face of classical cognitivism, Pacciolla noted that Frankl stood out in what is now called existential cognitivism, which

> should not be primarily understood as an extension of classical cognitivism (evidenced in the 1960s by Aaron Beck, George Kelly, etc.). The primordial concepts of cognitivism were already contained in Frankl's thinking, writings and clinical practice, in the 1950s and even before. (p. 23)

This unique place in which Frankl's theory finds itself was also built into discussions in the works of Freud, Adler, and others. Criticisms of Freud's ideas are found in several quotes, especially the risks of reductionism and determinism (e.g., Frankl, 2003, pp. 15, 18, 19, 45, 266, 335). Despite recognizing the greatness of Freud and his work, Frankl did not shy away from positioning himself emphatically for the presentation of a phenomenological anthropology that considered the noëtic aspects of human beings.

Frankl (2019a) appeared on the international scene as a fearless defender of existentialism. In 1959, he emphasized the words of Carl Rogers at an Existential Psychology Symposium in Cincinnati, when he stated that he came to believe again in the freedom of the human will when his student demonstrated statistically that it would not be possible to predict the chances of recidivism of a delinquent, except "through the understanding of oneself, the individual or, as we say, the ability to enter into oneself" (p. 58). Faced with human beings who question the meaning of life, Frankl added that "the doctor of our times must have the courage to get involved in these Socratic dialogues, to take seriously his mission to treat not only the sick, but all men" (p. 61).

Human beings distinguish themselves from other living beings by not only wanting meaning in their lives, but by having the conscience to perceive this meaning, the freedom to want to find and to realize meanings as well as the responsibility to respond to what life does. Individuals do this by coming out of themselves to meet the world, with the other, in a sense that manifests being outside of the personal self.

In dealing with suicide, logotherapy is a useful resource whether the individual is facing endogenous or psychogenic depression, as well as in cases of noögenic neurosis or an existential vacuum. This is especially true in situations in which the ego is weakened in the face of problems and other symptoms, or in which the tendency to lose the meaning of life from the horizon is amplified. With regard to suicide, Pacciolla (2015) considered that logotherapy:

> is capable of giving the best of itself, recognizing the role of the somatic dimension and the psychosocial dimension without putting the noëtic dimension in the background: the capacity for self-transcendence, to go beyond situations in which reason does not see a meaning. (pp. 14–15)

Yes to Life in Spite of Everything

Although no one says "yes to life" at the beginning, Frankl (2019a) stated that each person says "yes"

> constantly, says it at every moment of their current existence. He always says yes to life, to this incomplete life; "in spite of everything," he always says yes, despite his imperfections. "In spite of everything," he says yes. In spite of not having been questioned and having said nothing, in spite of not having chosen life but, on the contrary, having been "thrown" into existence, in spite of not having to agree with this or that of his hereditary disposition, and also he would never have agreed if he had been questioned, despite everything he continues, despite living. (p. 229)

Frankl (2019a) pointed out that the fact of existence is irrefutably a constant yes, precisely because human beings ultimately can say no to existence, and have the freedom to decide not to live anymore. It is this responsibility that brings freedom and it is, in a way, this freedom that gives meaning to responsibility. If we were forced to live, life would be a burden in the face of all the discomforts we face, and isn't that exactly what happens to many people in depression? If we were not free to decide about life, responsibility would have no meaning. Like the slave and the prisoner, we would live by fear, even though in slavery and in prison human beings do not necessarily let go of hope:

> In any case, he says yes to everything and so he is also, in any case, responsible for everything: for this responsibility also always includes a freedom, it has its freedom behind it; the freedom to say no—the freedom to say no to concrete life; to life in its facticity and heredity. I am not obliged to continue my life—I can throw it away." (p. 229)

If a person is capable of throwing away life, what is left? Frankl (2019a) presented a vision of human beings that denies the conditions that allow, in many cases, victimization in the face of life. Because individuals are not totally predetermined, they are constantly free to take a position in the face of their own conditions. Individuals can say that they feel obliged to stay alive, not because they really are, but because they have not allowed themselves to conceive the idea that, if they so choose, they have the power to end their own lives. In this way, the fact of being alive is a yes, a constant yes. Ultimately, one is never passive in the face of life:

In this manner, the theme of responsibility emerges as a foundation for human existence:

> Thus, I am ultimately responsible for everything—for my existence as a whole, as well as for my being-thus in particular. For man is always in agreement, his "I" is always in agreement with his id—even when he lets himself be guided by instinctual impulses—but also with "them," his parents, his ancestors. But this agreement is usually silent; that doesn't make it any less real. Finally, there is also, therefore, something like a hereditary responsibility. It is responsibility against the background of an ultimate, radical freedom, a radical "no": suicide. (p. 229)

This Franklian view of freedom puts the individual in charge of making decisions, even if influenced by instinctive impulses. The id does not rule, because what happens is that the self is always in agreement with this id, as it could not be otherwise. It is not that impulses command the "I," but that even when impulse allows itself to be guided by them, it is this "I" that "allows itself" to be led and allows itself to be led because its essence is spiritual, and its decision-making power is superior to the id. In this way, the "I" is never a victim of its own id, environmental conditioning, its own heredity, ancestors, or instinctual impulses. It is in this perspective that responsibility is reconfigured as power, the power that the person has to respond to what life proposes to him in all circumstances, in the face of all conditioning.

The fact that the agreement between the self and others, whether the id or the ancestors, is a silent agreement is another issue that marks the freedom of the self, since no one needs to know about this intimate decision. This place of healthy solitude is that in which only the self has all the possible variables to be able to decide for itself. Ultimate freedom also represents an ultimate responsibility: Because the self has the ability to deny its own life, it is solely responsible for maintaining this very life.

Suicide can also be seen as a message to others, to say something to someone, friends, family, a lost love, or even a social group. In this scenario, the first discourse seems noble, since death itself would have a meaning superior to the escape from something by not enduring a certain situation. However, the primary responsibility of the "I" is to the maintenance of itself. Without the "I" there is no freedom, nor the possibility of discourse.

The theme of responsibility in Frankl's writing was not based on a moral obligation to maintain one's own life, nor does it derive from social, ideological, or religious standards or rules, but rather on the facticity of existence and the search for meaning in life. Since a person is not determined by the environment, there is always a freedom to decide in spite of conditioning.

All dynamics of meaning in life, as the term itself expresses, is on the condition of existence; "not existing" means not seeking meaning. The healthy "me" movement is the movement towards life, in spite of everything. In this way, the search for death is therefore an unhealthy expression. The suicidal person may have a psychological disorder or a noögenic one in that their perception of freedom and responsibility may be distorted.

In his early years of medicine including his experience with the approximately 12,000 suicide-related cases in the 1930s, Frankl (1991) continued to work to promote a path to suicide prevention within the concentration camps, as reported in his book, *Man's search for meaning*. He also continued after the war. In 1946, Frankl (2019b) brought up the analogy of the game of chess to reflect on suicide:

> Let's imagine for a moment: A chess player is faced with a chess problem and he cannot find a solution, so—what does he do?—He hurls the pieces off the board. Is that a solution to the chess problem? Certainly not.
>
> But this is exactly how the suicide behaves: he throws his life away and thinks he has thereby found a solution for a seeminly insoluble life problem in life. He does not know that in doing so he has flouted the rules of life. (p. 42)

In his personal view, Frankl did not see human beings as incapable of dealing with the sufferings of life. For him, suffering had meaning, because life has meaning in all circumstances. In this way, even if there is a lot of suffering and frustration, each person is able to bear all suffering by finding meaning and being able to continue fighting for life.

There is a constant defense of the human capacity for overcoming and coping; Frankl's theory was focused on the capacity for resilience. In the dimensional ontology of logotherapy, the core of human essence is composed of its noëtic dimension. The concept of self-transcendence highlights the human capacity to go beyond oneself, to find the meaning of life through work, love, and deeds. Through these beliefs, Frankl encouraged the person to access core capabilities which invariably promoted the best response.

It is well known that stress affects cognitive abilities, but when a person believes that they are able to get out of a risky situation, their brain tends to decrease stress and is more able to find solutions to problems. The analogy of chess is an excellent example for overcoming suicidal ideation, because once the person accepts the stressing forces, he gives up thinking about finding solutions. But Frankl (2019b) insisted that life has meaning, even in the face of the highest level of stress and suffering. Frankl, who lived through the suicidal ideation and suicidal acts of people in the concentration camps, could safely say that "suicide also flouts the rules of the game of life; these rules do not require us to win at all costs, but they do demand from us that we never give up the fight" (p. 42).

When considering objections about the meaning of life, when one is sure that everything will end, whether due to a fatal illness or war, or any other circumstance, Frankl (2019b) proposed that we consider what life would be like if we were immortal. According to him, we could postpone everything and we could leave everything for later. But life does not lose meaning because it has an end:

> Conversely, the fact, and only the fact, that we are mortal, that our lives are finite, that our time is restricted and our possibilities are limited, this fact is what makes it meaningful to do something, to exploit a possibility and make it become a reality, to fulfill it, to use our time and occupy it. Death gives us a compulsion to do so. Therefore, death forms the background against which our act of being becomes a responsibility. (p. 43)

A Clinical Case—Ann: "Humanity Should Be Annihilated"

In the context of the pandemic, from August 2020 to September 2021, I (Elison Santos) had the opportunity to provide psychotherapeutic care to a university student who sought help, reporting suicidal ideation. The sessions took place weekly online through the Google Meet platform, lasting 50 minutes each.

This section is not intended to be a detailed presentation of psychotherapeutic sessions. On the other hand, it aims to demonstrate how logotherapy and Viktor Frankl's vision of people can positively influence the practice of clinical psychology in cases of suicidal ideation.

"Ann" was a graduate student in her early 20s in the master's degree program in mathematics. Smart, but born in a small town in the interior of northeastern Brazil and coming from a family with few financial resources, she stood out academically from her environment. She graduated from a local university and was accepted to the postgraduate program at the University of São Paulo. Eager to find new experiences in the great capital, she moved there in early 2020. After a few weeks of classes, she was confronted with the emerging Covid pandemic and the resulting need for social distancing. That experience was stressful, but she was still living with other young people and, therefore, had a social support system to help her deal with the stress.

Her treatment began with three initial meetings that were part of the intake process. Then she was offered continued treatment as part of a study that was conducted until the end of 2021, approved by the Ethics Council.[1] Ann agreed to be part of the study, signed the informed consent form, and we were able to continue the psychotherapeutic process that began with the intake.

Like many young people, Ann needed a scholarship to be able to survive in the big city. Not knowing how long the pandemic would last, she remained in the apartment she shared with a colleague. As the months passed, the colleague left the apartment and returned to her hometown. She experienced problems with her scholarship, to the extent that the university stopped depositing the money that supported her. Ann was forced to go to a nearby city and stay in the apartment of another friend who invited her. As the months passed, this friend also had to return home. Penniless,

[1] For reasons of confidentiality, the name and other personal information have been changed; the study was authorized by the Ethics Board of the University of São Paulo. Approval by the Ethics Committee under opinion No. 051165/2020 and CAAE: 32288820.6.0000.5561

struggling to find a place to stay, and unwilling to return to her hometown, Ann's psychological condition worsened.

It was in the midst of these changes brought about by the pandemic that Ann sought help. On the application form, she noted: "I am alone in another city, living with financial difficulties, often thinking about suicide. I am crying every day and feel frequent sadness and failure." To the prompt *I believe that an exclusively online therapy for me is…* she responded: "The only help possible right now."

The circumstances in which Ann began her therapeutic process were extraordinary. However, as with all occasions in life, Ann was also invited to find meaning, adapt to conditions, recover her inner strength, and move on. She wondered how to proceed if everything seemed to make no sense, if conditions seemed impossible, and if all that was inside her was weaknesses and defeat.

From the start of the intake process, noting the presence of suicidal ideation, my attitude was one of acceptance and positivity, seeking to perceive the healthy person behind the problems and convey my confidence in her and her ability to cope with the situation. In the dimensional ontology of logotherapy, the somatic and psychic dimensions are prone to illness, but the noëtic dimension is not. That is, even if there are noögenic neuroses, it is not the spiritual "I" that gets sick, but the somatic and/or psychic dimensions. In this way, the spiritual (noëtic) part of the person, which is healthy, must be accessed as soon as possible so that there is a successful therapeutic process. In practice, the therapist can look at the person beyond the illness, as in this case, and see a capacity within the person to face suicidal ideation and to find meaning in the presence of suffering. This attitude of the psychologist is reflected in body language, in gestures, and in the choice of words. It is an attitude of trust that translates into a message: "You may not be seeing that you are capable of overcoming this moment, but I am seeing it and I believe that you are capable."

In the sessions, Ann spoke of her family; she said that her parents were very simple people and lived in a very small town in the countryside. She reported that her parents were very religious. She was the only child who had managed to go to college. I showed my admiration for this fact, reinforcing her statement, "So, you're the only one in the family to go to college! This is something very important!" She smiled and replied that she felt good about it. Gradually, we established a relationship of trust and Ann opened up more.

In her first session, Ann spoke of feelings of anger, an anger that was directed towards social media, corruption, and the pandemic, that directed her aggression towards human existence. She stated:

> The greatest plague is the human being. I am in favor of voluntary extinction. I feel mutual hatred for all human beings. It's a bad thing, as a whole, but I'm not in favor of suffering, or wars, or viruses. I do think a comet could fall and end everything for humanity and there will be no more children.

This wording caught my attention because it did not just represent an impetuous reaction to a situation, it was a well-thought-out statement. She spoke of online communities that defend "anti-natalism," the extinction of humanity. This disbelief in people, absence of the possibility of goodness, and the lack of concern for humanity itself have been particularly challenging for people of all ages. From a psychogenic point of view, this stance can be interpreted as a hysterical reaction that could easily produce symptoms that support a diagnosis and need for treatment. But there was something else in her words: There was a healthy person who, since childhood, analyzed the world through a different prism than that of her family and friends and who yearned for something more, even if she was wrong in how she went about it.

In the same session, she added: "At school, when I was little, a boy fell out of a tree; I was the only one who didn't go there to look." Not only did she see no point in seeing the suffering of another, but she also felt bad and said she was very sensitive; she did not like to watch movies with themes of torture, rape, or violence. She reported being very sensitive to social injustices. Therefore, there was not only a sensitivity but also a capacity for empathy—valuable qualities that connected her with people and allowed her to perceive others and their feelings.

Ann said she sometimes felt naïve and dumb. She believed and trusted people, but felt colleagues lied to her just to make fun of her. She said she did not know if she loved her family or if what she felt was just for convenience. She was afraid of relationships that were not reciprocal. She did not know if caring about others was a good or bad thing. She noted: "One of the consequences of capitalism is caring more about money than others."

She had mixed feelings about these perceptions. On one hand, her internal capacities of sensitivity and empathy told her that she should care about people with their sufferings and anxieties and connect with their thoughts and feelings. On the other hand, her perception of the world, of people, and of society, revealed her perception that the world was somehow wild, human relationships were unreliable, people did not care about each other, and there was an intrinsic evil in every relationship.

From the point of view of some theories of development, such a picture represents an immaturity, characteristic of childhood, in which the person refuses to accept the fact that people are bad and thus leave the fantasy world of utopian ideations about life.

Her history of suicidal ideation and her complaints about the world denoted clear depressive traits but at the same time showed traces of an existential emptiness, as they demonstrated an "impediment to satisfaction in her own affect, work, and relational lives" (Pacciolla, 2015 p. 118). In this case, she was in search of meaning. In her childhood, she questioned evil, believed in people, and sought to break the limits imposed by her father's limiting beliefs. This search only took place because there was a mobilizing belief, a trust in life. This confidence had strengthened her to break boundaries. She left home, went to college in the capital and then went on to the best university in the country to attend graduate school. But this mobilization had a cost in her psychic structure.

On several occasions, in different sessions, Ann noted that her father always said, "Poor people don't go to college." Especially when she wasn't feeling well, this was a mandate that served as a driving force to prove him wrong. However, in moments of fragility, it served to nourish her doubts and insecurities, as if a voice inside said to her, "Is he right?" A neurosis intensified from time to time, in a way that sought to justify defeat, failure, and her inability to individuate from her parents.

Ann said that, when she was a child, "I never wanted to be a housewife or have children, I wanted to be something; I wanted to work at the mall," but she never did. It frustrated her that she was not using her master's degree as she had expected. Ever since she was a little girl, she did not want to become like so many others who got pregnant as teenagers. In this way, Ann remembered her strengths, desires, dreams, her will to meaning, and reminded herself of her "freedom of will" in search of something that actually made sense for her life.

Even far from home, Ann's contact with family, friends, teachers, and colleagues represented an encounter with her own inability to work. For a university student, this work was precisely her student obligation and, in the case of a graduate student, her research. The result of this dynamic of abysmal perception between being versus having to work was also manifested in her procrastination. This was not because she wanted to do the task later, but because she perceived it so deeply loaded with emotional meanings—and felt so deeply guilty for being incapable—that the task was considered impossible, at least for her, in that moment. These were constant accusations (Frankl, 2019a, p. 249) that she made to herself and heard from others.

Ann felt so guilty that she wished she had not been born. Not only did she wish she had not been born, but she held to the idea of annihilating humanity itself. A profound guilt underpinned her past suicide attempt and her present suicidal thoughts. With each exam on which Ann did not get an acceptable grade, she convinced herself that her whole life had no meaning. Reprimands—from self or others, according to Frankl (2019a), produce an unwanted paradoxical effect. Instead of producing motivation to improve, they can increase feelings of inadequacy and potentiate subjective guilt.

Faced with her inability to work, I did not present myself as a psychologist who could ease her tension directly. On the contrary, I proposed questions that led her to reflect on the importance that those tests had for her such as: "Are these tests very important to you?" and "Did you promise yourself that you would get good grades?" To both questions she answered affirmatively, which pointed to the importance of an instructor who had invested in her and given her a vote of confidence and had introduced her to her advisor. She felt indebted to him and also to herself. At that moment, the relational aspects of meaning were also highlighted, as the conscience presents its responsibilities not only towards itself but also towards the other.

Another component of the triad of failure was the inability to enjoy, because in the face of the inability to work and the consequent guilt, she did not see herself worthy of enjoyment. The abyss was so great that all that could exist is guilt and self-pity.

When Ann presented her account of her suicidal ideation, I asked, "And what keeps you alive? What's stopping you from carrying out your death thoughts?" Ann quickly replied:

> I keep thinking about my friend who is traveling, what would happen to her when she knew I did this at her house? I think about my parents, what it would be like for them, they don't deserve this, my friends from my city….

This question had the effect of stimulating thoughts of personal responsibility, provoking the voice of conscience and self-accountability. As Frankl (2019a) expressed it, this individual was not only accountable to herself but also to the doctors and nurses who provided her with a window to think about those who are part of her history and can have a satisfactory therapeutic effect in preventing suicide.

That is why the suffering presented by Ann when she did poorly on the tests should not be softened or belittled. In therapy, she was able to verbalize about the bond she had with her instructor. If she could suffer for him for not doing well on a test, she may consider it as part of her reasons for staying alive despite her sufferings, as he represents something important to her.

Therapy here does not always have as its objective the achievement of homeostasis, the absence of tension. The relationship is with the spiritual self, capable of taking action in the face of her challenges.

Final Considerations

A clinical psychology that seeks to face suffering and the causes of suicidal ideation must be able to understand the limits of human life. Viktor Frankl (2003) advocated a "height psychology" (p. 20); he understood that human beings can search for the meanings of life and can focus on the future and the possibility of fulfilling these meanings. Ewalds-Kvist and Lützén (2015) commented on Frankl's life: "As a survivor of four concentration camps, he [knew] that humans are capable of resisting and braving even the worst conditions through self-transcendence by detaching oneself, at least momentarily, from the situation" (p. 191).

In the Franklian code of ethics, the value of life must be preserved under any and all circumstances, even in the most adverse situations. Frankl's experience in the concentration camps demonstrated this as he implemented suicide prophylaxis measures, even under these inhumane conditions.

In addition to his professional and social curriculum, Frankl (1924) was interested in questioning theories and influencing them, even to the point of developing his own; for example, he questioned Freud in an article in the *Internationale Zeitschrift für Psychoanalyse*. He also attended Alfred Adler's meetings, as he was very interested in studies of individual psychology. Such events led to the formulation of his theses and to his accomplishments as a psychiatrist and neurologist, head of hospitals, organizer of youth centers, Holocaust survivor, husband, father, peacemaker, defender of life, scholar, and innovative theorist.

It is also important to highlight that Frankl did not dedicate himself only to the practical application of medicine, nor just to leadership roles in hospitals and universities. His life was marked by social initiatives, such as organizing the Youth Counseling Centers, where he offered free care to adolescents, and for being a volunteer in many other psychosocial initiatives. This says a lot about Frankl's humanity and how his vision of mental health was not limited to treatment but was deeply committed to an investment in the prophylaxis of psychic and existential problems.

The background against which human life is presented and interpreted by each person in its uniqueness is understood in different ways by various psychological schools of thought. Frankl (2003) criticized determinism and reductionism, instead pointing to the specifically human capacity for self-transcendence in which freedom and responsibility complement each other, producing a healthy balance in the psychic structure and enabling fulfillment and happiness.

In conclusion, Frankl's contributions to suicide prevention are yet to be fully understood, although they constitute a useful theoretical and practical construct that represents a solid foundation for clinical intervention.

References

Aquinas, T. (2011). *Summa theologiae* (A. J. Freddoso, Trans.). St. Augustine's Press.

Augustine, S. (1950). *The city of God* (D. B. Zema & G. G. Walsh, Trans.). Catholic University of American Press.

Bando, D. H. (2008). *Spatial patterns of suicide in the city of São Paulo and their socioeconomic-cultural correlates*. [Master's thesis, Universidade de São Paulo].

Bando, D. H., Brunoni, A. R., Fernandes, T. G., Benseñor, I. M., & Lotufo, P. A. (2012). Suicide rates and trends in São Paulo, Brazil, according to gender, age and demographic aspects: A joinpoint regression analysis. *Brazilian Journal of Psychiatry, 34*, 286–293.

Biller, K., Levinson, J. I., & Pytell, T. (2002). Viktor Frankl—Opposing views. *Journal of Contemporary History, 37*(1), 105–113.

Bowman, W. (2008). Despair unto death? Attempted suicide in early 1930s Vienna. *Austrian History Yearbook, 39*, 138–156.

Burton, R. (1857). *The anatomy of melancholy*. JW Moore.

Cutler, D. M., Glaeser, E. L., & Norberg, K. E. (2001). Explaining the rise in youth suicide. In J. Gruber (Ed.), *Risky behavior among youths: An economic analysis* (pp. 219–270). University of Chicago Press.

Durkheim, E. (1897/2011). *Suicídio, estudo de sociologia*. WFM Martins Fontes. (Original work published in French as *Le suicide: étude de sociologie* in 1897)

Ewalds-Kvist, B., & Lützén, K. (2015). Miss B pursues death and miss P life in the light of VE Frankl's existential analysis/Logotherapy. *OMEGA–Journal of Death and Dying, 71*(2), 169–197. https://doi.org/10.1177/0030222815570599

Frankl, V. E. (1924). Zur mimischen Bejahung und Verneinung. *Internationale Zeitschrift für Psychoanalyse, 10*, 437–438.

Frankl, V. E. (1978). *The unheard cry for meaning. Psychotherapy and humanism*. Touchstone.

Frankl, V. E. (1986). *The doctor and the soul. From psychotherapy to logotherapy*. Vintage Books.

Frankl, V. E. (1991). *Em busca de sentido* [Man's search for meaning]. Voices.

Frankl, V. E. (2000). *Man's search for ultimate meaning*. Basic Books.

Frankl, V. E. (2003). *Psicoterapia e Sentido da Vida* [Psychotherapy and meaning of life] (4th. ed.). Quadrant.

Frankl, V. E. (2007). *Escritos de juventud 1923–1942* [Writings of youth 1923–1942]. Herder.

Frankl, V. E. (2010). *O que não está escrito nos meus livros* [What is not written in my books]. It's Achievements.

Frankl, V. E. (2016). *Teoria e terapia das neuroses: Introdução à logoterapia e à análise existencial* [Theory and therapy of neuroses: Introduction to logotherapy and existential analysis]. It's Achievements.

Frankl, V. E. (2019a). *Sofrimento humano: Fundamentos antropológicos da psicoterapia* [Human suffering: The anthropological foundations of psychotherapy]. It's achievements.

Frankl, V. E. (2019b). *Yes to life: In spite of everything*. Beacon Press.
Frankl, V. E. (2020). *Psicoterapia na prática* [Psychotherapy in practice]. It's Achievements.
Freud, S. (1917). Mourning and melancholia. In *The standard edition of the complete psychological works of Sigmund Freud, 14*(1914–1916), 237–258.
Goethe, J. W. (1774/1987). *The sorrows of young Werther* (Original work published 1774 in German as *Die Leiden des jungen Werthers*) (M. Swales, Trans.). University Press.
Kühn, R. (2015). *Logothérapie et phénoménologie: Contributions à la compréhension de l'analyse existentielle de Viktor E. Frankl* [Logotherapy and phenomenology: Contributions to the understanding of Viktor E. Frankl's existential analysis]. L'Harmattan.
Loureiro, P. R. A., Moreira, T. B., & Sashsida, A. (2013). *Os efeitos da mídia sobre o suicídio: Uma análise empírica para os estados brasileiros* [The effects of the media on suicide: an empirical analysis for Brazilian states]. Institute of Applied Economic Research.
Pacciolla, A. (2015). *Psicologia contemporânea e Viktor Frankl: Fundamentos para uma psicoterapia existencial* [Contemporary psychology and Viktor Frankl: Foundations for an existential psychotherapy]. Cidade Nova.
Sonneck, G., Hirnsperger, H., & Mundschütz, R. (2012). Suizid und Suizidprävention 1938–1945 in Wien [Suicide and suicide prevention in Vienna from 1938 to 1945]. *neuropsychiatrie, 26*, 111–120. https://doi.org/10.1007/s40211-012-0032-8

Élison Silva Santos, is a licensed clinical psychologist in Brazil and licensed associate psychology in Washington DC, with over 16 years of expertise. Specialized in logotherapy and existential analysis from the Pontifical Catholic University of Parana, Brazil, with a master's in clinical psychology from the University of São Paulo, Brazil. Founder and director of the Sapiens Institute of Applied Psychology–IPSapiens and editor at the publisher Busca Sentido. Serving as director at large at the International Council of Psychologists–ICP and a member of the Steering Committee of the Global Network of Psychologists for Human Rights. He has authored books focusing on suicide prevention, the meaning of life, and human relationships.

Andrés Eduardo Aguirre Antúnez, is a psychologist with a doctorate in science and a postdoctoral fellowship at the Department of Psychiatry at the Federal University of São Paulo, Brazil. He is associate professor III in clinical psychology at the Department of Clinical Psychology, Institute of Psychology. He is also subsidiary professor at the Department of Psychiatry, University of São Paulo and a member of the International Society of Phénoméno- Structural Psychopathology, the Italian Center for Phenomenological Research, vice-president of the Brazilian Society of Rorschach and Projective Methods.

When the Angel Turns into a Demon: The Pathology of Psychopathology

Teria Shantall

A new approach in the use of logotherapy will be explored using case studies that bear painful witness to the anguish suffered by patients suffering from severe psychogenic neuroses. The illness submerges the essence of who these individuals are as spiritual, free-willed human beings in the sea of emotional turmoil and conflict. Not functioning on the supremely human level of meaning and purpose in life, they are held captive by distorted perceptions of themselves and the world. How can the stranglehold be broken of the pathology of psychopathology, the internalized lies about themselves and the world as a result of trauma suffered most often in the tender and formative stages of personality development during childhood? How to free these individuals from the pathologies still holding a tyrannical sway over the person in adulthood?

My question is: Can the tyranny of a life lost in what Frankl (2004) called the subhuman dimension of being be defied in going deeper and beyond the purely psychodynamic approach of traditional psychotherapies? Can logotherapy be practiced in a new, more comprehensive way?

The Provocation of Meaning

"Man is spiritual," Frankl (2010, p. 134) contended. By spiritual, Frankl meant *a freedom of thought* that intuitively evaluates everything that happens to us in terms of meaning. Does it make sense to us or not? Does it alert and awaken our interest, catch our attention, draw us in, make us reach out of ourselves toward what is being offered to us in the situation or encounter? Do we really connect to it? Does it, in

T. Shantall (✉)
Viktor Frankl Institute of Logotherapy of South Africa, Johannesburg, South Africa

C. L. McLafferty, Jr., J. I. Levinson (eds.), *Logotherapy and Existential Analysis*, Logotherapy and Existential Analysis: Proceedings of the Viktor Frankl Institute Vienna 2, https://doi.org/10.1007/978-3-031-48922-8_13

other words, enliven our spirits, call us forth, so to speak, by appealing to what we are seeking even beyond knowing, or not? *We intuit meaning.* Why? Because an appeal is made to what we inherently are geared to find in life: meaning! This core tendency or *will to meaning* (Frankl, 1969/1988) is essential to us as an inherent yardstick, one that directs us toward the meaning of every concrete situation or encounter in our lives, from the start to the end of it.

The Key Motivation

This key motivation in the human breast, Frankl (1975, 2000) also referred to as "the Unconscious God," that is, as an unconscious intentionality or outreach to connect or find ourselves in tune or harmony with something or someone outside of ourselves that *addresses us* and *calls us forth*. We are provoked into action. We are to *meet*, that is, *fulfil* the meaning of the moment.

Meaning is out there in the world, Frankl (1969/1988) contended, and inherent to our being is a will to find and bring our lives in alignment with it. We experience meaning when this connection, maybe to the very Source and Ultimate Destination of our lives, is made. Outside of this sense of connectedness at the heart of what we experience as meaningful, we feel cut off, alone, lost but yet restlessly searching.

A Search for Ultimate Meaning

It is a constituent of human existence that we need to experience our lives as meaningful, that is, as having a purpose, a direction, a vocation, and a goal. This sense of having something worthwhile to give to others—of having some kind of worthy place to fill in the world—is at the heart of a feeling of self-worth. We do not want to be left to ourselves. A disconnect, the feeling of being out of touch with others, is to feel out of touch with ourselves. We want to feel called upon, brought into relationship with others and, at a more evolved stage of being, directed to a destination held out to us.

In a deeper sense, we need to experience our lives as having intent; that is, our lives have been ordained or destined to be. Without this sense of inclusion or of being needed and ordained as part of a bigger picture, that is, by a world that summons us and a future that awaits us, human existence collapses into futility. Such a world has neither rhyme nor reason; it is arbitrary, heedless, and nonsensical.

Nothing short of finding meaning in life will satisfy!

Noödynamics

These *from within* and *from without* dynamics of meaningful living are called "*noödynamics*" (Frankl, 2010, p. 57), a fundamentally deeper, higher, and more holistic approach in therapy as opposed to psychodynamics, which confines itself only to the psychological dimension of being.

It must be acknowledged that, in focusing only on the furthest or mature stages of human development with clients suffering from childhood hurts and traumas, we, as logotherapists, may have designated those areas of repressed hurt and emotional turmoil as areas of explorations only to psychoanalytically orientated therapies. By separating psychodynamics from noödynamics, we may have left our own logotherapeutic methods of intervention unexplored and therefore incomplete.

The purpose of this chapter is to make the following point and to illustrate it with examples: If, from the very outset of our lives and through every phase of our lives, we have a fundamental outreach or will to find meaning in our lives, then it is the disturbance of this noödynamic between seeking and finding meaning in our lives, which is the deep anguish behind all mental and emotional afflictions. Mental illnesses can therefore be seen as a spiritual distress, and what caused them, whether constitutional, psychological, or noölogical in nature, as disruptions or ruptures of our natural leaning toward a life of optimal meaning and well-being.

The Golden Thread Running Through Our Lives: The Will to Connect

Encompassing All of Being

A new, or rather, more encompassing approach in logotherapeutic counseling is to incorporate, within clinical practice, the early manifestations of the will to meaning behind what may seem as only an urge toward need satisfaction—what Frankl (1946/1985) called "the will to pleasure" (p. 138)—in the earliest stages of growth, and the struggle for identity emerging in the later stages of personality development "the will to power" (p. 138).

"Your Eyes Saw My Substance, Being yet Unformed" (Psalms 139:16, New King James Version)

What do we see when we hold a newborn in our arms? What perceptions of the infant's perceptions are evoked in us? We feel called into an interaction with the yet-hidden person of the newborn baby, especially if our own; a child very much wanted by us.

A Basic Trust in Being

What earmarks the perceptual functioning of the infant? Developmental research has clearly and validly established the following fact: the need for connection, for bonding. The forming of an interactive attachment bond with the primary caregivers is essential for the healthy personality development of the child. Secure attachment, highlighted by the pioneering work of John Bowlby (1969, 1976a, b), is the infant's first experience of being connected to a world that the infant learns to trust. Frankl (2010) spoke about the need for a "basic trust in Being" (p. 190). "Underneath are the everlasting arms" (Deut 33:27, King James Version) is a scriptural definition of the Unconscious God in our experience of *unconditional love* and, with that, of *the unconditional meaningfulness* of our own lives. This realization may remain unconscious but become manifest in the realization, at a later stage in our lives, that there is meaning out there in the world and that it can be found in any situation, anywhere, and at all times. It is in the experience of *love, of being loved,* that we experience ourselves as worthy, of our lives as having meaning. It is the realization that struck Frankl (1946/1985) in the contemplation of his beloved wife while in the agony of the concentration camps, namely, that "*the salvation of man is in and through love*" (p. 37). Love puts a stamp of approval on our lives!

Love, like meaning, *is*! It is *found* or *experienced.* It cannot be demanded or made. The phrase "making love" is a misnomer. Love cannot be made or forced to happen. Love is an expression of the person behind the actions of love. In loving someone, you see the unique and singular person behind his or her appearance. In fact, the person *manifests themselves*; love is *shown.* That is why the infant experiences love in the way they are held, soothed, rocked, played with, fed and bathed, tucked in, and spoken to. *Love is sensed, intuited!* It is the manner of this primary caregiving and interaction with children that reaches down and touches the core of their person. They feel *responded to in meaning-enhancing ways.* The little persons prosper. Their will to life and meaning is evoked! Feeling loved, they entrust themselves to a loving other.

The developmental psychologist Erik Erikson (1963) was the first to speak about the formation of basic trust. He proposed that the infant has the first stirrings of a feeling of identity in being responded to in these connective ways. A bond is established. The meaning of meaning is this sense of connection, a sense of being meaningfully related to and of being in a securing, loving, and life-giving relationship. Meaning is in the *encounter.*

Frankl (2010, p. 81) contended that for meaning to be elicited or evoked, it must be illuminated. The illumination or the meaning of meaning, is nowhere stronger and clearer than in a profoundly personal experience of it. We need to experience meaning to come to believe in its existence! We want an affirmation and enhancement of what we, yet unconsciously, sense is what our whole being is reaching out toward.

A "Yes!" from Life

This natural or inherent leaning, or will to meaning, needs to be met. The developing child, from its very inception and throughout its life, needs to hear a "Yes!" from life to be fully able to say a "Yes!" to it in return.

Inherent to our very being, our essence, is the longing, the urge, the will, to say: "Yes!" to our lives that have been authenticated and affirmed as singularly worthy, embraced, sought out, and needed. Life awaits us and expects something from us. This gives us the dignity of *responsibility*; as Frankl (1946/1985) noted: "Thus, logotherapy sees in responsibleness the very essence of human existence" (p. 109).

Is being needed and responded to, and drawn into meaningful or life-giving interaction with a concerned, caring, or loving and acknowledging other, not the first expression of a sense of responsibility in children? Does it not draw them out of themselves into wanting to be pleasing, to provoke love-responses of acknowledgment from others?

Frances Tustin (1981), an early expert in the field of childhood autism, in her work with autistic children, clearly highlighted the essential need of the infant to experience a loving "Yes!" to its existence within the first 6 weeks of life. This affirmation of the uniqueness of its person enlivens the infant with a response-ability to say "Yes!" to others in its world and forms the foundation of a confident and adventurous spirit of *trust* in launching out into that world. How reminiscent this is of Frankl's (2020) famous challenge to us to say: "Yes!" to life! How descriptive this interchange is of the encounter between logotherapist and client which, to Frankl's (1969/1988) mind, was the strongest factor in the healing process. The client's sense of basic trust in life is restored. Enlivened by a sense of meaningful interaction, the client experiences a unique sense of identity; something the logotherapist strongly affirms and strengthens.

We help our clients to become fully themselves!

Awakenings

Bruno Bettelheim (1967), another early researcher in the field of childhood autism, wrote a book, *The Empty Fortress*, followed by two other pioneer researchers in the field, DesLauriers and Carlson (1969) with their book, *Your Child is Asleep*. Therapy with constitutionally hampered, emotionally disturbed, or dysfunctional children is, in fact, an awakening. The person of the child is awakened and assisted to come out or emerge from behind their dysfunction, handicap, or emotional affliction. Dormant capacities of the child or, in adulthood, of the client are awakened. They are, in fact, released into a meaningful, response-able interaction with their world.

In cases where this primary need to connect has been assailed through emotional abuse or neglect or, in the case of constitutionally handicapped or dysfunctional children where no remedial intervention could keep a sense of secure personhood intact in the child, the will to meaning is suppressed. This will result in insecure attachments, diffused or distorted perceptions of self as somehow unseen, unheard; in a sense non-existent, abandoned, or discarded. These perceptions are only a step away from feeling inferior, insignificant, or bad, and the world as fearful, untrustworthy, and something to withdraw from or to be defended against. The natural outreach toward meaning and worthy personhood in a life that calls upon the person to fill their assigned and unique destiny or place in this world, is thwarted, disrupted, even severed. The result is emotional trauma and anguish, a fearful withdrawal from the world, a defensive hiding away or submergence of the person who, in very essence, is suffering from *a spiritual distress, a crisis of meaning!*

It is clear from Frankl's writings, and his accent on self-transcendence as a prime feature of human existence, that we are most fully ourselves when we lose this state of being turned into ourselves or left only to ourselves but are, instead, meaningfully engaged with our world. The tragic severance of this life-giving bond gives rise to a state of supreme isolation and painful self-absorption—the hotbed of psychopathology and, with it, the mental anguish suffered by the one overwhelmed and taken over by it. The person is lost to us, to themselves, and to the world. A captive state on lower or *subhuman* levels of being is the outcome.

Going Deeper Than Depth Psychology

Man Is Spiritual

"Man is spiritual," Frankl (2010, p. 134) contended, and if he is, he is such from birth! From the outset, as immature as our thought and reasoning capacities may be, we are perceptively present in everything that happens to us and that we experience throughout our lives. This evaluation of our unscathed human spirit remains with us, no matter what happens to us at whatever stage of our lives or in whatever state of mind we find ourselves. Our quest is, and remains, a search for meaning in our lives. I, therefore, contend that psychogenic mental afflictions or neuroses, traditionally seen as psychological disturbances requiring psychologically based interventions, must be seen as a crisis of meaning requiring *a deeper and more intensive form of therapy: logotherapy.*

The Depth of Height Psychology

In addressing psychogenic neuroses from a logotherapeutic point of view, the therapy will be earmarked by the following phases, and not necessarily in the order given:

As noted, the will to meaning is the will to connect to another, to the world, in a meaningful way. It follows that the relationship between therapist and client is at the very heart of healing. It is a relationship peculiar to therapy, one most closely corresponding to the one relationship that is the Alpha and Omega of the client's life: the deep, ineradicable sense of belonging to the Divine. Divinity does not need us, but we are in absolute need of the Divine, the One Who has breathed the very spirit of life into us. There is no ultimate meaning to our lives without and outside of this context! This is the healing context of the logotherapeutic encounter. Any truly altruistic relationship of *unconditional love* is earmarked by a total devotion to and focus on the person and life of the one very much in need of it. Our clients need to experience a "Yes!" to their existence and person from us as therapists. This means that we are there for them; available to them in a total sense. The focus is on them, not on ourselves. It is this unique encounter between a caring and giving other and the one in need of it, that Frankl (1969/1988) stated is at the core of bringing a client out of his or her state of captivity on the lower and subhuman dimensions of being.

In this type of encounter, the client is made aware of being addressed in a meaning-focused way. It is not the problems to which they feel they are captive that are under consideration, but who they are, what their problems were and are doing to and saying to them and, in the final analysis, requiring of them.

This focus can be made evident by asking clients to consider why they came for therapy. Why are they there? Is it really only because they want their problems solved, or is it something much more? Does it not say that they are dissatisfied with their lives; that they want change in the direction of more meaning in their lives; that they want to experience greater purpose in their lives and, with that, want to experience a greater sense of self-worth in being more in line with what is truly good and valuable in life? The strength and power of their will to meaning will, in this way, be made clear to them.

Then it will be all important to highlight their strengths: their own tenacity in the face of what they have gone through; their strength in having survived and endured their traumas; their restless searching for what they know they really want; that they themselves came for help to live their lives in a way that would be more pleasing to themselves.

This will reflect on the person as inherently pure and good, and on the human spirit as unscathed in its capacity to keep on searching, struggling for and reaching out to secure what it most fundamentally needs. What is it that they really want in their lives? Spelling it out affirms the inherent goodness of their primary will to meaning in life.

From this platform of self-distancing and self-transcendence and awareness of meaning, in the therapy room, the actual trauma or hurt can begin to be explored, but and most importantly, *within a meaning context*. In so doing, the client's inherent search for meaning is taken to a stage prior to its developmental arrest. What happened to them? How did they feel about it? And how are they to understand those feelings? Hidden content through free association, dreams, flashbacks, and painful memories can then not only surface from their psychological unconscious, but also from their much deeper spiritual unconscious.

Clients are asked to explore more deeply how what they wanted was sharpened by experiencing what they in fact did *not* want; in what they had to endure, or are still suffering in their lives. The focus will be not on the nature of the trauma or conflict per se—this is just an aside—but on the *spiritual distress* that was suffered as a result of it.

It is imperative to realize that the client is doing this, with the therapist, from the *perspective of meaning*. This is vastly different from plunging into their hurtful experiences and blotting out a self-transcendent perceptiveness by indulging in the force of evoked emotions of lament, anger, blame, violent intent, bitterness, hysterical need, and overemotionality. No room for transference or countertransference is left in a meaning-centered approach to emotional trauma and psychological conflict! The accent is on boundaries. The lines are clearly drawn. The client is aware, and is kept aware, of their own boundaries in the interaction with the therapist as a person within his or her own sacred boundaries. No symbiotic entanglement or diffusion of boundaries is allowed. The client's efforts to manipulate the relationship in this direction is strongly discouraged and firmly resisted.

With this clarity of truthful self-reflection, the therapy will explore what has remained *intact* in their lives. This will include the recall of happy and good moments in their lives, the people who gave them a sense of worth and inspired their hope to find true fulfillment.

In so doing, clients will be asked to consider whether they were really abandoned in their lives. They will be made aware that they were never really alone; that meaning was always out there and to be found, despite the horrors they may have gone through. Not only was meaning always there, those moments of experiencing it consoled and encouraged them, gave them hope for the future, and somehow called upon them not to give up the struggle to come out of their states of emotional captivity.

This being so, what is the emotional captivity all about? Explored with the client will be what misperceptions and false images of themselves and the world they have formed as a result of what they suffered. They suffer *because* of the lies they started believing about themselves and the world! *This* is the source of their anguish, namely, that they lost touch with or never really discovered who they really are. Even so, life was always there, waiting for them to step into it and live it!

The pathology of psychopathology is also that it can take the client dangerously off course. They can land themselves in decadent and depraved situations. There can be deep shame and regret, a strong battle with their own conscience that can become weirdly distorted on the subhuman levels of being. Here the voice of conscience is *punitive*. It condemns, chastises, rebukes, and expresses disgust and strong rejection of the person of the client. This type of cold and oppressive superego disapproval can become unbearable. As its chastised victim, the person feels trapped in their wrongdoing, too afraid to come out and face it. The shame is too great; the fear of being found guilty, too overwhelming. Lies become a cover-up tactic; deceit and deviousness and angrily shifting the blame onto others, a way of life. The healthy defiance of the human spirit becomes an angry bravado in defiantly acting *against* the strict demands of a punitive conscience. This kind of god is appeased, feared, or defied. It certainly cannot be loved! "The heart is deceitful above all things and desperately wicked, who can know it?" (Jer 17:9–10, King James Version) is a saying in the book of Jeremiah to describe this type of fallenness from a state of grace: from the faith that one is worthy and that life is good. "The letter [of the law] kills, but the Spirit gives life" (2 Cor 3:4–6, New King James Version) is another Biblical saying. The world of dark distortions, even of hallucinations and delusions filled with angry or persecutory content, has the most viciously tenacious hold on the client caught up in neurotic guilt. The struggle to be freed from its evil grip is particularly fierce. In therapy, these clients are supersensitive to any form of censure or rebuke. Clients are, therefore, reassuringly and gently, sometimes even in a strongly supportive way, encouraged to face the destructive side of their behaviors. A great deal of unmasking of these distorted faces and false voices, speaking accusingly and relentlessly into the anguish mind of the client, may be necessary.

An important part of facing the demons in the client's tortured mind, is to unmask the so-called secondary gains or tempestuous pleasures and sense of bravado, or the power found in being rebellious that the pathologies have afforded the client. These are the compensations that are, in reality, self-destructive. Is pleasure for pleasure's sake, really pleasurable? Is power for power's sake, really powerful? These are questions that are explored with the client in a critical exposure of their pathological need for love and sense of identity by perhaps seeking it in sexual encounters, addictions, associations with what promises them specialness and gives them a sense of power, but which, in the end, leaves them empty, disappointed, disheartened, and disillusioned.

Clients are helped to *disassociate* themselves from what is false and very wrong in their lives. Intense self-reflection is provoked, as well as their sense of intuitive knowing as to what is good in life and what is destructive and bad, hurtful to themselves and others: Their true conscience is awakened. Strong regret and sincere repentance represent a breakthrough into the dimension of meaning. Seeking forgiveness, making restitution, and accepting responsibility are the surest ways of being able to forgive and accept themselves, to take up responsibility for their own lives!

The focus is on meaning, namely, on how the trauma or hurt can be understood from the viewpoint of what challenge it presents to the client, what the client is called upon to do about it, and why!

The trauma or hurt is seen not as something arbitrary, fateful, or senseless, for the very reason that the senselessness and cruelty, the injustice of it, is a call, even a commission, and in so many cases a future mission that the client is challenged to realize and embrace. The senselessness, cruelty, and injustice of the suffering only served to sharply illuminate what is to be done about it in order to turn it on its head. It is turned on its head when the client can take its painful lessons as a charge to combat the kind of suffering they have been subjected to.

What mission in life does it uniquely and singularly present to the client? Their particular area of suffering has equipped them with insights and sensitivities that they are provoked to use in helping others who have and are suffering in ways they have suffered. A victim of childhood sexual abuse can come to see it as a mission to use their first-hand expertise in qualifying themselves in the field of service to the sexually abused. What a triumph, what an overcoming of childhood hurts and traumas!

The client is left with a sense of mission. The conclusion of this type of logotherapy is the same conclusion that every other type of logotherapy accomplishes. Clients see their futures—their very lives—as awaiting them. It is a life filled with promise and hope. Every day is a new opportunity, another step forward. Every new insight into the noödynamics of their sufferings and traumas allows them to own and take possession of their emotions, of their physical needs and desires, and to exercise masterful, *spiritual control over them.* They begin to direct their own lives in the illuminated right direction!

A New Approach

A new look at pathology becomes possible with this approach. Pathology can be seen as a disruption and distortion of our fundamental will to meaning. The angel in us, our unscathed human spirit and its capacity to discern and realize its own personal path to a meaningful life, despite whatever assails this capacity, is turned into a demon. As a result of the failure to make sense of the hurtful and traumatic things that have happened to them, clients become overwhelmed by the force of powerfully evoked drives and emotions. Their capacities are concealed; their will to meaning is taken captive. They become slaves to torturous beliefs about themselves and terrorized by a world they can no longer perceive as their right and privilege to be part of. All their energies are consumed by self-defensive, self-protective, and self-compensatory behaviors.

Pathology lies to us; we become sick because of a lack of the truth of the worth and meaning of our lives and persons!

As a psychoanalytically trained clinical psychologist at the renowned Tavistock Clinic in London (the seat of Freudian analysis), and after my privileged meeting with Frankl and exposure to logotherapy at Frankl's first training center at the United States International University, I have had to rethink and re-evaluate everything I have learned about the psychodynamics of the mentally ill in the more encompassing context of logotherapy. What is the real truth behind the symptoms, the *real causes* behind the anguish of the mentally ill? What are they trying to tell us? Can we hear them? Do we understand them beyond the neat handling of their particular problems according to a certain diagnostic category and the particular method of treatment prescribed for it?

Let us explore all the questions and statements that have been made in this chapter by exploring the truths of it in the lives of four clients who have been thrown into the very depths of emotional turmoil and have fallen victim to the horror and despair of it. What was the real cause of their anguish? What is it that they struggled to achieve and could achieve through the help of this more intensive form of logotherapy?

Defying the Pathology of Psychopathology

Client 1: Never Give Up

Never give up! This is how a client described her life's orientation after her re-emergence from her own fall from the grace of being unconditionally loved; a love she sensed she needed in the very deprivation of it. She never had the love of her mother who rejected her, physically beat her—sometimes until she became unconscious—and, after some of the beatings, sexually molested her. She had no one to protect her. Her biological father divorced her mother; she was given main custody of her and her younger sister. His role was taken over by an abusive stepfather who raped and sexually abused her throughout her tender formative years. She often offered her own body to protect her younger sister from being raped.

Her world was a nightmare, a terrible daydream, one she projected outward by re-enacting, in adulthood, the trauma she suffered as a child. She perpetuated the struggle in marrying and divorcing two abusive husbands. At last, at the age of 50, she sought out therapy with a psychodynamically inclined therapist. After 4 years of delving into and bringing repressed childhood images to light to work through, they both got entangled in a transference and countertransference relationship. It was only in a last-ditch effort to break free of the demon of self-castigation and a state of emotional captivity that she found her release through logotherapy.

This is what she wrote about herself: She entitled it, "Lies told by the terrible dream." It was a dream she woke up from by letting the angel fight the demon that had come to possess her. She divided the two opposing sides; the first side was as follows:

> The lies the dream was telling me:
>
> I am stupid; I'm weak; I'm an idiot; I am useless; I cannot succeed; I may not succeed; I should not succeed; It's no use trying; I'm a loser.
>
> I am not important; I have no rights; my opinion doesn't count; my efforts will never be enough; I'm not good enough; I'm good for nothing.
>
> I am causing problems for others; I'm guilty; I am always being watched and judged; I must always listen to others; I must not fight back; I must comply; I must stay silent; I must be and do good; I must keep the peace.
>
> I'm invisible to the world; I have no voice; I don't deserve respect; I am not worthy; no one cares about me.
>
> No one will ever love me; I'm dirty and ugly; I deserve to suffer; I deserve pain; I deserve to be beaten; I deserve to be punished; I'm terribly bad; I don't deserve to live; I should not live; I should be dead.
>
> There is no peace; there is no rest; there's no escape; I'm trapped.
>
> My real crime is THAT I WAS BORN!

And yet, there was her unscathed human spirit, her self-distancing ability to be able to observe what was happening to her, and contrasting that to what she knew she really wanted. She wrote out a second column. These were the statements of the defiant power of her own human spirit:

> What "positives," I was saying to myself as I fought for my life in there!
>
> I must fight to survive; my life must have a reason; I must be worth more than this.
>
> I must believe in myself; I must endure; I must be strong; I must stay strong.
>
> I am strong! It is all up to me.
>
> There is always hope; I'm not the only one.
>
> I must survive the loneliness, pain, and fear; I must have courage.
>
> I am courageous!
>
> I must choose the right way; I must keep trying.
>
> I am not stupid! There is some goodness in the world.
>
> There must be an end to this.
>
> I will NEVER, EVER GIVE UP!

After completing two diplomates in logotherapy, one in research (educational/administrative) and the other in clinical work, she is now a logotherapist in her own right, doing wonderful and outstanding work among sexually abused women by way of workshops and counseling. She is soon to publish a book on the trauma of sexual abuse and on being healed of its devastating scars through the use of logotherapy. I have also appointed her as the secretarial administrator of the Viktor Frankl Institute of Logotherapy of South Africa. This is *her* story. She insisted that I use her name: Panayiota Ryall.

Client 2: Coming Out of Depression

The following are the perceptions of a severely depressed teenager after a successful course of logotherapy over a period of 4 months. She wrote:

> What depression is like:
>
> Uninvolvement. Involvement totally with yourself and negativity. Insecurity and worry and pain.
>
> Like a neutral color, it's almost nonexistent in a way. I was too scared to venture out. Too scared to do things for myself.
>
> The one thing that is true of depression is that there is more chaos than calm. There is more worry than peace and there is no harmony. In depression all you

have is yourself. When you are there you are not a person. You can't love and you can't live, because you are always anxious, you're always worried and you're always in a state of turmoil.

What healing is like:

Plans for the future; what I would like to become… something special that I would like to work towards; dreams and aspirations I have for the future; hope. It is like standing on a beach… if you were to watch a sunset… you dream… you think towards a future and you move away from the pain, the sorrow, the doubt, the fear.

I like to describe myself as someone who is full of surprises—the unexpected might arise and I feel in myself that I can rise to the occasion and meet whatever is required of me.

And then the creative self—the ability to make anew. There is growth and there is something positive happening.

And there is the regret; the remorse of what I have done to others; the call to make it up to them.

Client 3: From the Periphery to the Center of Being

The following quotations comes from the mouth of one of my most outstanding students of logotherapy. She cast new light on the other side of the shock and condemnation evoked by sexual promiscuity, drug taking, and alcohol abuse:

> Drinking eased my pain, helped me to talk to other people and pass the time rather than killing myself. It gave me something to look forward to. Drugs helped me see into spiritual vistas. Partying was a spiritual experience, where I could find people to philosophize with me and have deep conversations with—impossible for me in a sober state of mind as I was too self-conscious and had zero self-esteem.

Where was the focus in responding to her: on her drinking, drugging, sexual promiscuity as a result of this or that problem? The focus was on what she sought after in these deviations from healthy behavior: to have contact with people, to have something to look forward to, to reflect on the meaning of life, to find herself where she had lost herself—her sense of self-worth. There was a thwarting of her suppressed will to meaning; the ability to reach out to others, to experience the meaning that was there, out in the world. One of my responses as a logotherapist which broke through to her was this:

> Could all the humiliating experiences of your childhood which caused such self-loathing touch who you really were, concealed within an inner space that no outer violence could penetrate? Kept for its emergence when the shaping was

done, like a diamond unearthed but cut to perfection in the underground hiddenness of being, was the defiant power of the human spirit.

Her response, after further exchanges with me was:

> Now my journey is to wrap myself in the cocoon of self-love and kindness, and take whatever time it takes to transform into a butterfly who loves and values itself. I trust that my inner angel is reminding me and awakening me to who I really am while I "sleep" in safety.

Client 4: From Shame to Conviction

"I am ashamed. I have let myself down." This depiction of her fallen state given by another client illustrates the premise I have set out in this presentation. Caught in the pangs of psychological conflict, the spiritual person is submerged in a flood of emotional need and pressure. The angel in them turns into a demon. Their search for themselves, through the maze of psychological confusion, takes them into areas of darkness and despair where they lose touch with who they really are and become subject to the hellish anguish of being caught in the snares of self-destruction.

This client had a good-enough relationship with a father on whose lap she climbed as a little girl. Even then, she sought a sense of comfort in being in bodily contact with him because she knew that he only wanted boys, not a girl. She was even given a boy's name! When, in her teens, she began developing breasts and started to menstruate, her father rejected any physical contact with her. She felt she somehow disgusted him, even to the point that he would not allow her to use his shower cubicle. She sensed that her naked sexuality became a real problem for him. It turned out later that he had a promiscuous mother whom he despised, and had sexual problems of his own, repressed as they may have been. Our client felt the brunt of it, describing herself as some kind of alien creature, not wanted in the ordinary world of warm relationships. Her first sexual encounter at age 14 was a disaster. "A part of me shut down at that time," she confessed. She lost her sense of freedom, of feeling love-worthy. She felt she had lost herself and that she was given over to frustrated needs and desires. Her effort to still these raging emotions resulted in the development of sexual promiscuity. In all her consequent sexual encounters she never experienced orgasm. She felt her body was separate from herself, something she used as a tool or medium for what she was searching for: to be loved and needed.

Her first orgasm occurred when she actually felt some sense of friendship between herself and her much older partner. However, it did not last. The situation deteriorated until she started waitressing in a brothel and became a prostitute herself. In this free fall into the subterranean seas of a fully developed psychogenic neurosis, there was another awareness; one that made her cry bitterly in confessing it:

I have dishonored myself. At the time it didn't feel like sex but just about body parts, but there was something more, possibly more sacred than I had ever allowed; the realization that I had possibly not loved myself, showed myself no respect, that I just gave myself away. That was my sadness really.

But at the same time, she had lost all power to salvage herself: "I never saw that I could say no or yes; I never saw that I had that power." That was until she tried to get herself into another job and fell in love with her much older employer. She experienced it as a real friendship. Was this the father figure with whom she could at last come to love herself? But he was a married man and only kept her on as a mistress. The relationship dragged on for years until she at last came for therapy.

In therapy, she kept trying to understand the voices coming from her psychological unconscious where all the anguish of her conflict with her father was deeply buried. "I have to ask myself," she said, "what is the script running beneath?" She experienced a healing and restoring relationship with her therapist, who was one of my logotherapy students. Moments of deep insight and meaning miraculously surfaced from her spiritual unconscious along with psychological flashbacks emerging from her psychological unconscious. She expressed it as "a particular journey from the dance that I had with my father around sexuality. Somehow this has been a journey for me. The fact that I can feel (sexual) pleasure feels like there is still potential for something healthy."

Even though she gave herself over to sexual depravity, it never had her sanction: "It has always been a NO. It is wrong!" This conviction became so strong that she was able to say toward the end of the therapy:

"Now I must go. Now it's about getting out. It interferes with my relationship with God. I'm now prepared to lose the relationship, the friendship, and everything. It feels like I can't anymore. I'm a hypocrite, I can't. My relationship with God is stronger and bigger."

Her own emerged sanctity of spirit brought a breakthrough in conviction:

"I have kept myself locked up. Not anymore. I have a desire to not have any secrets, so I can't be in a secret relationship. There are many things that have made me want to get out, and also because I want to have an opportunity, as we've spoken about, to have a loving partnership, and I don't think that's available whilst I'm still in something like this."

What was most amazing was her confession of having found herself again:

"There's a deep sense of self that is not broken that I have not realized before. There is hope, it still feels intact. I feel that there is a lot intact. I feel quite optimistic, particularly where I am right now, and I think that it was there always: What's intact is change and the ability to change."

Conclusion: Homage to the Human Spirit

I want to end with one of the poems written by the first client, Panayiota Ryall, who had suffered sexual abuse for the greater part of her life. She is now a logotherapist of renown, especially in the area of dealing with sexually abused women:

BORN TO BE

How lovely this sweet spirit who lives within,
How beautiful is she,
She's true and wise and full of love
As she was born to be.
Her nature truly is divine,
For she was created so,
God the Father's Love for her,
He wants her to always know.
So He sent her to this world to live
And has given her tests and trials,
And though she's struggled very hard,
He's blessed her with His Smiles.
No trial could ever destroy her,
No one's cruelty,
Because her spirit who lives within
Is strong enough, you see.
And all those who've never believed in her,
Will not cause her to give in,
For her spirit who lives upon this earth,
Never forgets where she has been.
She keeps Heaven in her memory
And has carried it throughout her life,
It's been the strength she's held onto,
Through all her toils and strife.
How lovely this sweet spirit who lives within,
How beautiful is she,
She's true and wise and full of love,
As she was born to be.

Thank you!

References

Bettelheim, B. (1967). *The empty fortress: Infantile autism and the birth of the self*. The Free Press.
Bowlby, J. (1969). *Attachment and loss. Vol. 1: Attachment*. Hogarth Press.
Bowlby, J. (1976a). *Maternal care and mental health*. Shocken Books.
Bowlby, J. (1976b). *Child care and the growth of love*. Whitefriars.
DesLauriers, A. M., & Carlson, F. C. (1969). *Your child is asleep*. Dorsey Press.
Erikson, E. H. (1963). *Childhood and society*. W. W. Norton.
Frankl, V. E. (1975). *The unconscious God: Psychotherapy and theology*. Simon and Schuster. (Original work published in 1948 as Der unbewusste Gott)
Frankl, V. E. (1985). *Man's search for meaning* (3rd ed.). Washington Square Press/Pocket Books. (Original work published 1946)
Frankl, V. E. (1988). *The will to meaning: Foundations and applications of logotherapy*. Meridian. (Original work published 1969)
Frankl, V. E. (2000). *Man's search for ultimate meaning*. Perseus. (Original work published Der Unbewusste Gott, 1948; English translation, *The Unconscious God*, 1975)
Frankl, V. E. (2004). *On the theory and therapy of mental disorders: An introduction to logotherapy and existential analysis* (J. DuBois, Trans.). Brunner/Routledge. (Original work published *Theorie und Therapie der Neurosen Einfuhrung in die Logotherapie und Existenzanalys*)
Frankl, V. E. (2010). *The feeling of meaninglessness: A challenge to psychotherapy and philosophy* (A. Batthyany, & A. Tallon, Eds.). Marquette University Press.
Frankl, V. E. (2020). *Yes to life: In spite of everything*. Beacon Press.
Tustin, F. (1981). *Autistic states in children*. Routledge.

Teria Shantall, PhD, trained as a clinical psychologist in South Africa and studied psychoanalysis at the Tavistock Clinic in London. She trained as a logotherapist under the tutorage of the late Dr. Viktor Frankl at the United States International University in San Diego. Her doctoral research with Holocaust survivors was published by the Hebrew University in Jerusalem entitled: *Life's Meaning in the Face of Suffering*. She initiated logotherapy training courses at the University of South Africa, Israel, and Istanbul. She wrote *The Quest for Destiny: A Logotherapeutic Guide to Meaning-Centred Living, Therapy and Counselling* as a prescribed book for logotherapy students. She was nominated for a Jewish Achiever Award in South Africa in 2003 and won different awards at the 2005, 2007, 2009, 2011, 2013, 2015, and 2017 World Congresses in Logotherapy for distinguished service in promoting the work of Viktor Frankl by the Viktor Frankl Institute of Logotherapy of the United States and sat on their international board. She is president of the Viktor Frankl Institute for Logotherapy in South Africa and was vice-president of the Viktor Frankl Association for Logotherapy in Israel. Her latest book, published in 2020, is entitled: *The Life-changing Impact of Viktor Frankl's Logotherapy*. She is at present involved in running internet training courses in logotherapy by the Viktor Frankl Institute of Logotherapy of South Africa.

Truth, Meaning, and Attachment in Healing Combat Post-Traumatic Stress Disorder

Robert S. Brown Sr. and Charles L. McLafferty, Jr.

In 2005, I closed my psychiatric practice of 34 years in Charlottesville, Virginia, and moved to Fort Lee to help Soldiers returning from Iraq and Afghanistan. There was no logical reason for leaving a practice I loved, but a spiritual calling was compelling. For 11 years, from age 74 to 85, I served our Soldiers, and soon came to discover that I was on what I came to call "sacred ground."

I was permitted to know, admire, and respect our Soldiers, the most wonderful people in the world. I learned to know them by permitting them to get to know me as a person whose behavior they could come to predict. I intentionally satisfied their need to be treated consistently. It may sound silly, but I stuck to their unspoken first rule of conduct: "no surprises."

I wore a navy-blue blazer, shirt and tie, every day. I usually had a bottle of purified water and a cup of Twinings Irish Breakfast Tea within easy reach on my desk. I was attentive. Interruptions were minimized. I often felt there is no place on earth I'd rather be than with our Soldiers.

I made handwritten verbatim notes. Sometimes I read back to the Soldier exactly what they had just said to me. It let them know I was listening. It let them hear how they sounded. For many Soldiers, it was the first time they heard their own thoughts out loud as I read them their script. Too often, it was the first time their thoughts took on meaning and significance to someone who wanted to hear them. We were

R. S. Brown Sr.
United States Army Reserve (Retired), Charlottesville, VA, USA

Former Clinical Professor, University of Virginia, Charlottesville, VA, USA
e-mail: rsb6d@virginia.edu

C. L. McLafferty, Jr. (✉)
Purpose Research, Charlottesville, VA, USA

Viktor Frankl Institute of Logotherapy (USA) Stamford, TX, USA
e-mail: charles@purposeresearch.com

C. L. McLafferty, Jr., J. I. Levinson (eds.), *Logotherapy and Existential Analysis*, Logotherapy and Existential Analysis: Proceedings of the Viktor Frankl Institute Vienna 2, https://doi.org/10.1007/978-3-031-48922-8_14

establishing lasting attachments. Now, 7 years after I retired, I remain in an important, necessarily modified relationship of mutual respect with a number of these men and women.

The synopses of the following case histories have been approved for publication by the military members themselves, by the Department of the Army, and were published with full permission in *PTSD and Me: Healing Injured Minds* (Brown, 2017a), from which they have been excerpted.[1]

Case 1: The Captain's Picture

A 38-year-old Army Captain was haunted by a devastating visual image of two Soldiers, dragging a wounded Soldier, shouting, "Save our brother! Save our brother!" The captain knelt to examine the injured Soldier, but, in his words, he "froze for a moment… brain matter was leaking from the Soldier's head." Since his return from deployment to Iraq 3 months earlier, the captain had not slept: "When I close my eyes, I see the picture of the injured Soldier." The captain was able to sleep normally when he was helped to discover that he mistakenly believed he failed to save the injured Soldier's life by hesitating. He was able to replace that belief with the knowledge that no one could have saved the mortally wounded Soldier and that staying with the Soldiers who brought their "brother" to him was a meaningful, lasting experience for those two young Soldiers. The captain needed minimal follow-up treatment, having corrected the error in his thinking and identifying the truth of his situation and the meaningfulness he contributed to the Soldiers' "battle buddies."

Case 1: Commentary

Dr. Brown has no formal training in logotherapy, but Frankl noted that the principles of logotherapy were not exclusive; as far as these ideas contained basic truths, then individuals would discover these ideas in their own way. Brown was a psychiatrist, whose training was in attachment theory (Bowlby, 1969) and in cognitive behavior therapy (CBT). His therapeutic approach was to serve as an attachment figure for each of his patients—a steady, predictable "rock" on which they could lean as they healed. It was in reading his books that I discovered these powerful cases (in Brown, 2017a), and requested that he present them at the World Congress of Logotherapy in 2021. These narratives are detailed enough to see how he routinely appealed to meaning in the face of an unalterable fate (PTSD); in fact, it was this appeal to meaning that often created the pivotal point in healing.

[1] I have published two other books on PTSD (Brown, 2017b, c) as well as a number of YouTube videos.

In these tragic experiences, it is often vivid, graphic imagery that persists in those who report symptoms of PTSD. In this case, Brown addressed what Frankl (1984) called *hyper-reflection*—the persistent focus of the captain on the intense image of the mortally wounded comrade—and turned his attention to those who sought help. In this process, he indirectly addressed an important concept in logotherapy—that of *fate* versus *freedom* (Lukas, 2015). The captain was not free to save the life of the wounded man. Therefore, that was his fate, an area in which he had no freedom and was not *able to respond*—thus he was *not responsible* (response-able). But he did act on his area of freedom—to give support to the survivors, to those who had suffered the loss of their "battle buddy." Here the therapist refocused the captain's attention on his positive, active response in the context of the fate that befell him. In so doing, he relieved the captain from what Lukas (2015) called "unjustified guilt" (p. 164)—guilt that results from unavoidable circumstances (fate) and pointed to his fulfilment of "the meaning of the moment" (Fabry, 2013).

Case 2: "My Soldier Died in My Arms—Te amo Papa"

The command sergeant major (CSM) chose to join the Dream Interpretation Group. Small in stature, solemn in demeanor and facial expression, articulate in speech, mild in manner, he was physically exhausted from protracted insomnia. He was significantly depressed. He had a businesslike manner: a person, I deduced, unlikely to share his emotions or to value psychological phenomena.

Without visible emotion, he said:

CSM: One of my Soldiers died in my arms. Five of us were walking side-by-side. We had just left the mess hall. It was dark. An explosion… out of nowhere… seriously injured two of the five of us. We ran for the bunker, but I had to reach out and pull Suzy back into the bunker. She slumped forward in pain. I yelled for help and started CPR, but I could hear gurgling in her chest. I felt totally helpless.

A woman, not a Soldier but a civilian contractor, opened Suzy's blouse. Blood was pouring out of the left side of her chest. In Spanish, Suzy said, as she was dying, "Te amo Papa" [Tell my Papa I love him]. Suzy was one of my Soldiers… only 20 years old. It should have been me. If only I had walked in the front, it would have been me. It should have been me.

RSB: Where is it written that the injury and death should have been yours?

CSM: I just feel strongly it should have been me. It happened at the beginning of the war in Iraq, a long time ago, but it keeps coming back into my mind like a fresh memory.

We redeployed to Fort Lewis, Washington. I went to see her father in Arizona sometime later. I needed to do that for closure. Suzy's father is not American. He spoke very little English. I was able to tell him in Spanish what his daughter said before she died: "Her last words were for you: 'Te amo Papa.'" He fell to the ground; it broke him apart. He could not stop crying. The word Suzy used for "daddy" was the most intimate word in Spanish for "father."

Her high school honored her memory. The students built a 50-foot American flag design garden with flowers showing the red, white, and blue of our flag… in her honor.

I just can't get over feeling completely helpless as she died in my arms….

RSB: Are you thinking you should have saved her life?

CSM: Yes, I think that is what I have been thinking all these years. I think that is why I felt so helpless.

RSB: Could you have been there with Suzy for some other reason?

CSM: Like what…what other reason could there be?

RSB: You tell me if another reason comes to mind.

CSM: [His eyes filling with tears.] Do you mean was I there to take her message back to her father?

RSB: He will never forget you.

The Soldier wept. His depression and PTSD responded well to treatment over time. His protracted grief began to resolve when he corrected the error in his thinking and discovered the truth and meaning of the loving act of taking his dying Soldier's last words to her father.

Case 2: Commentary

This case is quite similar to the previous one, though the trauma to the Command Sergeant Major was magnified by the fact that he himself had experienced the blast and tried to save the life of one of his Soldiers, a difficult fate for anyone. In this case, differentiating between fate and freedom, resulting in a reframing of the officer's experience, was not enough—logotherapy must be uniquely applied to each unique person. His Soldier, as she died, gave him a meaning-task: "Tell my Papa I love him," one that could have been fulfilled in many ways—a phone call, a letter, a message through the casualty notification officers who convey news of the death to the family.

It is notable that Brown engaged spontaneously in a Socratic dialogue by challenging the Command Sergeant Major's assumption that he should have saved the Soldier's life. A key feature in this example is that Brown did not give him the answer, but provided the space for him to come to the realization himself. The application of logotherapy does not involve "giving meaning" to another person, but in providing the milieu in which the person can discover it.

In discussing these cases, Brown noted the confrontation of the patient's irrational beliefs in this dialogue; for example, "Where is it written that the injury and death should have been yours?" and "Are you thinking you should have saved her life?" This is a key part of cognitive behavior therapy: to challenge irrational beliefs and thoughts. Logotherapy parallels this process; as Lukas (2014) noted, the logotherapist leads the individual "gradually and purposefully, toward 'I don't have to take every nonsense from myself'" (p. 37). As Lukas noted, "The counselor seeks to change the unhealthy *I cannot because* to the healthy attitude of *I can in spite of*' (p. 37).

For this officer, his story pointed to something "left undone" that was resonating deep within. In examining the meaning of the moment—out of the entire galaxy of choices, which one was the best? (e.g., see Lukas, 2015, pp. 220–223)—he chose to visit the family to pay his respects and convey the last words of love from the Solider to the father. As Brown put it, in so doing, he "discovered the *truth and meaning* (italics added) of the loving act of taking his dying Soldier's last words to her father."

Case 3: "I Don't See How I Can Go on Like This"

The round sad Asian American face of the 26-year-old single Soldier sitting uncomfortably in front of me in my office could not have been more disheartened. Large black eyes, from which tears flowed endlessly, told me more about his sadness than his own few carefully chosen words. "Bataan" (his nickname) stood no taller than 5 feet 7 inches. His thick black hair was crew cut, short. By military standards, he might be judged somewhat overweight, but not disqualifying.

A combat medic, he did not want to recall his combat traumas, distracting himself by staying busy, avoiding reminders of combat, and preferring emotional numbness to all other human emotions. He was intelligent, articulate, and penultimately sensitive when the iron doors hiding his feelings were even slightly parted.

A month earlier, Bataan had been hospitalized for severe depression. He had suicidal thoughts and a detailed plan to end his life. He was released from the psychiatric hospital the day before I saw him. His anxiety was worse. His depression had not lifted. He still had suicidal thoughts, but he no longer had a plan to take his life.

"Every time I try to relax, my mind cannot erase my thoughts. I feel overwhelmed. I don't see how I can go on like this."

Reassuringly, I asked, "What is the 'this' you just referred to?"

To my great shock and approval, Bataan said, "Do you want to hear my story?"

By this time, I had been treating Bataan for 3 months. He had mostly talked about pain caused by stress fractures in his shins. Until today, he had no interest in talking about the inexpressible pain caused by his combat trauma.

"He Never Had Money on Paydays"

Bataan: Jack was my best friend. He was 17 and I was 18. We met at Fort Gordon, our first duty station. We were both combat medics. We became good friends. I don't know why. We were very different people. We came from very different backgrounds. Our friendship started with teasing. I always teased him about his lack of money. He never had any money, even on paydays. What do I do when I'm broke? I call my mother and dad.

"What are doing for your birthday, Jack?" He was doing nothing because he had no money. "It's your birthday, man. I have money. It'll be my treat," I said. We went out for dinner. We had a very nice time. I picked up the tab. Then we went bowling. We had a lot of fun. I picked up the tab.

That evening, Bataan learned why Jack had no money, even on paydays. Each payday, Jack sent his entire paycheck to his disabled parents who had four other children at home. He continued:

Bataan: At the end of that evening, Jack said, "Bataan, I haven't celebrated my birthday in 15 years. Thank you." That's when our friendship really started. From then on, each time we met we hugged and said, "I love you, brother."

Bataan Was on a Mission in My Office

Bataan cried in brief intervals. Each pause ended with vigorous blowing of his nose. He filled an entire small trash can next to his chair with Kleenex drenched with his tears. Each nose-blowing episode was like the end of a stanza of a mournful funeral dirge precisely played by a military band marching in cadence. Bataan was on a mission in my office. He perceived his mission, telling me his combat trauma story, as emotionally dangerous but as "mission essential."

"This is not easy," he said. "I'm afraid I'll completely lose control of myself. In the hospital, they kept telling me I had to tell my story. This is the third time I've tried to tell it."

Jack and Bataan, both in the same regiment, were deployed to Iraq from 2008 to 2009. Bravo and Alpha Companies were in the same sector in Iraq, close enough for Jack and Bataan to often meet and talk. When possible, they talked at length, once for 2.5 hours.

"I Came to Tell My Story"

Bataan's legs, by no means previously still, now really started rapidly moving up and down. From his appearance, it could have been a prisoner interrogation scene under blinding bright light. Mercilessly, the captive is demanded to disclose his secrets, but Bataan was the interrogator as well as the prisoner. Using the Soldier's nickname, I offered reassurance, suggesting he need not continue his report if he felt a later time would be less stressful.

Bataan: [In a raised voice] No. I came to tell my story today. [He continued.]

Jack was the youngest combat medic to win a CAB (Combat Action Badge). You only get that award if you have been engaged in the shooting war. Jack was the medic for Bravo Company. I was the medic for Alpha Company. Bravo Company went out on a night mission. I went to bed.

I was awakened in the middle of the night by a knock on my door. It was my Platoon Sergeant. He said, "I don't know how to tell you, Bataan, but Bravo Company was hit pretty bad. There were 3 deaths. There were scores of injuries. Jack is dead."

I didn't believe him. It must be a sick joke. "Don't fuck with me right now, Sergeant."

But this was no joke. I fell to my knees. My hands covered my face. I started throwing things around, yelling "I hate this place." My God, he was so young! I was furious! I still wanted to believe it was a joke. I kept expecting him to knock on my door. I kept expecting Jack to say, "Hey, let's go eat."

My Platoon Sergeant needed me as a medic to rush to the scene of the attack. I had to triage everybody to see who could be saved. One Soldier had disfiguring burns. We had to set up a perimeter to make sure no more attacks would take place.

[Bataan described the scene. It was too sickening and ghastly to ever be forgotten.] Bataan: "Doc, start bagging up body parts." It was an order from my Platoon sergeant.

I felt like a robot mechanically picking up anything resembling parts of a human being.

A long, silent pause filled my office. We could have been in a funeral home. Bataan was staring into space. Then he continued:

Bataan: Fifty yards away, I spotted a Soldier. There was a name tape on the flak vest [protective body armor] over an ACU [Army Combat Uniform].

I raced over to it. It was Jack's name tape. It was Jack's body. Thankfully and mercifully, he died instantly for his country.

I remember in training telling Jack I was afraid that I would fail as a medic.

Jack said, "What you wouldn't think of! You will do fine. If I can do it, you can do it, Brother."

I put Jack's body into a body bag. With help, I put the bag into the truck. I cried.

"Put those bags in the HUMWV [High Mobility Multipurpose Wheeled Vehicle, a four-wheel drive military automobile]!" the Platoon Sergeant shouted. "We only have six trucks. We will need the trucks to take the men back to our FOB [Forward Operating Base]."

I disobeyed orders. I got back into the truck and held Jack's remains all the way back to the FOB. I cried hysterically at his memorial service when they did the roll call. I cried the entire night. I cried the rest of the deployment. When I got home, I hoped they would send me right back to combat. He was such a good person to die. Every time I feel happy, I feel guilty.

Two years after Jack's death I visited [his grave]. I saw Jack's mother afterwards. We hugged for five minutes without a word. [Long pause.] I spoke on the phone to his mother. I said "I love you." She said, "I love you."

RSB: Bataan, this is the third time you have told your combat trauma story. It was not easy. It took courage to tell it today. I am honored by you to hear it. What meaning does the story have for you? [Bataan looked puzzled.] When you told your story the first two times, were you asked what the experience means to you?

Bataan: No sir, I've never thought about its meaning.

RSB: [Softly] It's the meaning we give to our experiences, Bataan, that determines their influence on us. [He pondered on my statement.] You helped him celebrate his birthday for the first time in 15 years. What can you celebrate now?

Bataan: [After a long pause] I always call his mom. I send gifts to his siblings on their birthdays. I was a bratty kid. I was given everything as a kid. [Bataan's legs were not bouncing now.]

RSB: You celebrated his birthday, what can you celebrate now?

Bataan: The Army has dedicated a Medical Aid Station to Jack.

RSB: What else can you celebrate?

Bataan: I never thought about it. [Another long pause] I can celebrate his life, but I miss him so much.

RSB: [Calmly] Jack is here in so many ways.

[Bataan looked up.]

RSB: Jack is here in you. Jack is here in his mother, his father, and in his four siblings. Jack was killed taking care of Soldiers. You picked up his remains on sacred ground. All of us need to celebrate Jack's life. Our nation needs to know the Jack you knew. Our nation needs to celebrate Jack's life. Jack showed you how to live. "If I can do it," Jack said, "you can do it, brother." That priceless encouragement came from Jack's heart.

Do not let death hold you captive. You were sent to Jack like a messenger, bringing him and his family good cheer. You brought celebration where poverty and disability held Jack and his family captive from his third birthday on. Do not let Jack's death for his country keep you from fully appreciating his life. Do not let Jack's death hold you captive. You have the spirit of generosity, Bataan. I will never forget Jack; I know him because you knew him. Jack's family will never forget you.

Sitting quietly, our stares of recognition comforted each other. "Regrettably," I said, "there are no more Kleenex left for either of us today." Bataan smiled.

Case 3: Commentary

Bataan experienced a blow of fate in the violent, sudden loss of his friend. This fate was magnified by a second cruelty—he was then required to go out into the sacred ground, where he discovered his friend's body and had to put it in a body bag. Against orders, he accompanied Jack's lifeless body—in loving arms—to the base.

Bataan was forced to transcend his own profound grief in order to provide a final act of kindness for Jack, to ensure his body was cared for in its return. Indeed, if there is a theme to this story, it is a growing brotherhood between the two Soldiers, exemplified in Bataan's spirit of giving (e.g., on his birthday and in his death).

In this case, Brown resonated with the idea of *temporality* in logotherapy, one that is presented in other chapters of this volume. Popielski, a Polish logotherapist, coined the term "*noëtic temporality*" (cited in Lukas, 2020), that is, the "place" each of us occupies in regard to our past, present, and future. Often, it is when we are fixated on our past (or the hazy, far-distant future) that we develop emotional or mental difficulties—we get "stuck," as symbolized in the story of Lot's wife in the Old Testament story in Genesis (19:24, King James Version), when she "turned to look back" and became a pillar of salt (crystallized).

Brown gently refocused Bataan's attention on his choices (his area of freedom) in the present and near future, rather than on the *tragic triad* (Frankl, 1969/1988) of the past—suffering, guilt, and/or death—which, for Bataan, was all three at once. But this was not just a refocus on the present to distract Bataan, it was pointing to a reservoir of love and meaning in his close friendship with Jack to support and connect with Jack's family members (who were also grieving). Bataan's profound loss opened a door of friendship with a whole clan; each needed the other for healing.

This love is at the heart of logotherapy; as Frankl (1984) recounted from a transcendent experience in the concentration camp:

> A thought transfixed me: For the first time in my life I saw the truth as it is set into song by so many poets, proclaimed as the final wisdom by so many thinkers. The truth—that love is the ultimate and the highest goal to which man can aspire. Then I grasped the meaning of the greatest secret that human poetry and human thought and belief have to impart: *The salvation of man is through love and in love*. (p. 37)

Reflections on Working with Veterans with PTSD

> Blessed *are* the peacemakers: for they shall be called the children of God (Matt 5:9, King James Version).

To our great misfortune, we have not learned to live at peace with each other, not even with ourselves. We have followed neither the guidance of our theologians nor our philosophers. William James (1901), both a philosopher and psychiatrist, insightfully observed in his *Varieties of Religious Experience* that "it is but giving our little private convulsive self a rest, and finding that a greater Self is there" (p. 53). When we find the Greater Self our work and our life will take on a sense of "lyrical enchantment" (p. 329). We would then be ready, as Freud and Breuer (2004) noted, to take on the common miseries of life.

Since my early childhood, I was called to be a physician and a Soldier. As my brother, 10 years my senior, wisely stated, "those ideas are silly; put them out of your head. They make no sense." After many twists and turns, a mother's prayers and her faith pollinated my life and eventually I became both a physician and a

Soldier. It was not until I was 74 years of age that the purpose of my calling was to be a physician to Soldiers. The sheer joy of fulfillment of sharing the sacred ground with suffering Soldiers confirmed my calling.

References

Bowlby, J. (1969). *Attachment and loss* (Vol. 1: Attachment). Hogarth Press.

Brown, R. S. (with Ruegsegger, G.). (2017a). *PTSD and me: Healing injured minds*. CreateSpace.

Brown, R. S. (2017b). *PTSD's a bear: A book for everyone*. Kindle Direct Publishing.

Brown, R. S. (2017c). *PTSD survival manual: The way and the truth and the life*. Kindle Direct Publishing.

Fabry, J. B. (2013). *The pursuit of meaning: Viktor Frankl, logotherapy, and life*. Purpose Research. (Original work published 1968)

Frankl, V. E. (1984). *Man's search for meaning* (3rd ed.). Pocket Books. (Original work published 1946)

Frankl, V. E. (1988). *The will to meaning: Foundations and applications of logotherapy*. Meridian. (Original work published 1969)

Freud, S., & Breuer, J. (2004). *Studies in hysteria* (N. Luckhurst, Trans.). Penguin. (Original work published in 1895 as *Studien über Hysterie*)

Lukas, E. (2014). *Meaning in suffering: Comfort in crisis through logotherapy*. Purpose Research.

Lukas, E. (2015). *The therapist and the soul: From fate to freedom*. Purpose Research.

Lukas, E. (2020). *Understanding Man's Search for Meaning: Reflections on Viktor Frankl's logotherapy (J. B. Fabry, H. T. Smith, B. Z. Hirsch, & J. O'Meara, Trans. C. L. McLafferty, Jr. Ed.). Purpose Research.*

Robert S. Brown, Sr., PhD, MD, COL (Ret. USAR) practiced psychiatry and forensic psychiatry in Charlottesville, Virginia. He was a Clinical Professor of Psychiatry and Professor of Education at the University of Virginia. He received the Distinguished Alumni Ward from UVA's School of Education and served 24 years in the US Army Reserve, volunteered during Operation Desert Storm, and taught forensic psychiatry at the Walter Reed Army Medical Center. He was awarded the Walter Reed Achievement Award by the UVA School of Medicine Alumni Association, 2017. He was also awarded the US Army Legion of Merit. He practiced military psychiatry at Fort Lee from 2005 to 2016. He was an Extramural Fellow under Aaron Beck and completed a 2-year mentorship under Judith Beck in cognitive behavior therapy (CBT). He is the author of six books, three of which focus on the effects and healing of PTSD among active-duty military. He has also produced 20 YouTube videos that focus on PTSD. Author's website: http://meaningfulwordswork.com

Charles L. McLafferty, Jr., PhD, has served on the faculties of the University of Virginia and the University of Alabama at Birmingham. He is the founder and president of Purpose Research, which seeks to incorporate meaning and purpose into the research, theory, and practice of the helping professions. McLafferty has edited and/or published more than a dozen books on logotherapy by authors such as Joseph Fabry, Elisabeth Lukas, Paul Wong, and Ann Graber. He has earned an educational diplomate from the Viktor Frankl Institute of Logotherapy (US). As a National Certified Counselor (US), he volunteered for five years at a regional crisis center as part of the National Suicide Prevention Lifeline network and for which he developed a logotherapeutic in-service training module.

Part IV
Research in Logotherapy: Empirical Studies

The Ontological Perception of Time Scale: Assessing Meaning in Life from a Temporal Perspective

Thiago A. Avellar de Aquino, Valdiney V. Gouveia, Pablo Lincoln Sherlock de Aquino, and Aureliano Pacciolla

No society can be sustainably developed without the awareness of its own civilization. Similarly, a person cannot be properly developed in society without the awareness of one's own *ontological time* (i.e., his/her personal history or place in one's life cycle). Perception, awareness, and the value of ontological time are key variables in the perception of the meaning of our lives and are essential for the normal development of a healthy and mature personality (Pacciolla, 2014).

In fact, it is possible to observe in the *Diagnostic and statistical manual of mental disorders* (5th ed., American Psychiatric Association, 2013) that in several psychopathologies time distortion is frequently present. For example, individuals who have neuroses often behave (think, perceive, and choose) as if they had failed in an earlier stage of life. Many of the psychopathological behaviors seen in adults may represent cognitive, emotional, and behavioral patterns of normal children or adolescents, as if they have been trapped in the past; other individuals with symptoms of psychopathology show a distorted ontological perception of present time, as if past or future did not exist. Individuals with some mental disorders show symptoms with an almost complete absence of roots in past; they live in the present as if it were already the future. For example, one can fear a future catastrophe as if it were already happening in the present. Thus, it seems justifiable to focus on the temporal dimension of existence for a better understanding of human perception of, especially by using the concept of meaning in life as an indicator of maturity and health (Pacciolla, 2014). The aim of this research is to gather psychometric evidence for the Ontological Perception of Time Scale (OPTS; Aquino, 2009).

T. A. A. de Aquino (✉) · V. V. Gouveia · P. L. S. de Aquino
Federal University of Paraíba, João Pessoa, Paraíba, Brazil

A. Pacciolla
Consorzio Universitario Humanitas, Rome, Italy

C. L. McLafferty, Jr., J. I. Levinson (eds.), *Logotherapy and Existential Analysis*, Logotherapy and Existential Analysis: Proceedings of the Viktor Frankl Institute Vienna 2, https://doi.org/10.1007/978-3-031-48922-8_15

Meaning in Life and Time

In recent years, the concept of *meaning in life* has acquired extensive relevance in clinical research. Instruments have been increasingly developed with the purpose of measuring and understanding its noölogical dimension. The first scale was the Purpose in Life (PIL) Test (Crumbaugh & Maholick, 1964), which defined meaning in life as "the ontological significance of life from the point of view of the individual experience" (p. 201). Subsequently, other instruments have been developed to assess the construct, such as the Life Purpose Questionnaire (LPQ) (Hablas & Hutzell, 1980), the Meaning in Suffering Test (Starck, 1983), the Logo-Test (Lukas, 1988), and the Life Attitude Profile—Revised (Reker, 1992). Moreover, in line with Frankl's theoretical framework, Steger et al. (2006) developed the Meaning in Life Questionnaire (MLQ) with two factors: Presence of Meaning and Search for Meaning, conceptualizing the meaning in life as "the sense made of, and significance felt regarding, the nature of one's being and existence" (p. 81).

Contemporary psychometric instruments have expanded the construct of meaning in life by including the dimension of human phenomena, not only the "will to meaning," but also self-distancing and self-transcendence. For example, Martinez et al. (2010) developed the Noëtic Resources Scale, which assesses six factors: Strength/Weakness, Distance from/Attachment to Self, Domination/Subjection of Self, Immanence/Transcendence, Caring/Indifference, and Self-Projection. By incorporating these dimensions, the Noëtic Resources Scale offers a more comprehensive assessment of the complex nature of meaning in life.

Frankl (2006) introduced the concept of noödynamics, which defined humans as being in "a polar field of tension where one pole is represented by a meaning that is to be fulfilled and the other pole by the man who has to fulfill it" (p. 105). This means that temporality is very important for a person to fulfill his/her obligations and become responsible. Frankl added: "In the past, nothing is irretrievably lost but everything irrevocably stored" (p. 143). Personal history is therefore an essential aspect to provide meaning in life, because the person constantly copes with the possibilities of meaning in the present, deciding actions while also considering the past and future. In fact, life flows from the past (i.e., from possibilities in the past to present realities), looking for future opportunities. Frankl noted that it is only in death that human beings lose the possibility to be, becoming one's own past, which is made up of one's essence and unicity (unrepeatability).

Despite Frankl's emphasis on the temporal perspective as a significant dimension of the concept of meaning in life, there has been limited effort to incorporate temporality into appropriate psychometric instruments. This perspective seems to be relevant in clinical settings, as it is oriented to the understanding of meaning in life as a perception built across one's lifespan. However, over the last few decades, there has been progress in this direction culminating with the development of the Ontological Perception of Time Scale (Aquino, 2009), which directly addresses this aspect.

From a psychometric perspective, the main emphasis on time perception has been provided by Zimbardo and his colleagues, stressing the importance of time orientation as a central dimension in life (Sircova et al., 2014; Zimbardo & Boyd, 1999). Previously, Reker (1992) considered a subscale that focused on time perception, assessing purpose in terms of life goals and a sense of direction from the past, in the present, and towards the future. Nevertheless, to the best of our knowledge, no specific instrument has been proposed to assess the ontological perspective of time as an independent construct.

An important contribution was made by Popielski (1994). In his findings, the concept of noëtic temporality involves the awareness of oneself as acting in and on the environment at a particular time, according to one's first-person perspective. It is distinct from autonoëtic awareness, which includes the ability to reflect upon oneself from a third-person perspective and engage in mental time travel through subjective re-experience of past events and projection into the future. His concept of noëtic temporality is closely related to the broader field of psychological time and time perception, and it is grounded in the context of human functioning and spirituality.

Ontological Perception of Time Scale

The OPTS includes three temporal dimensions as factors: Past, Present, and Future; in this scale, each category of time is measured with three items, with a General factor, composed of a single item, for assessing the temporal perspective of meaning in life. The measure was developed by Aquino (2009) in a study about attitudes towards suicide. The initial validation study was performed with undergraduate students ($N = 972$), with the scale presenting appropriate psychometric indices across a three-factor structure: [χ^2 (24) = 45.44, $p < .005$, $\chi^2/df = 1.89$, $GFI = .97$], adjusted goodness of fit = .94, comparative fit index = .98, $RMSEA = .054$, 90% CI [.029, .078]. Its reliability coefficients were considered acceptable (Past, $\alpha = .66$, Present, $\alpha = .76$, and Future, $\alpha = .75$; Kline, 2013), considering that each factor was composed by only three items. A General factor item (item 10) assesses the perception of one's life as a whole, through the following statement: "When looking to my life as a whole: I have to admit that there is a huge gap between who I am and who I could be."

Further, Pereira's (2012) study, which had a sample of 213 undergraduate students, did not find correlations between the three subscales of temporality and a measure of guilt. However, he found positive correlations between the general item and subjective ($r = .15$, $p < .05$) and temporal ($r = .23$, $p < .001$) guilt. Pontes (2012), in a sample of 115 patients with HIV/AIDS, also found positive correlations of the presence of meaning factor in the *MLQ* with scores on the OPTS on the subscales of Past ($r = .22$, $p < .05$), Present ($r = .47$, $p < .05$), and Future ($r = .51$, $p < .05$).

The Current Study

Overall, the OPTS has shown good psychometric results, highlighting temporality as a dimension of meaning in life and providing some evidence of construct validity and reliability. However, it was still premature to conclude that the scale is psychometrically adequate, as its applicability needs to be assessed through more diverse samples including participants from the general population. To provide further evidence regarding its psychometric properties, we assessed the OPTS structure through a range of analyses, while gathering evidence for its convergent validity and reliability. For this study, a mixed sample (general population and students) was considered in order to expand the applicability of the measure.

Method

Participants and Procedure

The convenience (nonrandom) sample was composed of 488 individuals (299 undergraduate students; 189 from general population) from João Pessoa, Brazil, with a mean age of 27.4 years (*SD* = 11.46; ranging from 16 to 75). Participants were mainly women (65.2%), and Catholic (65.6%). Each participant received a booklet composed of a series of instruments in a collective context (undergraduate students' classrooms), or in public spaces (general population). All participants were informed about the aims of the study as well as the voluntary and confidential nature of their participation; they signed an Informed Consent Form. On average, their participation required 20 minutes.

Measures

Ontological Perception of Time Scale As noted, Aquino (2009) developed this 10-item scale to assess the perception of Past, Present, and Future from a logotherapeutic perspective. Each category of time factor was measured by three items, and a General factor item was added for assessing one's temporal perspective in their meaning in life. Respondents were instructed to indicate their agreement with each item on a 5-point Likert scale (1 = Strongly disagree to 5 = Strongly agree). [Versions of this scale in English, German, Italian, Portuguese, and Spanish are available on request to the authors; the Appendix contains the English version.]

Meaning in Life Questionnaire (MLQ) Steger et al. (2006) constructed the MLQ with 10 items equally distributed between two factors of meaning in life: Presence of Meaning (e.g., "I have discovered a satisfying life purpose") and Search for

Meaning (e.g., "I am seeking a purpose or mission for my life"). They were rated using a 7-point Likert scale (1 = absolutely untrue; to 7 = absolutely true).

Data Analysis The study was conducted using Confirmatory Factor Analysis (CFA) with IBM SPSS Statistics, version 24.0 and Analysis of Moment Structures (AMOS) software. Good indicators were considered to be: CMIN/DF between <5; goodness-of-fit index (GFI) > 0.85; adjusted goodness-of-fit (AGFI) > 0.80; comparative fit index (CFI) > 0.90; and Root Mean Square Error of Approximation (RMSEA) < 0.08. To assess the superiority of the model, the Expected Cross-Validation Index (ECVI) and the Consistent Akaike Information Criterion (CAIC) were employed to evaluate improvements compared to alternative models. Statistically significant results indicating lower values in the χ^2 difference test, as well as lower ECVI and CAIC values, signify a better fit of the model.

Results

Factorial Structure and Reliability

Confirmatory factor analyses (maximum likelihood estimation) were used to assess the adequacy of the three-factor model underlying the OPTS, with an alternative one-factor structure. As shown in Table 1, results indicate a preference for the three-model structure, presenting a better fit. This was also corroborated when assessing the chi-squares [$\Delta\chi^2$ (3) = 146.00, $p < 0.001$], the indices of consistent Akaike information criterion, and expected cross-validation index. Figure 1 describes the three-factor solution. All factorial loadings (λs) were statistically different from zero ($\lambda \neq 0$, $z > 1.96$, $p < .05$).

The factor Past grouped three items (see Appendix for OPTS items), whose lambdas (λ) ranged from .57 to .69, presenting reliability (Cronbach's α) of .66 and homogeneity (mean inter-item correlation, $r_{i.i}$) of .39. The semantic analysis of its items confirmed that it can be named as "sense of meaning in the past." The factor Present was comprised of three items, presenting λ ranging from .66 to .73, $\alpha = .74$, and $r_{i.i} = .48$. These items clearly confirm a "sense of meaning in the present." Finally, the factor Future was also represented by three items. Its λs ranged from .59

Table 1 Fit indices for competing factorial models of the *OPTS*

Model	χ^2	*df*	χ^2/df	GFI	AGFI	CFI	RMSEA (CI90%)	CAIC	ECVI
M_1: Three-factor	98.27	24	4.10	0.95	0.91	0.94	0.08 (0.06–0.10)	249.27	0.29
M_2: One-factor	244.27	27	9.05	0.89	0.82	0.81	0.13 (0.11–0.14)	373.69	0.56

Note: *GFI* = Goodness-of-fit index; *AGFI* = Adjusted goodness-of-fit; *CFI* = Comparative fit index; *RMSEA* = Root mean square error of approximation; *CAIC* = Consistent Akaike information criterion; *ECVI* = Expected cross-validation index.

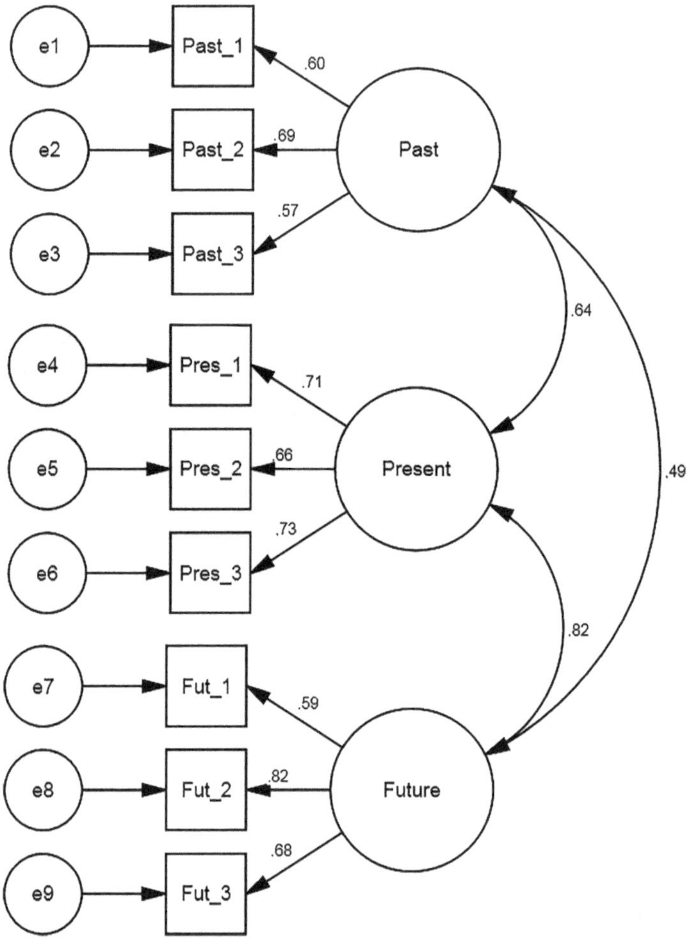

Fig. 1 Confirmatory factor analysis of the Ontological Perception of Time Scale

to .82, presenting a reliability coefficient α of .73 and homogeneity of .49. The pool of items comprising this factor corroborates the "sense of meaning in the future."

Convergent-Discriminant Validity

To assess the convergent-discriminant validity of the OPTS, we used two strategies: (a) the average variance extracted (*AVE*) (convergent validity) and comparing the square root of this variance ($\sqrt{AVE}$) with the correlation between each pair of factors (discriminant validity); and (b) correlating the three factors of ontological perception of time with the subscales of the MLQ. In the first strategy, all *AVE*s were

Table 2 Convergent validity of the *OPTS*

Indicators of meaning in life	2	3	4	5	6
1. Presence of meaning	−.47**	.29**	.55**	.48**	−.29**
2. Search for meaning		−.06	−.21**	−.12*	.26**
3. Perception of the past			.44**	.33**	.23**
4. Perception of the present				.60**	−.26**
5. Perception of the future					−.19**
6. Index of temporal perspective					

Note: *$p < .01$. **$p < 0.001$. (Two-tailed test).

higher than .50 (Past = .55; Present = .63; and Future = .63), and only the correlation between the factors (see Fig. 1) Present and Future was higher than their corresponding $\sqrt{AVE}$s, indicating limited discriminant validity of these factors. Results regarding the second strategy are presented in Table 2.

In line with the proposed theory, the three OPTS factors were positively correlated with the MLQ factor Presence of Meaning ($r_{\text{Mean}} = .44$, $p < .001$). An inverse correlation pattern was observed for the MLQ Search for Meaning factor, which was negatively correlated with the three temporal perspectives ($r_{\text{Mean}} = -.13$, $p < .05$). Nevertheless, the correlation for Past was not significant ($r = -.06$, $p > .05$). Moreover, the General Index of existential dissatisfaction was positively correlated with Search for Meaning ($r = .26$, $p < .001$), and negatively with Presence of Meaning ($r = -.29$, $p < .001$).

Discussion

This study was intended to provide further psychometric evidence of a new instrument to measure meaning in life, based on Viktor Frankl's (2006) theory. Specifically, evidence was gathered of factorial and convergent discriminant validities as well as internal consistencies (reliability and homogeneity) of the OPTS.

First, the three-factor (M_1) structure was compared with an alternative one-factor (M_2) model. Substantially, the first provided better fits, including lowest chi-square distribution, expected cross-validation index and consistent Akaike information criterion values. More importantly, the fit indices were close to those recommended in the literature (Byrne, 2010; Tabachnick & Fidell, 2013), corroborating the original findings of Aquino (2009).

The internal consistencies of the scales also presented satisfactory results. The reliability was assessed with Cronbach's alpha, and both Present and Future factors obtained values of the recommended cutoff (.70; Kline, 2013). Only the Past factor showed a marginally lower coefficient. In fact, alpha values of .60 or higher can be justified for research purposes (Peterson, 1994), as in this case. Moreover, for all the factors, the homogeneity levels (mean correlation between items by factor) were higher than .30, a recommended coefficient. So, these indicators were adequate despite the construct of past perspective, which is always perceived as more subjective as memory is susceptible to various interpretations depending on mood (Bower, 1981; Frankl, 1992). In order to minimize doubt, we computed the composite reliability for each factor, observing the following coefficients: Past, .66; Present, .74; and Future, .74, which are acceptable in expressing adequate measure consistency (Fornell & Larcker, 1981; Škerlavaj & Dimovski, 2009).

We also checked for evidence of convergent discriminant validity, using two strategies. The convergent validity of the OPTS was assessed through correlations with the factors of presence and search of meaning and through satisfactory levels of *AVE* coefficients (Fornell & Larcker, 1981; Hair et al., 2006). However, regarding discriminant validity, the factors Present and Future were strongly correlated with each other. In this case, their correlation was higher than the square roots of their *AVE*s, suggesting scarce evidence of this parameter. Yet, cognitively, one could expect that the future was a reflection on present time, which is coherent with Frankl's (2006) framework that considers the link between present and future.

Correlations between perceptions of time are consistent with Frankl's (2006) ideas; he noted that human beings act in the world according to the past (self) and change their past according to their choices in the present and future, therefore, turning any possibility into reality. The experience of existential vacuum or the frustration in the search for meaning would result in a dynamic tension between "who one is" and "who one could be." This gap is directly related to the perception of past, present, and future. In line with this, the results indicated an inverse relationship between the MLQ factor of Search for Meaning and perceived meaning of the OPTS factors of Past, Present, and Future. This is consistent with logotherapy, considering it asserts that the question of meaning emerges when people do not experience meanings. In these cases, when individuals are frustrated in their search, an existential emptiness emerges.

Future Studies, Limitations, and Conclusion

In line with Frankl's (2006) theory, we can comprehend meaning as the ontological significance of life from the point of view of the past, present, and future. Thus, the OPTS can be used as a complementary measure of meaning in life, to support the findings of Aquino (2009). For future study of this measure, three instruments could be used as reference: (1) the 14-item of the personality inventory to assess the degree of depression in the *Personality Inventory for DSM-5 (PID-5)—Adult* (Krueger et al., 2013); (2) the *PIL* (Crumbaugh & Maholick, 1964), a 20-item (Part A) to assess the degree of noögenic neurosis; and (3) the *Questionnaire on Personal Meaning (QIP)*; (Pacciolla et al., 2002), a 12-item instrument to estimate time in the context of the tragic triad of freedom and self-responsibility.

It is also important to check additional parameters of this instrument. For instance, its temporal stability (test–retest reliability) and discriminant validity regarding social desirability, which could cause bias in the participants' answers.

Additionally, it will be important to check the predictive validity of this measure with different constructs, such as the recurrence of mental disorders (e.g., depression and anxiety), as well as to explore potential correlates (e.g., human values, suicidal ideation) (Aquino, 2009).

The OPTS can offer information for psychotherapists to indicate which temporal dimension needs to be analyzed when finding new meanings and (simultaneously) to identify the origins of any existential emptiness. Furthermore, patients may become aware of their existential situation, taking temporality as a new reference, thus, broadening their horizon (Frankl, 2006). In fact, ontological time could be an important variable for diagnosis and prognosis. Addressing the ontological perception of time in psychotherapy may accelerate the healing processes. Growing up means changing over time and giving oneself the time to change.

This study was intended to identify evidence of the factor validity and internal consistency of the OPTS. Results confirmed the existence of three factors of time perception with suitable psychometric parameters in this sample. However, the sample cannot be considered representative of the general population, suggesting that future studies include broader and more diverse samples from other cultures, including from general populations and psychological/psychiatric inpatients. Finally, we believe that the OPTS can make a significant contribution to diagnosis and psychotherapy if administered along with other instruments, permitting helping professionals to understand the distortion of ontological time and indicating appropriate treatment.

Appendix: Ontological Perception of Time Scale (OPTS)—English Version

Instructions Please carefully read the following statements and, taking into account the response scale on the side, indicate to what extent you agree or disagree with each one. It is important that you consider the specific time frame (past, present, or future) and select the corresponding response alternative according to your personal experience.

	Strongly disagree	Disagree	Not sure	Agree	Strongly agree
When looking to the past:					
1. I have a sense of fulfillment with what I have accomplished.	1	2	3	4	5
2. I feel that I have evolved towards the kind of human being that I always wanted to be.	1	2	3	4	5
3. I would do everything once again.	1	2	3	4	5

(continued)

	Strongly disagree	Disagree	Not sure	Agree	Strongly agree
When looking to the present:					
4. I always see a reason to be in this world.	1	2	3	4	5
5. I feel that I am developing important tasks.	1	2	3	4	5
6. I always find a reason to wake-up in the morning.	1	2	3	4	5
When looking to the future:					
7. I see multiple possibilities to choose from.	1	2	3	4	5
8. I sense a reason to live for.	1	2	3	4	5
9. I sense that I have an ideal or a dream to be fulfilled.	1	2	3	4	5
When looking to my life as a whole:					
10. I have to admit that there is a huge gap between "who I am" and "who I could be."	1	2	3	4	5

References

American Psychiatric Association. (2013). *Diagnostic and statistical manual of mental disorders: DSM-5* (5th ed.). American Psychiatric Association.

Aquino, T. (2009). *Atitudes e intenções de cometer o suicídio: Seus correlatos existenciais e normativos* [Attitudes and intention to commit suicide: Existential and normative correlates]. Unpublished doctoral dissertation. Federal University of Paraíba, João Pessoa, Brazil.

Bower, G. H. (1981). Mood and memory. *American Psychologist, 36*(2), 129–148. https://doi.org/10.1037/0003-066X.36.2.129

Byrne, B. M. (2010). *Structural equation modeling with AMOS: Basic concepts, applications, and programming*. Taylor and Francis.

Crumbaugh, J. C., & Maholick, L. T. (1964). An experimental study in existentialism: The psychometric approach to Frankl's concept of noogenic neurosis. *Journal of Clinical Psychology, 20*(2), 200–207.

Fornell, C., & Larcker, D. F. (1981). Evaluating structural equation models with unobservable variables and measurement error. *Journal of Marketing Research, 18*(1), 39–50. https://doi.org/10.1177/002224378101800

Frankl, V. E. (1992). *Teoría Y Terapia de las Neurosis*. Herder.

Frankl, V. E. (2006). *Man's search for meaning*. Beacon Press. (Original work published 1946)

Hablas, R., & Hutzell, R. (1980). The life purpose questionnaire: An alternative to the purpose-in-life test for geriatric, neuropsychiatric patients. In *Analecta Frankliana: The proceedings of the First World Congress of Logotherapy* (pp. 211–215). Strawberry Hill.

Hair, J., Jr., Black, W., Babin, B., Anderson, R., & Tatham, R. (2006). *Multivariate data analysis* (6th ed.). Pearson Prentice Hall.

Kline, P. (2013). *Handbook of psychological testing*. Routledge.

Krueger, R., Derringer, J., Markon, K., Watson, D., & Skodol, A. (2013). *The personality inventory for DSM-5 (PID-5)-adult (Full Version)*. Retrieved from https://www.psychiatry.org/File%20

Library/Psychiatrists/Practice/DSM/APA_DSM5_The-Personality-Inventory-For-DSM-5-Full-Version-Adult.pdf

Lukas, E. (1988). Para validar la logoterapia [Validation of logotherapy]. In V. Frankl (Ed.), *La volundad de sentido* [The will to meaning] (pp. 255–284). Editorial Herder.

Martinez, E., Díaz del Castillo, J., & Jaimes, J. (2010). Validación de la prueba Escala de Recursos Noölógicos Aquí Y Ahora para personas mayores de 15 Años [Validation of the scale of noölogical resources here and now for people older than 15 years]. *Revista Argentina de Clínica Psicológica, 3*, 257–272.

Pacciolla, A. (2014). *DSM-5 e temi esistenziali* [DSM-5 y cuestiones existenciales]. Laurus Robuffo.

Pacciolla, A., Allegrucci, F., & Carucci, T. (2002). Questionario sulle capacità di produzione metaforica [Questionnaire on capacity of producing metaphor]. In A. Pacciolla, & N. Natoli (Eds.), *Metafora e psicologia* (Metaphor and psychology) (pp. 261–276). Laurus Robuffo.

Pereira, G. D. A. (2012). *A culpa e suas relações com a religiosidade e o sentido da vida* [Guilt and its relationship with religiosity and the meaning of life]. Unpublished master's thesis. Federal University of Paraíba, João Pessoa, Brazil.

Peterson, R. A. (1994). A meta-analysis of Cronbach's coefficient alpha. *Journal of Consumer Research, 21*(2), 381–391.

Pontes, A. M. (2012). *Proposta de um modelo teórico para explicar a noopsicossomática em pacientes com HIV* [Proposal of a theoretical model to explain the noösomatopsychic in patients with HIV]. Unpublished master's thesis. Federal University of Paraíba, João Pessoa, Brazil.

Popielski, K. (1994). W Kierunku Psychoterapii "o Ludzkim Obliczu": Logoterapia i nooteoria. *Roczniki Filozoficzne*, 13–31.

Reker, G. (1992). *Life attitude profile-revised manual*. Student Psychologists Press.

Sircova, A., Van De Vijver, F. J., Osin, E., Milfont, T. L., Fieulaine, N., Kislali-Erginbilgic, A., et al. (2014). A global look at time: A 24-country study of the equivalence of the Zimbardo Time Perspective Inventory. *SAGE Open, 4*(1). https://doi.org/10.1177/2158244013515686

Škerlavaj, M., & Dimovski, V. (2009). Organizational learning and performance in two national cultures: A multi-group structural equation modeling approach. In W. King (Ed.), *Knowledge management and organizational learning* (pp. 321–367). Springer.

Starck, P. L. (1983). Patients' perceptions of the meaning of suffering. *International Forum for Logotherapy, 6*(2), 110–116.

Steger, M. F., Frazier, P., Oishi, S., & Kaler, M. (2006). The meaning in life questionnaire: Assessing the presence of and search for meaning in life. *Journal of Counseling Psychology, 53*(1), 80.

Tabachnick, B. G., & Fidell, L. S. (2013). *Using multivariate statistics* (6th ed.). Allyn & Bacon.

Zimbardo, P., & Boyd, J. (1999). Putting time in perspective: A valid, reliable individual-differences metric. *Journal of Personality and Social Psychology, 77*, 1271–1288.

Thiago A. Avellar de Aquino, Ph.D. in Social Psychology. Associate Professor at the Federal University of Paraíba (UFPB–Brazil) at the Education Center; Department of Sciences of Religions; leader of the LAPLAE group: Laboratory for Research in Logotherapy and Existential Analysis (CNPq); Professor of the Graduate Program in Sciences of Religions (UFPB–Brazil).

Valdiney V. Gouveia, Ph.D. in Social Psychology. Professor of Social Psychology and President of the Federal University of Paraíba (UFPB–Brazil). Researcher on Human Values, Pro and Antisocial Behaviors, and Personality Traits. Author of the Functional Theory of Human Values.

Pablo Lincoln Sherlock de Aquino, Master in Learning Organizations. Psychologist of Student Assistance and Promotion at the Federal University of Paraíba (UFPB–Brazil). Clinical Psychologist. Organizational Logotheory researcher. Member of LAPLAE (Laboratory for

Research in Logotherapy and Existential Analysis (CNPq). Labor court expert psychologist in Paraíba–Brazil.

Aureliano Pacciolla, Doctor of Research—Ph.D. Qualifications to teach at the undergraduate, graduate, and post-graduate levels; qualifications as a psychotherapist and psycho-juridical consultant—consultant in sports psychology. Psychotherapy instructor at the following schools of psychotherapy: APC, Humanitas, Master of Criminology, Master of Psychology of Emergencies, LUM, Unisalus. Forensic expert psychologist, serving the Prosecutor and the Civil, Criminal, and Juvenile Tribunals of various cities. Expert, Ecclesiastical Tribunal of the Diocese of Rome, Italy.

The Noëtic Orientations Test (NOT): A Multiscale Russian Modification of the Purpose-in-Life Test

Dmitry A. Leontiev and Evgeny N. Osin

The Purpose-in-Life Test (PIL; Crumbaugh & Maholick, 1964) was one of the first assessment tools based on Viktor Frankl's (1969) theory of logotherapy and the will to meaning; Crumbaugh and Maholick intended to validate a number of Frankl's (1969, 1973) theoretical constructs, specifically the concepts of the *existential vacuum* and *noögenic neuroses*. Frankl asserted that the failure to find meaning in life (*existential frustration*) and the resulting feeling of meaninglessness (existential vacuum) are a cause of a specific category of mental disorders, which he termed "noögenic neuroses" (Frankl, 1973, p. xviii), which differed from traditional categories of neurotic disorders. Crumbaugh and Maholick initially planned to show that: (a) their test is a valid assessment of the extent of existential vacuum, (b) the latter is characteristic of mentally ill individuals, and (c) the presence of an existential vacuum is not indicative of mental pathology (p. 201). They defined "purpose in life," the target construct, as the experience of ontological significance of an individual's life.

The original test in its final version consisted of 20 items, in the form of a beginning statement with two opposite variants of its ending with seven preference gradations. Crumbaugh and Maholick (1964, p. 201) showed a sample item:

I am usually:

1	2	3	4	5	6	7
completely bored			(neutral)			exuberant, enthusiastic

D. A. Leontiev (✉)
HSE University, Moscow, Russia

E. N. Osin
HSE University, Moscow, Russia

Laboratory LINP2, University of Paris Nanterre, Paris, France

C. L. McLafferty, Jr., J. I. Levinson (eds.), *Logotherapy and Existential Analysis*, Logotherapy and Existential Analysis: Proceedings of the Viktor Frankl Institute Vienna 2, https://doi.org/10.1007/978-3-031-48922-8_16

The participants are instructed to circle a number that reflects the answer that is most nearly true to them. The Likert-scale items use an ascending or descending sequence of numbers (ranging from 1 to 7), with the largest number (7) always corresponding to the pole of the presence of purpose in life and the smallest one (1) to its absence. The test score is the sum of the 20 numbers circled.

Together with this formalized quantitative part A, the PIL included parts B and C. Part B consists of 13 incomplete sentences concerning the meaning and meaninglessness of life, and in part C the participant is asked to give a brief but specific account of their aspirations and purposes in life and tell how successfully they are brought into life. The authors stress that parts B and C are not necessary for research but are useful in individual work in clinical settings, provided that they are evaluated by a psychiatrist, a clinical psychologist, or a counseling psychologist (Crumbaugh & Maholick, 1981).

Crumbaugh and Maholick (1964, 1981) reported findings that showed high internal consistency, which supported the validity of the PIL. In a comparative study of five participant groups ranging from postgraduate students of Harvard Summer School (deemed to be highly purposeful) to clients of psychological counseling services and hospitalized patients with alcohol addiction ($n = 225$), the mean group scores showed a progressive decrease in PIL scores from the first to the fifth group, indicating criterion validity. The difference between clinical and nonclinical samples was significant; gender differences were not significant but notably interacted with the clinical status. Additional evidence of the validity of the PIL was demonstrated by its high correlation with the results of another questionnaire constructed by Crumbaugh and Maholick (1964) on the basis of Frankl's informal clinical interview questions, which he used to determine the degree of existential vacuum in his clinical practice. Another typical finding was the negative correlations of PIL with various measures of depression and anomie.

Further validation studies with 1151 participants from four nonclinical and six clinical groups revealed lower scores in the clinical groups with the lowest scores observed in psychotic and alcoholic patients, whereas the highest scores were found in active parishioners and successful professionals (Crumbaugh, 1968). Individuals who abused substances of various kinds also demonstrated much lower scores on the PIL than the general population (for a review of several early studies, see Frankl, 1978, pp. 26–27). PIL scores were not significantly associated with sex, age, education level, religious beliefs, or income. Frankl (1985, p. 274) interpreted these findings as a confirmation of his idea that the meaning of life can be found by any person. At the same time, PIL scores were significantly associated with the Crowne-Marlow Social Desirability scale (Crumbaugh & Henrion, 1988, pp. 80–82).

Shek et al. (1987) performed an exploratory factor analysis of the PIL test using a sample of 480 Hong Kong students with a Chinese version of the test that proved as internally consistent as the original English-language version. Five factors were singled out, which seem fuzzy from a theoretical viewpoint:

- quality of life (seven items)—the general evaluation of an individual's satisfaction with the life they live;

- the meaning of existence (six items)—the presence of meaning and purpose in life, the belief in the possibility of finding them;
- the obstacles to existence (two items)—attitude towards death and personal choice;
- Answers to the questions of existence (three items)—the possibility of finding a solution of existential problems, absence of fear, and embarrassment in front of them; and
- future life and responsibility (two items)—the attitude towards retirement and self-reported responsibility.

Various factor analytic studies using exploratory and confirmatory methods have yielded inconsistent results with over 15 different factor models published, typically finding between two and five factors (Harlow et al., 1987; Morgan & Farsides, 2009; Schulenberg & Melton, 2010; Zhang et al., 2021).

Later, Crumbaugh (1977) created a scale he considered to be complementary to the PIL, the Seeking of Noëtic Goals test (SONG) with 20 items. Crumbaugh noted that it was intended to measure the power of the motivational tendency towards seeking the meaning of life. Thus, the scale was expected to have a moderately negative correlation with the PIL score and the results were expected to be higher in clinical vs nonclinical groups. The results from his research confirmed these hypotheses.

In addition, Crumbaugh (1977) reported that the negative correlation between the PIL and the SONG was stronger in healthy subjects than in clinical groups. He explained this difference by assuming that the low level of meaningfulness of life should entail a high motivation for seeking noëtic goals. This is the case of healthy examinees; however, in clinical groups, this motivation is lower due to various pathogenic influences, thus lowering the association between the scales (pp. 903–904). An additional confirmation of the validity of the scale was the noticeable decrease of SONG scores in patients with alcohol dependence who have undergone a logotherapy course, while in the control group of patients without any logotherapeutic intervention, an opposite tendency was observed.

Russian Adaptation of the PIL

The first adaptation of the PIL test in Russian was carried out by sociologist Kuanyshbek Muzdybayev (1981), who reproduced the form of the original test without alteration, but substituted several items for different ones: Items 6, 11, 15, and 16 dealing with the topics of death or suicide were replaced with different formulations. The resulting instrument placed more emphasis on the experiences of fulfilling and purposeful life and was less heterogeneous, which was intended to allow for a clearer factor structure.

The main sociological study by Muzdybayev (1981) used a sample of 540 employees of three Leningrad factories. The item-total correlations were moderate.

PIL scores were much higher in men than in women, higher in married than in unmarried and divorced individuals; having children was also correlated positively with PIL scores. Some age differences in PIL scores were revealed with the highest scores in the age groups of 25–30 and over 50 years old, the lowest scores in under 25, and a low plateau between 30 and 50.

As the first author of this paper, I continued this work in 1986–1993 (Leontiev, 1992a, b; Leontiev et al., 1993). Muzdybayev's (1981) translation was taken as the starting point and somewhat modified, in particular:

1. The formulations of some items were simplified with their general sense retained.
2. Instead of the common beginning of the sentence with two variants of the ending, a pair of complete alternative sentences with the same beginning was formulated.
3. The asymmetrical scale (1 2 3 4 5 6 7) was changed to a symmetrical one (3 2 1 0 1 2 3) in order to facilitate the understanding of the items, to reduce the diagnostic "transparency" of the scale, and to remove the positional effects, although the procedure of calculating the sum score became more complex.

At the same time, the SONG test (Crumbaugh, 1977) was also translated into Russian. The only change as compared with the original version of the methods was in substituting the seven-point Likert scale with a five-point one ("never—seldom—sometimes—often—constantly") for convenience.

The adapted Russian PIL revealed better internal consistency compared to Muzdybayev's (1981) version and showed good test–retest reliability. Criterion validity established by comparison of a nonclinical group with several groups of patients with alcoholic and drug addiction was also in line with the theoretical expectations. An additional bonus of the modified version was a nonsignificant correlation with the social desirability measure (Leontiev, 1992a). In contrast, the Russian version of the SONG test was not reliable enough and revealed some unexpected correlations, so that the further attempts to adapt it were canceled.

Leontiev et al. (1993) conducted a special study aimed at revealing the factor structure of the Russian-language version of the test. The participants were 77 engineers from Moscow, men and women from 23 to 36 years old, most of them with a university degree. Exploratory factor analysis allowed the identification of six factors, which accounted for 64% of the variance (as compared to 53.3% in the Shek et al., 1987 study); in the latter study, the proportion was distributed more evenly across factors. Five of those six factors had loadings of .40 or more on four to six items (with some shared loadings) and allowed a very meaningful theoretical interpretation, revealing the structure of human life meaning.

Three of these five meaningful factors referred to different sources of meaningfulness, referring to temporal dimensions. Factor 1 (six items) referred to life goals, calling, and intentions (foreseen or planned future outcomes). Factor 2 (six items) referred to the actual emotional experiences of interest and emotional fullness of life (the present). Factor 3 (five items) referred to satisfaction with self-realization related to past events. It is easy to see that these three categories correlate with the goal (the future), the process (the present), and the result (the past). Indeed, one can find the meaning of life in any of these three components of life or in all of them. This confirmed Frankl's (1985) contention that the meaning of life can always be found and laid the foundation for theoretical and empirical typologies of meanings of life.

Two other factors referred to control beliefs as regards one's life. Factor 4 (four items) expressed the feeling of one's capacity of influencing the course of one's own life. Factor 5 (five items) expressed the belief that life is controllable, in principle, and allows one to make and implement one's own choice. It was not surprising, in view of previous data, that control beliefs were strongly associated with the meaning of life, but rather amazing that these two factors diverged, one of them characterizing the general belief that control is possible, and the second one reflecting the belief in one's own capacity for such a control (self-efficacy). This divergence may have been due to the historical context at the time the data were collected: Early 1990s in Russia was the time of collapse of the Soviet social order and a rather chaotic transition full of frustration, dangers, and uncertainty; most people felt unable to control their lives the way they had been able to only a few years earlier. As we will demonstrate, later, in a more stable period, these two factors converged into one.

On the basis of these results, the PIL test was transformed into the multiscale NOT, which included a general index of meaningfulness of life and five subscales reflecting three specific noëtic orientations (goals in life, fullness of life, and satisfaction with self-realization) and two control beliefs (Leontiev, 1992b).[1]

Noëtic Orientations Test: 30 Years Later

Since 1992, the NOT has become a very popular instrument in Russian-language psychological studies with over 5000 publications mentioning it as of early 2022, according to the Russian Index of Scientific Citations. Over the years, the authors have accumulated empirical data that has allowed investigation of the structure, psychometric properties of the measure, as well as demographic correlates of its scores using larger and more diverse samples.

The most important methodological work was carried out by Osin and Kosheleva (2020) and used two samples: a sample of volunteer participants who were invited to complete the measure online (N = 9876) using a popular-psychology themed website aimed at a general population (87% female and 13% male participants aged 16–64, mean age 26) and a combined sample of students and professionals who completed the paper-based version of the measure (N = 3402) as part of various research studies (65% female and 35% male participants aged 14–77, mean age 22).

[1] The Russian title, "Test smyslozhiznennykh orientatsii" translates literally into English as "Test of orientations referring to life meaning"; in different publications using the test, this name has been translated into English in varied ways. The only authorized English name is the "Noëtic Orientations Test."

One of the goals of the analysis by Osin and Kosheleva (2020) was to reinvestigate the structure of the NOT, as it had been established in a small sample and included numerous cross-loadings (seven items were assigned to two scales and one item to three scales): This could be an artifact of the orthogonal rotation used, which could undermine the discriminant validity of the subscales. To explore the structure of the measure anew, a stratified random subsample with equal proportions of male and female participants was created from the online group ($N = 2520$). The resulting structure was subsequently cross-validated in the paper-based sample ($N = 3402$). The items were modeled as ordered categorical. Given the theoretical expectation of a multifaceted single construct, bifactor models were used to separate the general dimension from the specific variance of item groups (subscales). Exploratory graph analysis identified four groups of items interpreted as a fulfilling process of life (five items), future purpose and goals (five items), satisfaction with self-realization in the past (four items), and belief in the controllability of life (four items). Exploratory factor analysis (maximum likelihood with bifactor rotation) has corroborated these findings quite well. Parallel analysis and the investigation of the scree plot have supported five dimensions. Bifactor rotation has produced a general factor and four specific factors with the same substantive interpretation. Two items with more specific content (6 and 13) only loaded on the general dimension.

For parsimony, Osin and Kosheleva (2020) opted not to include cross-loadings into the model. Apart from the general dimension interpreted as general meaningfulness of life, the model included for specific dimensions: (a) Goals (items 3, 4, 16, 16, 18 of the original 20-item scale), reflecting the presence of and commitment to important goals and purpose in life; (b) Process (items 1, 2, 5, 9, 20), reflecting the emotional experiences of interest and importance associated with one's daily activities and fulfilment; (c) Result (items 7, 8, 10, 11), reflecting satisfaction with self-realization and the evaluation of the past periods of life as productive and meaningful; and (d) Locus of Control (items 12, 14, 15, 19), reflecting belief in the possibility of carrying out one's choices and controlling the course of one's life; based on the item content, the subscales were similar, but emerged as more theoretically clear and distinct, compared to the original study of Leontiev (1992b).

The only substantial difference found by Osin and Kosheleva (2020) from the previously established structure concerned lack of separation between the aspects of locus of control related to oneself and to life in general: Instead of two different subscales, there emerged only one. The splitting of the two control scales in the initial study could be, as mentioned, an artifact caused by the specific context of the highly turbulent period in Russia immediately preceding the collapse of the Soviet Union, when the vast majority of the population felt disoriented and helpless, hardly capable to control their lives, in contrast to a few years earlier. This is why the general belief in the controllability of life and the confidence in the capacity to control one's life formed different dimensions. A few decades later, when people's lives had again become more stable and predictable, this split disappeared from the factor structure of the NOT.

Using confirmatory factor analysis, a bifactor model with one General factor and four specific factors—as noted earlier, Goals, Process, Result, Locus of

Control—showed good fit in both samples. The instrument, however, has emerged as essentially unidimensional, as 71% of the item variance was explained by the general dimension, according to the explained common variance index (Rodriguez et al., 2016), whereas the contribution of the subscales was relatively minor. The scales were highly reliable, with omega coefficients ranging from .77 to .88 for the subscales and .94 for the general dimension. The proportion of unique variance explained by the subscales was fairly modest, but substantial enough to suggest some discriminant validity (omega subscale in the .17–.26 range).

The demographic differences were investigated in the balanced online subsample ($N = 2520$). Male participants had slightly lower scores on the process ($d = .14$), result ($d = .20$), and the general index of purpose in life ($d = .12$). The differences associated with age alone (9 age groups, minimum $N = 50$) were not significant, apart from age–gender interactions indicating lower meaning for male participants aged 18–19 ($d = .34$), 24–25 ($d = .30$), and 30–34 ($d = .37$), compared to female participants. Education was positively associated with life meaning; however, this association, again, was only significant for male, but not for female participants. It should be noted that these demographic differences were all quite weak, with gender, age, and education explaining less than 1% of the variance in life meaning and it is only due to the large sample size that they could be detected. Thus, the results are consistent with Frankl's (1985) insistence that meaning can be found by any person.

Participants in the online sample ($N = 9876$) also indicated their occupation. Based on content analysis, 51 professional groups were identified (minimum $N = 25$). Professional differences were somewhat stronger, explaining nearly 5% of the variance in meaning. The highest meaning was reported by individuals working in occupations that offer more autonomy, require higher competence, and involve relationships, such as psychology, management, business, creative or performing arts, science, etc. The lowest scores were reported by individuals who identified as unemployed, housekeepers, clerks, assistants, in professions that do not require advanced training (such as cleaning), or in accounting. Nevertheless, professional differences were still quite weak compared to the individual differences, suggesting that meaning can potentially be found within any profession, with some occupations making the process only somewhat easier or more difficult.

Data from some subgroups of participants who completed other measures of meaning and well-being was used to establish convergent and discriminant validity of the NOT. Predictably, scores on the NOT were positively associated with subjective happiness ($r = .62$), positive affect ($r = .64$), satisfaction with life ($r = .62$), and negative affect ($r = -.47$). At the level of subscales, the strongest associations with positive affect and happiness were shown by the Process subscale, whereas the strongest associations with negative affect and satisfaction with life were revealed by the Result subscale.

Scores on the NOT were also positively associated with the presence of meaning scale of the Meaning in Life Questionnaire (Steger et al., 2006) ($r = .61$), which was mainly due to the Goals subscale ($r = .74$). The association of the NOT with the Search for Meaning factor of the Meaning in Life Questionnaire was not significant, apart for the Goals subscale ($r = -.15$). Predictably, the strongest associations were found with the Test of Existential Motivations (Shumskiy et al., 2017) ($r = .70$) which operationalizes Alfried Längle's (2004) model of existential fundamental motivations stemming from Frankl's theory. Predictably, the strongest association was found with the scale measuring the fourth existential fundamental motivation—Meaning ($r = .77$).

A recent validation study (Bolotova & Leontiev, 2016) used the NOT and the Sources of Meaning inventory by Schnell (2009). The Sources of Meaning embraces 25 primary scales referring to different possible sources of meaning in life; they are organized into 4 secondary (more general) scales. The inventory also includes two main scales: Meaningfulness, referring to the general experience of meaning in life, and Crisis of Meaning, referring to existential frustration and lack of meaning. In the cross-validation study of a sample of 97 university students, we found that the Meaningfulness scale of the Sources of Meaning had a significant positive correlation, whereas the Crisis of Meaning scale had a significant negative correlation ($p < .01$), with both the General factor and all the subscales of NOT. Weaker associations were also found between the NOT and specific sources of meaning (Self-Actualization, Order, Well-being).

Additional evidence in favor of validity of the NOT has been obtained in studies comparing the groups of existential psychologists (students of training programs or attendees of thematic conferences) with psychologists of nonexistentialist orientation. Several comparative studies (Leontiev & Osin, 2007; Leontiev et al., 2016) have consistently revealed higher levels of meaningfulness in groups of existential psychologists, compared to those with a nonexistentialist orientation; effect sizes varied from small to substantial.

Boniwell et al. (2010) investigated the associations of the NOT with the Zimbardo Time Perspective Inventory (Zimbardo & Boyd, 1999) in a sample of university students ($N = 289$) from three regions of Russia. Using correlation and regression, the authors found that the scores on the Process and Control subscales were most strongly predicted by the two time-perspective dimensions reflecting the attitudes towards the present (positive associations with Present-Hedonistic and negative ones with Present-Fatalistic). The scores on the Goals subscale were most strongly predicted by the Future and Present-Fatalistic (negative association) aspects of time perspective. The scores on the Result subscale were only associated with Past-Negative (negative association) and Future. The R^2 coefficients ranged from .18 to .32, suggesting a moderate proportion of shared variance with the Zimbardo Time Perspective Inventory by the NOT scales. Altogether, these findings indicate strong convergent validity of the NOT and provide some evidence of the discriminant validity of its subscales.

Conclusion

The PIL test and the NOT, developed on the foundational basis of logotherapy, remain promising research tools. They are particularly pertinent within the emerging context of eudaimonic well-being, which is commonly understood as an effortful process of self-realization in pursuit of purpose or meaning (Huta & Waterman, 2014). The aspects of the meaning of life related to the future, present, and the past provide a more complete insight into the process of self-transcendence.

Acknowledgements The paper was prepared within the framework of the HSE University Basic Research Program.

Appendices

Appendix 1: Noëtic Orientation Test Items (Back-Translated from Russian)

1. I'm usually very bored ...3 2 1 0 1 2 3... I'm usually full of energy
2. Life seems always thrilling and exciting to me ...3 2 1 0 1 2 3... Life seems completely calm and routine to me
3. I don't have definite goals and intentions in life ...3 2 1 0 1 2 3... I have very clear goals and intentions in life
4. My life seems to me extremely meaningless and aimless ...3 2 1 0 1 2 3... My life seems to me quite meaningful and purposeful
5. Every day seems to me always new and different ...3 2 1 0 1 2 3... Every day seems to me quite similar to every other day
6. When I retire, I will do the interesting things I have always dreamed of doing ...3 2 1 0 1 2 3... When I retire, I will try not to burden myself with any worries
7. My life has turned out the way I dreamed it would ...3 2 1 0 1 2 3... My life has not turned out the way I dreamed it would
8. I have not been successful in fulfilling my life plans ...3 2 1 0 1 2 3... I have accomplished much of what I had planned for my life
9. My life is empty and dull and uninteresting ...3 2 1 0 1 2 3... My life is filled with interesting pursuits
10. If I had to sum up my life today, I would say it has been quite meaningful ...3 2 1 0 1 2 3... If I had to sum up my life today, I'd say it had no meaning
11. If I could choose, I would have lived my life very differently ...3 2 1 0 1 2 3... If I could choose, I would live my life again the way I live it now
12. When I look at the world around me, it often makes me confused and anxious ...3 2 1 0 1 2 3... When I look at the world around me, it does not cause any anxiety and confusion for me
13. I am a very dutiful person ...3 2 1 0 1 2 3... I am a person who is not dutiful at all
14. I believe that a person has the ability to make life choices at will ...3 2 1 0 1 2 3... I believe that a person is deprived of the ability to choose because of the influence of natural talents and circumstances

15. I can certainly call myself a goal-oriented person …3 2 1 0 1 2 3… I cannot call myself a goal-oriented person
16. I have not yet found my mission and clear goals in life …3 2 1 0 1 2 3… I have found my mission and goals in life
17. My views on life have not established themselves yet …3 2 1 0 1 2 3… My views on life have become quite definite by now
18. I believe that I have been able to find a vocation and interesting goals in life …3 2 1 0 1 2 3… I am barely able to find a vocation and interesting goals in life
19. My life is in my hands and I control it myself …3 2 1 0 1 2 3… My life is beyond my control and it is governed by external events
20. My daily activities bring me pleasure and satisfaction …3 2 1 0 1 2 3… My daily activities bring me nothing but troubles and worries

Appendix 2: Interpretation of Noëtic Orientation Test Subscales

1. *Goals in life.* Scores on this subscale reflect the presence or absence of personally important future goals, which can give life meaning, direction, and future prospects. Low scores on this subscale even with a high general PIL score might be characteristic of a person living in the present or the past. At the same time, very high scores on this subscale may characterize not only a purposeful person, but also a dreamer whose plans are not grounded in reality and are not supported by a sense of personal responsibility for carrying them out. These two cases can be distinguished from each other by taking into consideration the scores on the other subscales.
2. *Process of life (interest and emotional fullness of life).* The content of this subscale corresponds to the popular idea that the only meaning of life is in the process of living itself. This subscale shows whether the respondent perceives their own process of life as interesting, emotionally fulfilling, and meaningful. High scores on this subscale combined with low ones on the other subscales may characterize a hedonist living for the present day. Low scores on this subscale reflect a person who is not satisfied with their own life in the present but may experience meaning thanks to recollections of the past or goals for the future.
3. *Result of life (satisfaction with self-realization).* The scores on this subscale reflect the evaluation of the past periods of life as productive and meaningful. High scores, combined with low scores on other subscales, may characterize a person living the remainder of their life, where everything important has happened in the past, which is the main source of meaning for the rest of their life. Low scores reflect a lack of satisfaction with one's self-realization and/or one's life lived in the past.
4. *Control beliefs (The mastery of life).* High scores on this subscale reflect the view of oneself as a strong personality with a sufficient freedom of choice to shape one's life in accordance with one's goals and ideas of its meaning. Low scores reflect disbelief in one's ability to control the events of one's own life.

References

Bolotova, A. V., & Leontiev, D. A. (2016). Russkoyazychnaya adaptatsiya oprosnika istochnikov smysla T. Schnell [Russian adaptation of T. Schnell's Sources of Meaning and Meaning in Life Questionnaire (SoMe)]. In D. Leontiev, & A. Fam (Eds.), *Shestaya vserossiiskaya nauchno-prakticheskaya konferentsiya po ekzistentsial'noi psikhologii, 4–6 maya 2016 g. Materialy soobshchenii* [Proceedings of the 6th National research and practical conference in existential psychology, May 2–6, 2016] (pp. 77–82). Smysl.

Boniwell, I., Osin, E., Alex Linley, P., & Ivanchenko, G. V. (2010). A question of balance: Time perspective and well-being in British and Russian samples. *The Journal of Positive Psychology, 5*(1), 24–40. https://doi.org/10.1080/17439760903271181

Crumbaugh, J. C. (1968). Cross-validation of purpose-in-life test based on Frankl's concepts. *Journal of Individual Psychology, 24*(1), 74–81.

Crumbaugh, J. C. (1977). The seeking of noëtic goals test (SONG): A complementary scale to the purpose in life test (PIL). *Journal of Clinical Psychology, 33*(3), 900–907.

Crumbaugh, J. C., & Henrion, R. (1988). The PIL test: Administration, interpretation, uses theory and critique. *International Forum for Logotherapy, 11*(2), 76–88.

Crumbaugh, J. C., & Maholick, L. T. (1964). An experimental study in existentialism: The psychometric approach to Frankl's concept of noogenic neurosis. *Journal of Clinical Psychology, 20*(2), 200–207.

Crumbaugh, J. C., & Maholick, L. T. (1981). *Manual of instructions for the purpose in life test*. Psychometric Affiliates.

Frankl, V. E. (1969). *The will to meaning*. World Publishing Company.

Frankl, V. E. (1973). *The doctor and the soul* (R. Winston, & C. Winston, Trans.). Penguin Books. (Original work published 1946 as *Ärztliche Seelsorge*)

Frankl, V. E. (1978). *The unheard cry for meaning: Psychotherapy and humanism*. Simon and Schuster.

Frankl, V. E. (1985). Logos, paradox, and the search for meaning. In M. J. Mahoney & A. Freeman (Eds.), *Cognition and psychotherapy* (pp. 259–275). Springer.

Harlow, L. L., Newcomb, M. D., & Bentler, P. (1987). Purpose in life test assessment using latent variable methods. *British Journal of Clinical Psychology, 26*(3), 235–236. https://doi.org/10.1111/j.2044-8260.1987.tb01355.x

Huta, V., & Waterman, A. S. (2014). Eudaimonia and its distinction from hedonia: Developing a classification and terminology for understanding conceptual and operational definitions. *Journal of Happiness Studies, 15*, 1425–1456. https://doi.org/10.1007/s10902-013-9485-0

Längle, A. (2004). The search for meaning in life and the existential fundamental motivations. *International Journal of Existential Positive Psychology, 1*(1).

Leontiev, D. A. (1992a). Test osmyslennosti zhizni (Purpose in life test). In *Praktikum po psichodiagnostike. Prikladnaya psikhodiagnostika* [Psychological assessment practicum: Applied assessment] (pp. 9–20). Lomonossov Moscow State University Press.

Leontiev, D. A. (1992b). *Test smyslozhiznennykh orientatsii* [Noëtic orientations test]. Smysl.

Leontiev, D. A., & Osin, E. N. (2007). Pechat ekzistentcializma: Empiricheskie korrelyaty ekzistentsialnogo mirovozzreniya [The mark of existentialism: Empirical correlates of existentialist worldview]. *Ekzistentsialnaya traditsiya: filosofiya, psikhologiya, psikhoterapiya, 1*(10), 121–130.

Leontiev, D. A., Kalashnikov, M. O., & Kalashnikova, O. E. (1993). Faktornaya struktura testa smyslozhiznennykh orientatsii [The factorial structure of Noëtic orientations test]. *Psikhologicheskii zhurnal, 14*(1), 150–155.

Leontiev D. A., Miyuzova A. E., Mospan A. N., & Osin E. N. (2016). Lichnostnye osobennosti ekzistentsialnykh psikhologov [Personality features of existential psychologists]. In D. Leontiev, & A. Fam (Eds.), *Shestaya vserossiiskaya nauchno-prakticheskaya konferentsiya po ekzistentsial'noi psikhologii, 4–6 maya 2016 g. Materialy soobshchenii* [Proceedings of the 6th National research and practical conference in existential psychology, May 2–6, 2016] (pp. 69–74). Smysl.

Morgan, J., & Farsides, T. (2009). Measuring meaning in life. *Journal of Happiness Studies, 10*, 197–214. https://doi.org/10.1007/s10902-007-9075-

Muzdybayev, K. (1981). Udovletvorennost zhiznyu, oshushenie schastya, perezhivanie smysla sobstvennogo bytiya [Satisfaction with life, subjective happiness, experiencing meaning of one's existence]. In L. A. Gordon (Ed.), *Rabochii klass SSSR na rubezhe 80-kh godov (Working class of the USSR on the verge of 1980s)* (pp. 181–198). Institute of world workers' movement of the USSR Academy of Sciences.

Osin, E. N., & Kosheleva, N. V. (2020). Test smyslozhiznennykh orientatsii: novye dannye o structure i validnosti [Noëtic orientations test: New data on the structure and validity]. *Voprosy Psikhologii, 66*(6), 150–163.

Rodriguez, A., Reise, S. P., & Haviland, M. G. (2016). Evaluating bifactor models: Calculating and interpreting statistical indices. *Psychological Methods, 21*(2), 137–150. https://doi.org/10.1037/met0000045

Schnell, T. (2009). The sources of meaning and meaning in life questionnaire (SoMe): Relations to demographics and well-being. *The Journal of Positive Psychology, 4*(6), 483–499. https://doi.org/10.1080/17439760903271074

Schulenberg, S. E., & Melton, A. M. (2010). A confirmatory factor-analytic evaluation of the purpose in life test: Preliminary psychometric support for a replicable two-factor model. *Journal of Happiness Studies, 11*, 95–111. https://doi.org/10.1007/s10902-008-9124-3

Shek, D. T., Hong, E. W., & Cheung, M. Y. (1987). The purpose in life questionnaire in a Chinese context. *Journal of Psychology, 121*(1), 77–83. https://doi.org/10.1080/00223980.1987.9712646

Shumskiy, V., Osin, E., & Ukolova, E. (2017). Psychometrics in pursuit of existence: A new version of the test of existential motivations. *Existenzanalyse, 34*(2), 123–138.

Steger, M. F., Frazier, P., Oishi, S., & Kaler, M. (2006). The meaning in life questionnaire: Assessing the presence of and search for meaning in life. *Journal of Counseling Psychology, 53*(1), 80–93. https://doi.org/10.1037/0022-0167.53.1.80

Zhang, L., Lin, J., Liu, K., Cai, Y., & Tu, D. (2021). Factor structure and psychometric properties of the purpose in life test (PIL) in a sample of Chinese college students: An application of confirmatory factor analysis and item response theory. *Current Psychology, 42*, 11049–11068. https://doi.org/10.1007/s12144-021-02356-5

Zimbardo, P., & Boyd, J. (1999). Putting time in perspective: A valid, reliable individual-differences metric. *Journal of Personality and Social Psychology, 77*, 1271–1288.

Dmitry A. Leontiev, PhD, DrSc, is a tenured professor of psychology and head of the International Laboratory of Positive Psychology of Motivation and Personality at the Higher School of Economics, Moscow, Russia. He strives to integrate existentialist approaches to the human person with a culturalhistorical activity theory approach and synergetic views on human self-regulation and self-organization in the research domain of positive psychology. Both his PhD and habilitation works were focused on the problem of personal meaning. He is the author of over 600 publications in Russian, including book titles such as Psychology of Personal Meaning, Personality Potential: Structure and Assessment, Psychology of Choice, Hardiness and its Assessment, and over 80 publications in English, including the edited books Motivation, consciousness, and self-regulation and Positive psychology in search for meaning. Dmitry is a recipient of the Promotional Award of Viktor Frankl Foundation of the city of Vienna (2004), honorary lifetime member of Society for Logotherapy and Existential Analysis of the Viktor Frankl Institute (Vienna), and national representative of Russia in European Network of Positive Psychology.

Evgeny N. Osin, Ph.D., from Moscow State University and a professional degree in Existential Analysis from HSE University. He has taught positive psychology at HSE University and the University of Paris Nanterre. His research combines existential psychology, positive psychology, and psychometrics, focusing on the meaning of life, alienation, and existential aspects of well-being.

Life Meaning Versus Intelligence: An Analysis of Three Qualities of Meaning Among Gifted Adults

Bernadette Vötter and Tatjana Schnell

"Nothing in this world can empower a person more to overcome exterior difficulties or interior trouble than an awareness of having a purpose in life" (Frankl, 1942–1944). Based on the recent evidence from our project on meaning in life among the highly gifted (Pollet & Schnell, 2017; Schnell, 2021; Vötter & Schnell, 2019a, b), we propose that gifted adults might find it taxing to experience meaning in life. Following Frankl's quote, this means that individuals who are gifted might have particular problems overcoming difficulties, exterior or interior. Thus, this research aimed to shed light on the meaning in life among gifted adults who are hypothesized to bear a higher risk of suffering from an existential crisis.

To date, no universally accepted definition of giftedness exists. However, one widely used approach to distinguish gifted individuals from the rest of the population is to use the results of an IQ test. Thus, individuals who reach or surpass the 98th percentile can be classified as highly intellectually gifted (e.g., Bortz & Weber, 2005; Rost, 2013; Wirthwein & Rost, 2011a). As an alternative to this criterion of high general intelligence, giftedness is often operationalized as superior (academic) achievement or performance (e.g., Preckel & Vock, 2020; Rost, 2013; Wirthwein & Rost, 2011b; Ziegler & Raul, 2000). The present study takes both approaches into account when exploring the distribution of different qualities of meaning among gifted adults.

Regarding psychosocial and emotional characteristics of gifted individuals, two diverging assumptions have emerged: the harmony hypothesis versus the disharmony hypothesis (e.g., Baudson, 2016; Neihart, 1999). The former postulates that

B. Vötter (✉)
Institute of Psychology, University of Innsbruck, Innsbruck, Austria

T. Schnell
Institute of Psychology, University of Innsbruck, Innsbruck, Austria

MF Specialized University, Oslo, Norway

C. L. McLafferty, Jr., J. I. Levinson (eds.), *Logotherapy and Existential Analysis*, Logotherapy and Existential Analysis: Proceedings of the Viktor Frankl Institute Vienna 2, https://doi.org/10.1007/978-3-031-48922-8_17

the gifted are similar or even superior to their nongifted peers with regards to these characteristics (e.g., Mönks, 1963; Plucker & Callahan, 2008; Terman, 1925). However, the hypothesized higher risk of crisis of meaning among the gifted could be evidence for the converse disharmony hypothesis, which postulates that gifted individuals have an increased vulnerability as well as a higher risk of the development of disorders (e.g., Neihart, 1999).

Qualities of Meaning

Schnell (2009, 2010) has classified three qualities of meaning: meaningfulness, crisis of meaning, and existential indifference. A *meaningful life* is experienced as a fundamental sense of meaning, based on an appraisal of one's life as coherent, significant, directed, and belonging (Schnell, 2009). It is related to a plethora of resources and indicators of health as well as well-being, and eudaimonic well-being in particular (Park, 2010; Roepke et al., 2014; Schnell, 2021; Vos, 2016; Winger et al., 2016). In contrast, individuals who suffer from a *crisis of meaning* judge their lives as frustratingly empty. They often experience anxiety and depression; they report low degrees of life satisfaction, resilience, self-efficacy, and self-regulation (Damásio & Koller, 2015; Hanfstingl, 2013; Sørensen et al., 2019). Moreover, crisis of meaning has been found to be a strong predictor of suicidality among youth, comparable to the predictive power of depression (Schnell et al., 2018). The third measurable quality of meaning in life is known as *existential indifference*, a state that is characterized by an absence of meaningfulness and absence of crisis of meaning (Schnell, 2010). Existential indifference is comparable with Frankl's (1955) state of an "existential vacuum," which is classified by a lack of commitment to values. Individuals who are classified as existentially indifferent are in general content with their lives. They do not report significant degrees of distress, even though they have a low internal locus of control and do not believe their actions to have relevant consequences (Schnell, 2010). They are further characterized by generally low commitment, particularly low degrees of self-knowledge and self-transcendence (Damásio et al., 2013; Schnell, 2021).

Hypotheses

Earlier studies have linked giftedness to self-criticism, hypersensitivity, and perfectionism (Brackmann, 2010; Holahan & Holahan, 1999; Miller et al., 2009; Silverman, 1999), as well as a vulnerability to depression (Jackson & Peterson, 2003; Wraw et al., 2016). *Self-criticism* refers to feelings of worthlessness, failure, shame, and critical self-examination (Beutel et al., 2004). It has been linked to low social support; for example, parental rejection, a strict parenting style (Zuroff et al., 1994), as well as introversion, an avoiding attitude towards social interactions, perfectionism, and neuroticism (Beutel et al., 2004). *Hypersensitivity* is characterized by a heightened sensory processing sensitivity (Aron & Aron, 1997). Highly sensitive people process and respond to social as well as environmental stimuli more intensely, are easily overstimulated, and/or show stronger (positive and negative) emotional, and empathic responses (Acevedo et al., 2014; Aron & Aron, 1997; Aron et al., 2012). *Perfectionism* refers to dysfunctional perfectionistic attitudes paired with hyper-conscientiousness; for example, negative reactions to mistakes, performance-based self-evaluation, concerns about doing things in the right way, and the aspiration to the self to be perfect as well as accurate (Flett & Hewitt, 2015; Frost et al., 1990). These traits hamper a positive outlook on life, draw attention to others' and one's own deficiencies as well as shortcomings. Hyper-reflection might thus be amplified, a form of excessive attention to oneself which was described by Frankl (1985) as a major cause for neurosis.

We proposed that these traits would be particularly frequent among those gifted individuals who were suffering from a crisis of meaning, especially because a crisis of meaning is associated with depression, low degrees of resilience, and self-regulation (Damásio & Koller, 2015; Hanfstingl, 2013). Additionally, we hypothesized that those among the gifted population who experienced their lives as meaningful were more resilient, that is, able to bounce back and recover quicker from adversity (Leppert et al., 2008), and might therefore be less affected by the traits mentioned above. Thus, differences between the three qualities of meaning pertaining to resilience, perfectionism, depression, self-criticism, and hypersensitivity were analyzed. Furthermore, associations between the qualities of meaning and school experiences as well as aspects of family life were examined, since these factors are known to be important dimensions for general life satisfaction and well-being in the lives of the gifted (Ash & Huebner, 1998).

Throughout the following three studies, we examined if gifted individuals experienced lower levels of meaningfulness and more crises of meaning compared to a nongifted population. Therefore, the distribution of the three qualities of meaning—meaningfulness, crisis of meaning, and existential indifference—among the gifted and a control group from the general population were analyzed. Furthermore, we aimed to investigate whether the aforementioned internal and external factors—which are assumed to be of particular significance for the gifted population—differed within the three qualities of meaning.

Study I: Experiences of Meaning in Intellectually Gifted and High Academic Achievers

The aim of the first study was to examine the distribution of the three qualities of meaning among two preselected gifted samples: highly intellectually gifted (HIQ) and high academic achievers (HAA). Furthermore, differences in resilience, hypersensitivity, subjective well-being, as well as positive family and school experiences were analyzed for both groups based on the three qualities of meaning.

Method

Participants and Procedure Gifted participants were recruited through two main sources. Firstly, the HIQ group was recruited through a link to an online survey which was transmitted to members of the German and Austrian high IQ society Mensa. All recipients had already participated in a previous study (Pollet & Schnell, 2017) and given their permission to be contacted for a follow-up study. Of these, 100 members of Mensa participated. Since an IQ of at least 130 is a premise to qualify as a member of Mensa, this group can be classified as intellectually gifted (e.g., Preckel & Vock, 2020).

Secondly, we recruited the HAA group by contacting Austrian academic award winners who obtained their doctorate *sub auspiciis praesidentis rei publicae.* This is the highest possible academic honor one can achieve in Austria up to PhD level. To qualify, all grades from high school up to the end of tertiary education must be excellent, and thus, the candidate has to have graduated with highest honors at every level. Again, all contacted individuals had participated in a previous study (Pollet & Schnell, 2017) and had given their permission to be contacted for a follow-up study; 52 of them agreed to participate.

Among the HIQ sample (55 women, 45 men, M_{age} = 43 years, age range: 24–63 years), 25% were single, 22% were in a relationship, 51% were married, and 2% were divorced. Two percent of the sample had completed general education, 4% had completed an apprenticeship or vocational secondary school, 19% were high school graduates, 62% had graduated from university, and the remaining 13% were holders of a doctoral degree.

Among the HAA sample (18 women, 34 men, M_{age} = 57 years, age range 32–87 years), 6% were single, 11% were in a relationship, 77% were married, and 6% were divorced. All HAA participants held a doctoral degree.

Until recently, German-speaking countries were skeptical about surveying race or ethnicity, as this might encourage essentializing and exclusionary categorization (Baumann et al., 2018). Race or ethnicity was therefore not surveyed in the present studies.

Measures *Meaning in life* was assessed by the German version of the respective scales for meaningfulness and crisis of meaning of the Sources of Meaning and Meaning in Life Questionnaire (SoMe; Schnell, 2009; Schnell & Becker, 2007). They provide independent and reliable assessments of both meaningfulness (α = .78–.81) and crisis of meaning (α = .94–.95). Each participant was assigned to one of the three qualities of meaning (meaningful, crisis of meaning, existential indifferent) by using a combination of these two scales. Schnell (2010) recommended the following computation: (a) individuals who tended to agree with the items of the meaningfulness scale ($M \geq 3$) and to disagree with the crisis of meaning items ($M < 3$) were classified as experiencing their lives as meaningful; (b) those who reported reverse values were classified as suffering from a crisis of meaning; and (c) individuals who disagreed ($M < 3$) on both scales were classified as existentially indifferent.

Resilience was assessed by the German version of the Resilience Scale, Short Form (RS-13; Leppert et al., 2008; $\alpha = .81–.89$). It measures an individual's ability to cope with and bounce back from adversity. *Hypersensitivity* was measured by the German version of the High Sensory Processing Scale (HSP; Körnung, 2015; $\alpha = .85–.87$), which assesses an individual's sensory processing sensitivity. *Subjective well-being* was assessed by means of the five-item World Health Organization Well-Being Index in its German version (WHO-5; Brähler et al., 2007; $\alpha = .80–.82$). The scale measures a subjective account of well-being, based on positive mood and vitality. *School and family experiences during childhood* were assessed by a German version of the Child and Youth Resilience Measure (CYRM-28; Liebenberg et al., 2012; $\alpha_{family} = .88$; $\alpha_{school} = .59–.75$), which explores individual and communal resources in school and family life that may support resilience. Additionally, two single-item measures were included to assess a retrospective evaluation of school experiences: (1) We asked participants to rate the demands put on them during their years in school as either (a) unchallenging, (b) adequately demanding, or (c) overextending; and (2) we also asked if their intellectual potential had been (a) unnoticed, (b) appreciated, or (c) appreciated and promoted.

Analysis Descriptive and inferential statistical analyses were performed with IBM SPSS Statistics, version 24.0 (IBM Corporation, 2016).

Results

Descriptive Statistics Descriptive statistics (Pearson correlations, means, standard deviations, and scale reliabilities of all variables) for both groups are shown in Table 1. Multivariate analysis of covariance (MANCOVA) was conducted to test for group differences (HIQ versus HAA) within the observed variables using Wilks' lambda (Λ). Demographics (age and gender) were included as covariates. A statistically significant main effect (Tabachnick & Fidell, 2013) was found for the group variable, $\Lambda = .651$, $F(7, 142) = 10.86$, $p < .001$, $\eta^2 = .349$, gender, $\Lambda = .766$, $F(7, 142) = 6.21$, $p < .001$, $\eta^2 = .234$, and age, $\Lambda = .897$, $F(7, 142) = 2.34$, $p = .027$, $\eta^2 = .103$. Between-subjects effects were significant for the following variables: meaningfulness, $F(1, 148) = 10.60$, $p = .001$, $\eta^2 = .067$, crisis of meaning, $F(1, 148) = 7.44$, $p = .007$, $\eta^2 = .048$, positive family experiences, $F(1, 148) = 32.29$, $p < .001$, $\eta^2 = .179$, and positive school experiences, $F(1, 148) = 60.56$, $p < .001$, $\eta^2 = .290$. Thus, the HAA group showed higher levels of meaningfulness, lower levels of crisis of meaning, and more positive family as well as school experiences than the HIQ group. No significant group differences were found for the following variables: subjective well-being, $F(1, 148) = 2.47$, $p = .118$, $\eta^2 = .016$, resilience, $F(1, 148) = 2.03$, $p = .156$, $\eta^2 = .014$, and hypersensitivity, $F(1, 148) = 0.91$, $p = .343$, $\eta^2 = .006$.

Table 1 Correlations, means, standard deviations, and reliabilities

	1. MF		2. CoM		3. RES		4. HS		5. SWB		6. PFE		7. PSE	
	HIQ	HAA	HIQ	HAA	HIQ	HAA	HIQ	HAA	HIQ	HAA	HIQ	HAA	HIQ	HAA
1. MF	(.78)	(.81)												
2. CoM	−.62***	−.63***	(.94)	(.95)										
3. RES	.43***	.67***	−.46***	−.70***	(.81)	(.89)								
4. HS	.09	.01	.21*	.10	−.25*	−.14	(.87)	(.85)						
5. SWB	.56***	.59***	−.62***	−.59***	.58***	.67***	−.23*	−.13	(.82)	(.80)				
6. PFE	.24*	.05	−.17	.00	.24*	−.01	.22*	.05	.36***	.25	(.88)	(.88)		
7. PSE	.08	.31*	−.05	−.11	.09	.19	−.15	.07	.10	.26	.36***	.38**	(.75)	(.59)
M	2.74	3.58	1.34	0.41	4.34	4.67	4.48	4.15	2.71	3.32	2.20	3.51	2.59	3.93
M_{diff}*	***		***		**		*		***		***		***	
SD	1.01	1.02	1.33	0.89	0.72	0.82	0.81	0.72	0.88	0.84	1.25	1.05	0.97	0.71

Note: *HIQ* Highly Intellectually Gifted ($N = 100$), *HAA* High Academic Achievers ($N = 52$). M_{diff}* significance level of mean difference. *$p < .05$, **$p < .01$, ***$p < .001$; Cronbach's alphas are provided in parentheses on the diagonal. *MF* meaningfulness, *CoM* crisis of meaning, *RES* resilience, *HS* hypersensitivity, *SWB* subjective well-being, *PFE* positive family experiences, *PSE* positive school experiences

Correlational results indicated that meaningfulness was positively related with resilience and subjective well-being. Retrospectively elicited positive family experiences were positively associated with meaningfulness only among the HIQ group, whereas positive school experiences were positively related to meaningfulness in the HAA group. In both groups, resilience and subjective well-being were inversely related to crisis of meaning. Hypersensitivity did not show a significant relation to meaningfulness in either group, but was positively related to crisis of meaning in the HIQ group.

The retrospective evaluation of school experiences showed the following results for the HIQ group: 74% reported that school was unchallenging, 20% felt adequately challenged, and 6% experienced demands in school as overextending. Moreover, 59% reported that their intellectual potential had not been noticed, 35% experienced appreciation, and 6% reported that their potential was appreciated and promoted during school years. In contrast, 21% of the HAA group experienced school years as unchallenging, whereas 77% felt adequately challenged, and only 2% reported overextending demands during school years. Additionally, 10% reported that their intellectual potential had not been noticed, 46% experienced appreciation, and 44% reported that their potential was appreciated and promoted during school years.

Distribution of the Qualities of Meaning To explore the distribution of the three qualities of meaning among the gifted populations, we utilized a combination of the meaningfulness and crisis of meaning scales as explained in the Method section. Results showed that 41% of the HIQ group experienced their lives as meaningful, 15% suffered from a crisis of meaning, and 44% were classified as existentially indifferent. In contrast, 71% of the *HAA* group experienced their lives as meaningful, 6% suffered from a crisis of meaning, and 23% were classified as existentially indifferent.

Differences Between the Qualities of Meaning Multivariate analyses of covariance (MANCOVA) were conducted using Wilks' lambda (Λ) to test the hypotheses that resilience, hypersensitivity, subjective well-being, as well as positive family and school experiences differed based on the three qualities of meaning. Age and gender were included as covariates.

Analyses Among the HIQ Group A statistically significant main effect was obtained for the three qualities of meaning, $\Lambda = .58$, $F(10, 182) = 5.68$, $p < .001$, $\eta^2 = .24$ and gender, $\Lambda = .66$, $F(5, 91) = 9.23$, $p < .001$, $\eta^2 = .34$. Additionally, post-hoc analyses (Bonferroni) were performed to examine mean differences across the three qualities of meaning and the other variables. Bonferroni corrected post-hoc comparisons indicated that there were significant mean differences (see Table 2) in subjective well-being, $F(2, 95) = 26.16$, $p < .001$, $\eta^2 = .36$, resilience, $F(2, 95) = 6.24$, $p = .003$, $\eta^2 = .12$, and positive family experience scores, $F(2, 95) = 4.41$, $p = .015$, $\eta^2 = .09$ between the three qualities of meaning. Thus, HIQ participants who experienced a meaningful life showed significantly higher resilience scores compared to

Table 2 Means and standard deviations of the observed variables, clustered by the qualities of meaning

	Highly Intellectually Gifted (HIQ)			High Academic Achievers (HAA)		
	MF	CoM	EI	MF	CoM	EI
RES	4.63* (0.65)	4.08* (0.66)	4.15* (0.72)	4.91* (0.56)	2.28* (0.44)	4.53* (0.48)
HS	4.56 (0.83)	4.69 (0.78)	4.34 (0.80)	4.15 (0.68)	4.27 (0.62)	4.15 (0.90)
SWB	3.26* (0.75)	1.84* (0.71)	2.49* (0.71)	3.52* (0.72)	1.33* (0.12)	3.20* (0.59)
PFE	2.55* (1.46)	1.75* (0.82)	2.03 (1.09)	3.50 (1.08)	3.87 (0.42)	3.47 (1.10)
PSE	2.61 (0.90)	2.70 (1.01)	2.54 (1.04)	4.09* (0.50)	3.56 (0.48)	3.50* (1.07)

Note: *$p < .05$. *MF* meaningfulness, *CoM* crisis of meaning, *EI* existentially indifferent, *RES* resilience, *HS* hypersensitivity, *SWB* subjective well-being, *PFE* positive family experiences, *PSE* positive school experiences

those who had a crisis of meaning ($p = .035$) or those who were classified as existentially indifferent ($p = .005$). Moreover, those among the HIQ group who experienced meaningful lives had significantly higher subjective well-being scores than both other meaning types ($p < .001$). Additionally, those who were classified as existentially indifferent experienced significantly more subjective well-being than those who suffered from a crisis of meaning ($p = .013$). HIQ participants who classified as meaningful reported significantly higher scores for positive family experiences during childhood than those who suffered from a crisis of meaning ($p = .32$). Furthermore, results indicated that there were significant differences between men and women regarding hypersensitivity, $F(1, 95) = 26.87$, $p < .001$, $\eta^2 = .22$, subjective well-being, $F(1, 95) = 11.82$, $p = .001$, $\eta^2 = .11$, and positive family experiences, $F(1, 95) = 10.65$, $p = .002$, $\eta^2 = .10$. Thus, hypersensitivity scores of HIQ females ($M = 4.82$, $SD = .76$) were significantly higher than those of HIQ males ($M = 4.07$, $SD = .67$). Whereas, subjective well-being ($M = 2.48$, $SD = 0.86$) and positive family experience scores ($M = 1.90$, $SD = 1.29$) among HIQ females were significantly lower than those among HIQ males (SWB: $M = 2.98$, $SD = 0.84$; PFE: $M = 2.56$, $SD = 1.11$).

Analyses Among the HAA In the HAA group, a statistically significant main effect was obtained for the three qualities of meaning, $\Lambda = .33$, $F(10, 86) = 6.37$, $p < .001$, $\eta^2 = .43$ and age $\Lambda = .72$, $F(5, 43) = 3.41$, $p = .011$, $\eta^2 = .28$. Furthermore, Bonferroni-corrected post-hoc comparisons indicated that there were significant differences (see Table 2) in resilience, $F(2, 47) = 30.96$, $p < .001$, $\eta^2 = .57$, subjective well-being, $F(2, 47) = 13.57$, $p < .001$, $\eta^2 = .37$, and positive school experience scores $F(2, 47) = 3.81$, $p = .029$, $\eta^2 = .14$ between the three qualities of meaning, but differences in hypersensitivity and family experiences were not significant. Thus, HAA who suffered from a crisis of meaning showed significantly lower scores in resilience than those who experienced their lives as meaningful ($p < .001$) and those who were classified as existentially indifferent ($p < .001$). A similar direction was found regarding the subjective well-being scores: Those who suffered from a crisis of meaning showed significantly lower scores on subjective well-being than those who experienced their lives as meaningful ($p < .001$) and those who were classified as existentially indifferent ($p = .001$). HAA who experienced a meaningful life reported better school experiences than those who were classified as existentially indifferent ($p = .036$). Furthermore, there was a significant association between age and subjective well-being, $F(1, 47) = 12.16$, $p = .001$, $\eta^2 = .21$ in that subjective well-being increased with age.

Study II: Experiences of Meaning in a Nonpreselected Gifted Sample

The aim of the second study was to investigate the distribution of the three qualities of meaning in a nonpreselected gifted sample. Again, we analyzed differences in resilience, perfectionism, depression, self-criticism, and subjective well-being based on the three qualities of meaning.

Method

Participants and Procedure Participants ($N = 519$) were invited to an online survey via a university mailing list and social media channels. Data collection took place between May and June 2017. The questionnaire included a standardized measure of intelligence, the multiple-choice vocabulary intelligence test in its German version (MWT-B; Lehrl, 2005), allowing us to identify a nonpreselected gifted group high ($\geq$ 130) in crystallized—verbal—intelligence (HVIQ; $N = 65$, 40 women, 25 men, $M_{age} = 38$, age range = 18–70). Crystallized intelligence is the ability to put acquired knowledge to use (e.g., vocabulary). Twenty-five percent of the respondents were single, 49% were in a relationship, 23% were married, and 3% were divorced. Three percent of the sample had general education, 26% were high school graduates, 62% had graduated from university, and the remaining 9% were holders of a doctoral degree. Eighty-eight percent of the participants had a verbal IQ score between 130 and 140; the remaining 12% had a verbal IQ score higher than 140. As noted in Study I, ethnicity/race was not assessed.

Measures Three of the measures were the same as in Study 1: *Meaningfulness and crisis of meaning*, SoMe (Schnell, 2009; Schnell & Becker, 2007), *subjective well-being*, WHO-5 (Brähler et al., 2007), and *resilience*, RS-13 (Leppert et al., 2008).

Perfectionism was measured by the German version of the Multidimensional Perfectionism Scale (MPS-F; Altstötter-Gleich & Bergemann, 2006; $\alpha = .88$), which measures dysfunctional perfectionistic attitudes; for example, negative reactions to mistakes, performance-based self-evaluation, and concerns about doing things in the right way.

Depression was assessed by the German version of the NEO Personality Inventory—Revised (NEO-PI-R; Ostendorf & Angleitner, 2004; $\alpha = .88$), which operationalizes depression as a facet of neuroticism. It is characterized by feelings of severe despondency, sadness, and inadequacy as well as a lack of energy and the tendency to blame oneself. *Self-criticism* was assessed by the German version of the Depression Experiences Questionnaire (DEQ; Beutel et al., 2004; $\alpha = .77$), which measures a self-critical or introjective depression with feelings of worthlessness, failure, shame, and critical self-examination.

Analysis Descriptive and inferential statistical analyses were conducted with IBM SPSS Statistics, version 24.0 (IBM Corporation, 2016).

Results

Descriptive Statistics Descriptive statistics (Pearson correlations, means, standard deviations, and scale reliabilities for all variables) are shown in Table 3. Meaningfulness was positively associated with resilience and subjective well-being, and negatively with depression. Perfectionism and self-criticism were not significantly correlated with meaningfulness, but had a significant positive association with crisis of meaning. Resilience and subjective well-being were inversely related to crisis of meaning. Conversely, depression was much higher when crisis of meaning was high.

Table 3 Correlations, means, standard deviations, and reliabilities

Variables	1. MF	2. CoM	3. RES	4. PERF	5. DEP	6. SCri	7. SWB
1. MF	(.75)						
2. CoM	−.58**	(.92)					
3. RES	.41**	−.60**	(.84)				
4. PERF	−.19	.46**	−.45**	(.88)			
5. DEP	−.32*	.73**	−.60**	.64**	(.88)		
6. SCri	−.13	.57**	−.51**	.61**	.80**	(.77)	
7. SWB	.53**	−.64**	.63**	−.43**	−.63**	−.52**	(.80)
M	3.07	1.23	4.31	2.46	2.55	3.03	2.89
SD	1.02	1.25	0.79	0.58	0.58	1.17	0.77

Note: $N = 65$. $^*p < .05$, $^{**}p < .001$; Cronbach's alpha provided in parentheses on the diagonal. *MF* meaningfulness, *CoM* crisis of meaning, *RES* resilience, *PERF* perfectionism, *DEP* depression, *SCri* self-criticism, *SWB* subjective well-being

Table 4 Means and standard deviations of the observed variables, clustered by the qualities of meaning

	Meaningfulness	Crisis of meaning	Existentially indifferent
Depression	2.33* (0.81)	3.67* (0.98)	2.63 (0.96)
Subjective well-being	3.11* (0.67)	2.13* (0.82)	2.70 (0.76)
Resilience	4.53* (0.66)	3.55* (1.14)	4.15 (0.75)
Perfectionism	2.38 (0.54)	2.91 (0.69)	2.49 (0.60)
Self-criticism	2.91 (1.09)	3.98 (1.10)	2.98 (1.24)

Note: $N = 65$; $*p < .05$

Distribution of the Qualities of Meaning To explore the distribution of the three qualities of meaning, we again utilized a combination of the meaningfulness and crisis of meaning scales as noted in the Method section of Study I. Results indicated that 59% of the HVIQ group experienced their lives as meaningful, 9% suffered from a crisis of meaning, and 32% were classified as existentially indifferent.

Differences Between the Qualities of Meaning A multivariate analysis of covariance (MANCOVA) was conducted using Wilks' lambda (Λ) to test for differences between the three qualities of meaning with regard to resilience, perfectionism, self-criticism, and subjective well-being. Age and gender were included as covariates. Means and standard deviations within the qualities of meaning are presented in Table 4. A statistically significant main effect was obtained for age, $\Lambda = .80$, $F(5, 56) = 2.74$, $p = .028$, $\eta^2 = .20$. Additionally, Bonferroni-corrected post hoc comparisons indicated that there were significant differences in depression, $F(2, 60) = 4.07$, $p = .022$, $\eta^2 = .12$ and subjective well-being scores, $F(2, 60) = 3.91$, $p = .025$, $\eta^2 = .16$ between the three qualities of meaning. Thus, gifted individuals who experienced a meaningful life showed significantly lower scores in depression compared to those who suffered from a crisis of meaning ($p = .018$). Moreover, compared to those who suffered from a crisis of meaning, individuals who experienced meaningful lives had significantly higher subjective well-being scores ($p = .045$) and reported more resilience, $F(2, 60) = 3.09$, $p = .053$, $\eta^2 = .09$. Finally, the data suggested a positive relationship between age and depression, $F(1, 60) = 6.34$, $p = .003$, $\eta^2 = .14$.

Study III: Experiences of Meaning in the General Population

The aim of the third study was to investigate the distribution of the three qualities of meaning in a control group taken from the general population. In a final step, differences between the distribution of the qualities of meaning across all four groups (from Study I to Study III) were analyzed.

Method

Participants and Procedure Participants ($N = 134$, 59 women, 75 men, $M_{age} = 47$, age range = 18–83) were randomly chosen from the national telephone directory and subsequently received a letter with an invitation to take part in the study. Data collection took place between April and July 2013. Both online and paper-pencil surveys were offered. Only two participants asked for postal delivery of the material. Fifteen percent of the respondents were single, 19% were in a relationship, 59% were married, 5% were divorced, and 2% were widowed. Seven percent of the sample had general education, 25% had completed apprenticeship or vocational secondary school, 34% were high school graduates, 29% had graduated from university, and the remaining 5% were holders of a doctoral degree. Ethnicity/race was not assessed.

Measures *Meaningfulness and crisis of meaning* were assessed by the SoMe (Schnell, 2009; Schnell & Becker, 2007), as in the previous studies.

Analysis Descriptive and inferential statistical analyses were run with IBM SPSS Statistics, version 24.0 (IBM Corporation, 2016).

Results

Distribution of the Qualities of Meaning To explore the distribution of the three qualities of meaning, we again utilized a combination of the meaningfulness and crisis of meaning scales as noted in the Method section of Study I. Results indicated that 71% of the control group sample experienced their lives as meaningful, 4% suffered from a crisis of meaning, and 25% were classified as existentially indifferent.

Qualities of Meaning Across All Four Groups Chi-square tests of independence were performed to analyze differences in the frequencies of the qualities of meaning across the four groups. As expected, the HIQ group differed significantly from the control group regarding all three qualities of meaning: HIQ experienced less meaningfulness, χ^2 $(1, N = 234) = 22.15$, $p < .001$, $\phi = .31$, more crises of meaning, χ^2 $(1, N = 234) = 9.30$, $p = .002$, $\phi = .20$, and more existential indifference, χ^2 $(1, N = 234) = 9.74$, $p = .002$, $\phi = .20$. Furthermore, the HIQ group differed significantly from the HAA group regarding two qualities of meaning: HIQ experienced less meaningfulness, χ^2 $(1, N = 152) = 12.45$, $p < .001$, $\phi = .29$ and more existential indifference, χ^2 $(1, N = 152) = 6.44$, $p = .011$, $\phi = .21$. Although the nonpreselected HVIQ group had the second highest prevalence of crises of meaning, and the second lowest percentage of people reporting a meaningful life, the analyses did not establish significant differences from the HAA or the control group. The HAA and the control group did not show significant differences with respect to the frequency of qualities of meaning.

Discussion

The current paper aimed to investigate whether experiences of meaning differ among individuals with different forms of giftedness and in comparison to the general population. Therefore, cross-sectional data of three gifted groups—HIQ, HVIQ, and HAA—and a control group were analyzed.

In line with our hypothesis, evidence was found for an association between high intellectual giftedness and problems in finding meaning in life. The HIQ group (Study I) reported significantly lower meaningfulness than the control group as well as the HAA group. Furthermore, the HIQ group had a higher risk of suffering from a crisis of meaning. Interestingly, the HVIQ group (Study II) showed a similar pattern, that is, less meaningfulness and more crises of meaning in life. However, these group differences did not reach statistical significance.

Moreover, interesting findings regarding differences between the qualities of meaning emerged from our studies. As expected, depression was more prevalent among those who were suffering from a crisis of meaning than among those who had a meaningful life. In general, subjective well-being and resilience were higher when life was experienced as meaningful and lower when the gifted were suffering from a crisis of meaning. While positively remembered family experiences were associated with the current sense of meaning among the HIQ group, positively remembered school experiences were associated with the current sense of meaning among the HAA group. This suggests that for HAA individuals, achievement-related contexts, and memories thereof, might be of particular relevance to their sense of meaning. Some of our assumptions—that perfectionism, self-criticism, and hypersensitivity were related to the experience of meaningfulness, crisis of meaning, or existential indifference—were not confirmed by the data. In this respect, however, we found a gender effect among the HIQ women, who reported more hypersensitivity, lower subjective well-being, and worse family experiences than HIQ men, thus suggesting the well-being of HIQ women might be even more vulnerable than that of men.

When comparing individuals characterized by HIQ with those characterized by HAA, we found these groups to differ regarding several variables that we had posited to be crucial for their well-being and mental stability. The HAA group reported significantly lower levels of crisis of meaning, higher levels of meaningfulness, as well as more supportive family and school experiences during their childhood than the HIQ group.

Our findings of a higher risk of negative psychological states in this particular sample of German and Austrian Mensa members tie in with recent results from Karpinski et al. (2018) who reported a higher prevalence for certain disorders among an American Mensa population. This also partially supports the disharmony hypothesis (e.g., Neihart, 1999), which suggests a higher risk of certain vulnerabilities among the gifted. Adding important nuances, our study provided evidence on their challenge of experiencing meaning in life. Moreover, it suggests that such vulnerability seems to apply primarily to HIQ individuals—but not to HAA individuals, who excel in academic performance.

Furthermore, the importance of differentiated schooling was highlighted by our results. Negative experiences at school (e.g., low appreciation and promotion of intellectual potential) were significantly prevalent in the reports of the HIQ group. These findings are in line with the results of other scholars (Perrson, 2010; Stålnacke & Smedler, 2011) who reported predominantly negative school experiences among Swedish Mensa samples. Further research would be needed to investigate whether a lack of recognition, appreciation, and promotion of talent in childhood and youth could have a long-lasting negative effect on gifted adults' lives and their experienced existential fulfillment.

Strengths and Limitations

Recent findings (Pollet & Schnell, 2017; Wirthwein, 2010) have indicated the necessity to differentiate between different groups of gifted individuals, which had rarely been done so far. In the present studies, we thus targeted several gifted samples as well as a control group from the general population to test for differences in meaning in life. Since gifted individuals are a small minority and respective samples are therefore hard to acquire, the diversity of our groups is one of the studies' strengths. Due to the cross-sectional study design, our results cannot claim to show causality. Thus, the variables used could still be causally unrelated, with unmeasured variables impacting on the reported associations.

Another limitation is that the majority of participants were residents of Austria or Germany and were for the most part highly educated. Thus, generalizability to other cultures, or segments of the population, cannot be assumed. Future studies would be needed to test whether the reported results can be replicated in a more diverse population, other cultures, or ethnic groups. Finally, we surveyed and considered high intellectual giftedness and high academic achievement as two separate groups. Although it is reasonable to assume that there is overlap between the two groups, the data indicate substantial differences with respect to meaning in life. Further studies are needed to understand what specific factors cause these differences.

Conclusion

Our findings are consistent with the assumption that highly intellectually gifted adults may be at higher risk of existential crises and lower meaningfulness in life. These findings should be considered in future research, therapy concepts, as well as interventions. Additionally, more (longitudinal) research is necessary to shed light on how internal (e.g., self-compassion, cf. Vötter & Schnell, 2019a) and external factors contribute to life meaning among the gifted in their adult lives.

Viewing our findings from Frankl's perspective, we could conclude that individuals with particularly high intellectual capacities might tend to hyper-reflect as well as question and criticize themselves, their actions, and their environments. The step towards trusting self-transcendence might therefore be especially challenging, resulting in more frequent crises of meaning, problems of finding meaning, and related low well-being. It is therefore vital to provide guidance in the form of meaning-centered as well as personality-developing therapy and coaching. The aim of such therapy or coaching should be to strengthen individual resources and self-efficacy, to foster soft skills such as self-compassion and resilience, and to increase the ability to cope with difficult feelings as well as critical social situations. Through such support, gifted individuals could be enabled to live up to their high potential.

Acknowledgments This research was made possible by the award of a Talent Austria Doctoral Research Scholarship of the OeAD–GmbH to the first author, supported by the Austrian Federal Ministry of Science and Research (BMWFW) and the Austrian Research and Support Centre for the Gifted and Talented (ÖZBF). The authors would like to thank all participants who dedicated their time and energy to participate in this study.

References

Acevedo, B. P., Aron, E. N., Aron, A., Sangster, M. D., Collins, N., & Brown, L. L. (2014). The highly sensitive brain: An fMRI study of sensory processing sensitivity and response to others' emotions. *Brain and Behavior: A Cognitive Neuroscience Perspective, 4*(4), 580–594. https://doi.org/10.1002/brb3.242

Altstötter-Gleich, C., & Bergemann, N. (2006). Testgüte einer deutschsprachigen Version der Mehrdimensionalen Perfektionismus Skala von Frost, Marten, Lahart und Rosenblate (Mps-F) [Test quality of a German-language version of the Multidimensional Perfectionism Scale by Frost, Marten, Lahart and Rosenblate]. *Diagnostica, 52*(3), 105–118. https://doi.org/10.1026/0012-1924.52.3.105

Aron, E. N., & Aron, A. (1997). Sensory-processing sensitivity and its relation to introversion and emotionality. *Journal of Personality and Social Psychology, 73*(2), 345. https://doi.org/10.1037/0022-3514.73.2.345

Aron, E. N., Aron, A., & Jagiellowicz, J. (2012). Sensory processing sensitivity: A review in the light of the evolution of biological responsivity. *Personality and Social Psychology Review, 16*(3), 262–282. https://doi.org/10.1177/108886831143421

Ash, C., & Huebner, E. S. (1998). Life satisfaction reports of gfted middle-school children. *School Psychology Quarterly, 13*(4), 310. https://doi.org/10.1037/h0088987

Baudson, T. G. (2016). The mad genius stereotype: Still alive and well. *Frontiers in Psychology, 7*, 368. https://doi.org/10.3389/fpsyg.2016.00368

Baumann, A.-L., Egenberger, V., & Supik, L. (2018). *Erhebung von Antidiskriminierungsdaten in repräsentativen Wiederholungsbefragungen* [Collection of anti-discrimination data in regular representative surveys]. Antidiskriminierungsstelle des Bundes. Retrieved from https://www.antidiskriminierungsstelle.de/SharedDocs/Downloads/DE/publikationen/Expertisen_Studien/Datenerhebung.html

Beutel, M. E., Wiltink, J., Hafner, C., Reiner, I., Bleichner, F., & Blatt, S. (2004). Abhängigkeit und Selbstkritik als psychologische Dimensionen der Depression-Validierung der deutschsprachigen Version des Depressive Experience Questionnaire (DEQ) [Dependence and self-criticism as psychological dimensions of depression—Validation of the German language version of the Depressive Experience Questionnaire (DEQ)]. *Zeitschrift für Klinische Psychologie, Psychiatrie und Psychotherapie, 52*(1), 1–14.

Bortz, J., & Weber, R. (2005). *Statistik für Human-und Sozialwissenschaftler* [Statistics for the humanities and social sciences]. Springer.

Brackmann, A. (2010). *Ganz normal hochbegabt: Leben als hochbegabter Erwachsener* [Just normally gifted: Life as a highly gifted adult]. Klett-Cotta.

Brähler, E., Mühlan, H., Albani, C., & Schmidt, S. (2007). Teststatistische prüfung und normierung der deutschen versionen des EUROHIS-QOL lebensqualität-Index und des WHO-5 wohlbefindens-index [Test evaluation and standardization of the German version of the EUROHIS-QOL Quality of Life Index and the WHO-5 Well-Being Index]. *Diagnostica, 53*(2), 83–96. https://doi.org/10.1026/0012-1924.53.2.83

Damásio, B. F., & Koller, S. H. (2015). Complex experiences of meaning in life: Individual differences among sociodemographic variables, sources of meaning and psychological functioning. *Social Indicators Research, 123*(1), 161–181. https://doi.org/10.1007/s11205-014-0726-3

Damásio, B. F., Koller, S. H., & Schnell, T. (2013). Sources of Meaning and Meaning in Life Questionnaire (SoMe): Psychometric properties and sociodemographic findings in a large Brazilian sample. *Acta de Investigación Psicológica, 3*(3), 1205–1227. https://doi.org/10.1016/S2007-4719(13)70961-X

Flett, G. L., & Hewitt, P. L. (2015). Measures of perfectionism. In G. J. Boyle, D. H. Saklofske, & G. Matthews (Eds.), *Measures of personality and social psychological constructs* (pp. 595–618). Elsevier.

Frankl, V. E. (1942–1944). *Handschriftliche Ankündigung von Vorträgen Viktor Frankls im Lager Theresienstadt* [Handwritten announcement of Viktor Frankl's lectures in the Theresienstadt camp] (T. Schnell, Trans.). Retrieved from http://www.viktorfrankl.at/Theresienstadt2.jpg

Frankl, V. E. (1955). *Pathologie des zeitgeistes: Rundfunkvorträge über Seelenheilkunde* [Pathology of the zeitgeist: Radio lectures on mental health]. Deuticke.

Frankl, V. E. (1985). *Man's search for meaning* (3rd ed.). Washington Square Press/Pocket Books. (Original work published 1946)

Frost, R. O., Marten, P., Lahart, C., & Rosenblate, R. (1990). The dimensions of perfectionism. *Cognitive Therapy and Research, 14*, 449–468. https://doi.org/10.1007/BF01172967

Hanfstingl, B. (2013). Ego and spiritual transcendence: Relevance to psychological resilience and the role of age. *Evidence-Based Complementary and Alternative Medicine, 2013*. https://doi.org/10.1155/2013/949838

Holahan, C. K., & Holahan, C. J. (1999). Being labeled as gifted, self-appraisal, and psychological well-being: A life span developmental perspective. *The International Journal of Aging and Human Development, 48*(3), 161–173. https://doi.org/10.2190/CLU1-DEUK-XAFB-7

Jackson, P. S., & Peterson, J. (2003). Depressive disorder in highly gifted adolescents. *Journal of Secondary Gifted Education, 14*(3), 175–186. https://doi.org/10.4219/jsge-2003-42

Karpinski, R. I., Kinase Kolb, A. M., Tetreault, N. A., & Borowski, T. B. (2018). High intelligence: A risk factor for psychological and physiological overexcitabilities. *Intelligence, 66*, 8–23. https://doi.org/10.1016/j.intell.2017.09.001

Körnung, R. L. (2015). *Die latente Struktur von Hochsensibilität—Eine taxometrische Untersuchung von Sensory-Processing Sensitivity* [The latent structure of high sensitivity: A taxometric study of sensory-processing sensitivity]. Dissertation. Bielefeld University.

Lehrl, S. (2005). *Mehrfachwahl-Wortschatz-Intelligenztest MWT-B* (5th ed.) [Multiple choice vocabulary intelligence test MWT-B]. Spitta Verlag.

Leppert, K., Koch, B., Brähler, E., & Strauss, B. (2008). RS-13 Resilienzfragebogen [Resilience questionnaire]. *Klinische Diagnostik und Evaluation, 1*, 226–243.

Liebenberg, L., Ungar, M., & Van de Vijver, F. (2012). Validation of the Child and Youth Resilience Measure-28 (CYRM-28) among Canadian youth. *Research on Social Work Practice, 22*(2), 219–226. https://doi.org/10.1177/1049731511428619

Miller, N. B., Falk, R. F., & Huang, Y. (2009). Gender identity and the overexcitability profiles of gifted college students. *Roeper Review, 31*(3), 161–169. https://doi.org/10.1080/02783190902993920

Mönks, F.-J. (1963). Beiträge zur begabtenforschung im kindes-und jugendalter [Contributions to research on giftedness in childhood and adolescence]. *Archiv für die Gesamte Psychologie, 115*, 362–382.

Neihart, M. (1999). The impact of giftedness on psychological well-being: What does the empirical literature say? *Roeper Review, 22*(1), 10–17. https://doi.org/10.1080/02783199909553991

Ostendorf, F., & Angleitner, A. (2004). *NEO-Persönlichkeitsinventar nach Costa und McCrae* [NEO Personality Inventory according to Costa and McCrae] (Manual; Rev ed.). Hogrefe.

Park, C. L. (2010). Making sense of the meaning literature: An integrative review of meaning making and its effects on adjustment to stressful life events. *Psychological Bulletin, 136*(2), 257. https://doi.org/10.1037/a0018301

Persson, R. S. (2010). Experiences of intellectually gifted students in an egalitarian and inclusive educational system: A survey study. *Journal for the Education of the Gifted, 33*(4), 536–569. https://doi.org/10.1177/016235321003300405

Plucker, J. A., & Callahan, C. M. (2008). *Critical issues and practices in gifted education: What the research says*. Prufrock Press Inc.

Pollet, E., & Schnell, T. (2017). Brilliant: But what for? Meaning and subjective well-being in the lives of intellectually gifted and academically high-achieving adults. *Journal of Happiness Studies, 18*, 1459–1484. https://doi.org/10.1007/s10902-016-9783-4

Preckel, F., & Vock, M. (2020). *Hochbegabung: Ein Lehrbuch zu Grundlagen, Diagnostik und Fördermöglichkeiten* [Giftedness. A textbook on theory, assessment and support options]. Hogrefe Verlag.

Roepke, A. M., Jayawickreme, E., & Riffle, O. M. (2014). Meaning and health: A systematic review. *Applied Research in Quality of Life, 9*, 1055–1079. https://doi.org/10.1007/s11482-013-9288-9

Rost, D. H. (2013). *Handbuch intelligenz* [Handbook of intelligence]. Beltz.

Schnell, T. (2009). The Sources of Meaning and Meaning in Life Questionnaire (SoMe): Relations to demographics and well-being. *The Journal of Positive Psychology, 4*(6), 483–499. https://doi.org/10.1080/17439760903271074

Schnell, T. (2010). Existential indifference: Another quality of meaning in life. *Journal of Humanistic Psychology, 50*(3), 351–373. https://doi.org/10.1177/0022167809360259

Schnell, T. (2021). *The psychology of meaning in life*. Routledge.

Schnell, T., & Becker, P. (2007). *Fragebogen zu Lebensbedeutungen und Lebenssinn: LeBe* [Questionnaire on Sources of Meaning and Meaning in Life: SoMe]. Hogrefe.

Schnell, T., Gerstner, R., & Krampe, H. (2018). Crisis of meaning predicts suicidality in youth independently of depression. *Crisis, 39*, 294–303. https://doi.org/10.1027/0227-5910/a000503

Silverman, L. K. (1999). Perfectionism: The crucible of giftedness. *Advanced Development, 8*, 47–61.

Sørensen, T., la Cour, P., Danbolt, L. J., Stifoss-Hanssen, H., Lien, L., DeMarinis, V., et al. (2019). The Sources of Meaning and Meaning in Life Questionnaire in the Norwegian context: Relations to mental health, quality of life, and self-efficacy. *The International Journal for the Psychology of Religion, 29*(1), 32–45. https://doi.org/10.1080/10508619.2018.1547614

Stålnacke, J., & Smedler, A.-C. (2011). Psychosocial experiences and adjustment among adult Swedes with superior general mental ability. *Journal for the Education of the Gifted, 34*(6), 900–918. https://doi.org/10.1177/0162353211424988

Tabachnick, B. G., & Fidell, L. S. (2013). *Using multivariate statistics* (6th ed.). Allyn & Bacon.

Terman, L. M. (1925). *Genetic studies of genius*. Stanford University Press.

Vos, J. (2016). Working with meaning in life in mental health care: A systematic literature review of the practices and effectiveness of meaning-centred therapies. In P. Russo-Netzer, S. Schulenberg, & A. Batthyany (Eds.), *Clinical perspectives on meaning: Positive and existential psychotherapy* (pp. 59–87). Springer.

Vötter, B., & Schnell, T. (2019a). Cross-lagged analyses between life meaning, self-compassion, and subjective well-being among gifted adults. *Mindfulness, 10*, 1294–1303. https://doi.org/10.1007/s12671-018-1078-x

Vötter, B., & Schnell, T. (2019b). Bringing giftedness to bear: Generativity, meaningfulness, and self-control as resources for a happy life among gifted adults. *Frontiers in Psychology, 10*. https://doi.org/10.3389/fpsyg.2019.01972

Winger, J. G., Adams, R. N., & Mosher, C. E. (2016). Relations of meaning in life and sense of coherence to distress in cancer patients: A meta-analysis. *Psycho-Oncology, 25*(1), 2–10. https://doi.org/10.1002/pon.3798

Wirthwein, L. (2010). *Mehr Glück als Verstand? Zum Wohlbefinden Hochbegabter* [More luck than brains? On the well-being of highly gifted people]. Dissertation. Marburg University.

Wirthwein, L., & Rost, D. H. (2011a). Giftedness and subjective well-being: A study with adults. *Learning and Individual Differences, 21*(2), 182–186. https://doi.org/10.1016/j.lindif.2011.01.001

Wirthwein, L., & Rost, D. H. (2011b). Focussing on overexcitabilities: Studies with intellectually gifted and academically talented adults. *Personality and Individual Differences, 51*(3), 337–342. https://doi.org/10.1016/j.paid.2011.03.041

Wraw, C., Deary, I. J., Der, G., & Gale, C. R. (2016). Intelligence in youth and mental health at age 50. *Intelligence, 58*, 69–79. https://doi.org/10.1016/j.intell.2016.06.005

Ziegler, A., & Raul, T. (2000). Myth and reality: A review of empirical studies on giftedness. *High Ability Studies, 11*(2), 113–136. https://doi.org/10.1080/13598130020001188

Zuroff, D. C., Koestner, R., & Powers, T. A. (1994). Self-criticism at age 12: A longitudinal study of adjustment. *Cognitive Therapy and Research, 18*(4), 367–385. https://doi.org/10.1007/BF02357511

Bernadette Vötter, is a clinical psychologist and postdoctoral researcher. Her work is driven by a deep fascination with the complexities of the human psyche and its exceptional capacity to adapt to and overcome adversity. Vötter's research focuses on key aspects of mental health including well-being, self-regulation, resilience, and meaning in life, with a specific interest in young adults, high achievers, and highly gifted individuals. Her clinical practice specializes in fostering nervous system regulation, somatic awareness, and emotional resilience.

Tatjana Schnell, is professor of existential psychology at MF Specialized University, Oslo, Norway and associate professor at the University of Innsbruck, Austria, where she established the Existential Psychology Lab. Her research focuses on existential issues such as meaning in life, suffering, and religious/spiritual/secular worldviews and their practical significance for individuals, organizations, society, and the environment. Schnell's measures of meaning in life (the Sources of Meaning and Meaning in Life Questionnaire, SoMe; The Meaning and Purpose Scales, MAPS; and Meaning in Work, ME-Work) have been translated into numerous languages. Her research is regularly covered by the media. She is a former coeditor for the Journal of Happiness Studies and has contributed to numerous international publications, collaborations, functions, and talks. Her latest book is The Psychology of Meaning in Life (Routledge, 2021).

Altruism, Motivation to Serve, and Purpose in Life Among College Students

William F. Evans, Lindsey Umstead, and Cynthia M. Evans

The undergraduate collegiate experience provides students with many opportunities to gain academic knowledge and skills as well as to explore interests, abilities, and life purpose. An important part of student identity development is attaining a sense of purpose, which often involves vocational plans and aspirations in addition to personal interests (Moran, 2001). Since many colleges and universities aim to prepare students to lead productive and meaningful lives (Langridge et al., 2012), it is essential to understand which aspects of the collegiate experience influence and prepare them for meaningful living.

Previous research suggests that student involvement may facilitate the development of life purpose (Moran, 2001). Moran (2001) proposed that a student's desire to participate in social activities and engage in service experiences positively influences their sense of life purpose. Langridge et al. (2012) explored relationships between life meaning and the collegiate experience by examining students' service motivation with their perceived purpose in life. Such findings support evidence that the collegiate experience itself may influence one's meaning in life. The present study aims to expand upon the findings of Astin (1993), Moran (2001), and Langridge et al. (2012) by exploring the relationships between altruism, motivation to serve, and life purpose among undergraduate students.

Altruism has been defined as "the motivation to increase another person's welfare" (Batson & Powell, 2003, p. 463). Rushton et al. (1981) argue for the existence of an altruism trait of personality based on the fact that, "some people are consistently more generous, helping, and kind than others" (p. 296).

W. F. Evans (✉) · L. Umstead
James Madison University, Harrisonburg, VA, USA
e-mail: evanswf@jmu.edu; lindsey@threebirdscounseling.com

C. M. Evans
Liberty University, Lynchburg, VA, USA
e-mail: cmevans2@liberty.edu

C. L. McLafferty, Jr., J. I. Levinson (eds.), *Logotherapy and Existential Analysis*, Logotherapy and Existential Analysis: Proceedings of the Viktor Frankl Institute Vienna 2, https://doi.org/10.1007/978-3-031-48922-8_18

A college student's degree of involvement in cocurricular activities predicts altruistic values or behaviors (Pascarella et al., 1988; Pascarella & Terenzini, 1991), so one might expect students with higher levels of motivation to serve to be more actively involved in these activities and to display higher levels of altruism. Further investigation of altruism as an influential factor in service motivation is needed to better understand the role it plays in students' service involvement.

Research on service engagement has examined several features of service, including types of service, the benefits of engagement, persistence of commitment, and factors influencing participation (Bowman et al., 2010; Trudeau & Devlin, 1996). Many colleges and universities are offering more courses that "promote students' understanding and commitment to local, national, and global communities" (Sax, 2004, p. 66). Examples of such courses are service-learning and community-based learning courses that are designed to promote civic responsibility and facilitate student citizenship. Despite the evidence describing many of the influences on people's decisions to engage in service activities, little is known about the differences in service motivation among college students pursuing different academic majors.

Research shows positive relationships between an individual's degree of service motivation and healthy vocational outcomes. Duffy and Raque-Bogdan (2010) explored motivation to serve in college students as a possible influence of healthy vocational development. The researchers found a significant positive relationship between students' desire to serve others and their level of excitement towards their future careers. These findings suggest that individuals planning to serve others through their careers are more likely to show optimism towards their future vocations. Thus, motivation to serve positively impacts students' attitudes and beliefs about certain facets of their futures. These findings support the notion that service motivation has the potential to contribute positively to students' overall purpose in life.

Much research on the concept of purpose in life is based on Viktor Frankl's theoretical framework (e.g., see Batthyány & Guttmann, 2005; Batthyány & Levinson, 2009; Moran, 2001). Frankl (1959, 2006) maintained that finding meaning in life is the primary motivational force in human beings. An inability to achieve meaning and purpose may result in a condition that Frankl referred to as an "existential vacuum," or a state of emptiness that often results in feelings of boredom (Crumbaugh & Henrion, 1988, p. 76). Ultimately, the existential vacuum results in feelings of apathy and leads to a loss of joy in living (Frankl, 2006).

College major choice impacts one's career opportunities and rewards (Pascarella & Terenzini, 1991). Personal values often influence the choice of a major. Students demonstrating high levels of social activism are more likely to major in the social sciences or education (Astin, 1993). Our study sought to verify any differences between students in seven college majors regarding altruism, motivation to serve, and purpose in life.

Method

The dependent variables (altruism, motivation to serve, and purpose in life) were assessed in terms of the independent variable, the motivation to select a particular major. Seven majors were compared in the analysis: psychology, social work, interdisciplinary liberal studies (IDLS), accounting, marketing, computer science, and nursing. These majors were selected based on the idea that many students in these majors may have selected their major either to seek job and financial security or from a desire to help others. Three majors, psychology, social work, and IDLS demonstrated similar motivation, mostly to help others, so we labeled this group the "others-directed" majors. Three others, accounting, marketing, and computer science, demonstrated similar motivation toward job and financial security, so they were labeled as the "jobs-directed" majors. Nursing majors were the most distinct group, showing even greater motivation to help others than those in the others-directed majors (see Table 1).

Instruments

Rushton et al. (1981) developed a self-report measure to assess patterns of individual differences in altruistic behavior, called the Self-Report Altruism (SRA) Scale; it allows individuals to rate the frequency of their engagement in certain behaviors that reflect an altruistic personality trait and provide evidence for a broad-based trait of altruism. The authors reported high internal consistency, with an alpha level of .89. For our sample, we found an alpha level of .88.

Langridge et al. (2012) integrated two well-established measures of service-learning in a study measuring service motivation and life purpose. Seven items from the Civic Action subscale were utilized to evaluate students' intentions to become involved in community service in the future (Moely et al., 2002). Seven items from the Social Justice Responsibility subscale were used to measure students' attitudes towards helping and changing society (Wang et al., 2005). These combined subscales identify students' motivation for service engagement. Moely et al. (2002) found the reliability coefficient for the Civic Action subscale to be .86 and .88 for two separate samples. In our sample, the alpha level was .91. Wang et al. (2005) reported alpha levels for the Social Justice subscale to be .82; for our study, the alpha level was .89. The combined subscales (Civic Action and Social Justice) in our sample had an alpha level of .92.

Table 1 Motivation for major choice

	Others-directed		Jobs-directed		Nursing	
Motivation	*n*	%	*n*	%	*n*	%
Job security	6	2.7	19	26.4	1	3.1
Financial success	3	1.4	23	31.9	1	3.1
Opportunity to help others	183	82.4	0	0.0	28	87.5
Opportunity for advancement	4	1.8	8	11.1	0	0.0
Influence from peers	1	0.5	2	2.8	0	0.0
Influence from parents	1	0.5	0	0.0	0	0.0
Other	24	10.8	20	27.8	2	6.3
Total	222	100.0	72	100.0	32	100.0

Note. Frequencies and percentages of students' main motivation for choosing a certain type of major are presented above. Others-directed = psychology, social work, and IDLS; jobs-directed = marketing, accounting, and computer science; nursing = nursing

Crumbaugh and Maholick (1964) developed the Purpose in Life (PIL) scale to measure Frankl's existential construct of meaning in life. This measure also assesses an individual's existential vacuum, or lack of meaning (Crumbaugh & Henrion, 1988). The reliability coefficient for the PIL was initially found to be .85; however, this coefficient was later corrected to .92 using the Spearman-Brown formula (Batthyány & Guttmann, 2005; Batthyány & Levinson, 2009; Crumbaugh & Henrion, 1988). For our sample, we found an alpha level of .89 for the PIL.

Hypotheses

We predicted positive correlations between all dependent variables: altruism, motivation to serve, and purpose in life, consistent with Clemmons and Fields (2011) and Logue et al. (2005). We predicted that students pursuing others-directed majors would exhibit higher levels of altruism, motivation to serve, and purpose in life than students pursuing jobs-directed majors, consistent with Debats et al. (1995) and Clemmons and Fields (2011). We also predicted that students pursuing the nursing major would exhibit higher levels of altruism, motivation to serve, and purpose in life than students pursuing either others-directed or jobs-directed majors. Lastly, we predicted that students who served, regardless of the motivation for their service, would score higher on altruism, motivation to serve, and purpose in life when compared with those who did not serve.

Participants and Procedures

Participants were undergraduates at a mid-size, mid-Atlantic university. Undergraduates from the targeted majors [psychology, social work, IDLS, accounting, marketing, computer science, and nursing] were recruited via mass email. The email invitation included a link to items relating to the variables of interest (SRA, MTS, and PIL) and 17 demographic questions. The survey was active for 3 weeks.

Of the 413 students who opened and began the survey, 326 students completed all items (freshmen: $N = 58$, 17.8%; sophomores: $N = 65$, 19.9%; juniors: $N = 85$, 26.1%; seniors: $N = 113$, 34.7%; fifth year or above: $N = 5$, 1.5%). The participants were 84% female; 16% male; they reported race/ethnicity as 3.1% Black/African American, 4.6% Asian, 0.9% Hispanic, 1.5% Native American, 82.5% White/Caucasian, and 7.1% multiracial. The participants reported majoring in psychology 39.6%, social work 6.4%, IDLS 22.1%, marketing 9.5%, accounting 6.7%, computer science 5.8%, nursing 9.8%.

Results

The initial analysis involved comparing the overall group means for each variable among the various majors chosen by the students. The reasons for choosing their respective major were also analyzed. To ensure that the clusters of majors were valid (i.e., there were no significant differences in mean scores of the dependent variables (SRA, MTS, and PIL) among majors in their assigned groups), a one-way ANOVA was performed to test for significant differences among majors. The Bonferroni correction was applied to reduce the risk of Type I error. All post hoc analyses for majors within the same clusters yielded statistically non-significant results ($p > .05$). After confirming differences between students in these various majors, participants were clustered into larger groups by their stated motivation for their selected major, whether more *jobs directed*, *others directed*, or distinctively different from the others, *nursing*. The frequencies and percentages for these motivations are noted in Table 1.

The vast majority of others-directed and nursing majors reported opportunity to help others as their main motivation for choosing their selected major. More than two-thirds of students majoring in jobs-directed majors cited either financial success, job security, or opportunity for advancement as their main motivation for choosing their major.

Table 2 shows the means and standard deviations for each variable by each major group.

Correlations between all variables among all subjects revealed significant positive relationships. The relationship between altruism and purpose in life resulted in a correlation of $r = .218$, significant at the .01 level (two-tailed). The correlation between motivation to serve and purpose in life showed a relationship of $r = .400$, significant at the .01 level (two-tailed). The relationship between altruism and motivation to serve showed a correlation of $r = .455$, also significant at the .01 level (two-tailed).

An independent-samples *t*-test was performed to compare altruism (SRA), motivation to serve (MTS), and purpose in life (PIL) between all major groups: nursing, jobs-directed, and others-directed. Significant differences were found in SRA between: nursing majors ($M = 36.66$, $SD = 10.27$) and jobs-directed majors ($M = 29.30$, $SD = 10.22$); $t(102) = 3.381$, $p = .001$ (two-tailed); between nursing majors ($M = 36.66$, $SD = 10.27$) and others-directed majors ($M = 32.26$, $SD = 10.98$); $t(252) = 2.135$, $p = .034$ (two-tailed); and between others-directed majors ($M = 32.26$, $SD = 10.98$) and jobs-directed majors ($M = 29.30$, $SD = 10.22$); $t(292) = 2.014$, $p = .045$ (two-tailed).

Significant differences were found in MTS scores between nursing majors ($M = 67.47$, $SD = 10.98$) and jobs-directed majors ($M = 62.17$, $SD = 13.47$); $t(102) = 1.954$, $p = .05$ (two-tailed) as well as between others-directed majors ($M = 70.86$, $SD = 9.46$) and jobs-directed majors ($M = 62.17$, $SD = 13.47$);

Table 2 Means and standard deviations for all variables by major motivation

	Job-directed		Others-directed		Nursing		Total	
N	72		222		32		326	
	M	*SD*	*M*	*SD*	*M*	*SD*	*M*	*SD*
SRA	29.30	10.22	32.26	10.98	36.66	10.27	32.04	10.89
MTS	62.17	13.47	70.86	9.46	67.47	10.99	68.61	11.17
PIL	104.22	16.10	109.12	14.37	106.53	13.87	107.78	14.82

Note. Means and standard deviations of measures of student motivation are presented above. *SRA* Self-Report Altruism scale, *MTS* Motivation to Serve subscales, *PIL* Purpose in Life test

$t(292) = 6.059, p < .001$ (two-tailed). The difference between MTS scores in nursing majors ($M = 67.47$, $SD = 10.98$) and others-directed majors ($M = 70.86$, $SD = 9.46$); $t(252) = 1.86$. $p = .065$ (two-tailed) did not reach significance.

The differences in PIL scores between nursing majors ($M = 106.53$, $SD = 13.87$) and jobs-directed majors ($M = 104.22$, $SD = 16.10$); $t(102) = .703$, $p = .484$ (two-tailed), as well as between nursing majors ($M = 106.53$, $SD = 13.87$) and others-directed majors ($M = 109.11$, $SD = 14.37$); $t(252) = .954$, $p = .341$ (two-tailed) were not significant. However, there was a significant difference in PIL scores between others-directed majors ($M = 109.11$, $SD = 14.37$) and jobs-directed majors ($M = 104.22$, $SD = 16.10$); $t(292) = 2.435$, $p = .015$ (two-tailed).

Utilizing a one-way ANOVA, students who did service within the past year were compared with those students who did no service over the past year. A comparison was also made between students regarding their reason for serving, with students stating whether their service occurred with an organization they were involved with, because it was a class requirement, or whether they did the service simply because they wanted to. Differences were found between the groups of participants who had served compared with those who had not served in each comparison, regardless of their reason or motivation for their service. Those students who served scored higher on average than those who had not served on purpose in life in each comparative analysis. Table 3 displays the results of each one-way ANOVA.

Discussion

The data supported several of the hypotheses. First, the correlations between all three dependent variables were found to be significant, consistent with existing research (Pascarella et al., 1988; Pascarella & Terenzini, 1991). Second, significant differences were found on all three dependent variables related to whether one had done service within the past year, service with a class, service with an organization, or served simply because they wanted to.

However, the results of our study failed to fully support two of our hypotheses, and these results were inconsistent with previous research by Debats et al. (1995). While others-directed majors did score higher on purpose in life than jobs-directed majors, no differences were found on purpose in life between nursing majors and either jobs-directed majors or others-directed majors. Differences between nursing and the other two groups were not significant, indicating that no conclusions can be

Table 3 ANOVA by service or no service during the past year

Served during the past year? Yes = 253, No = 73
Yes/No by PIL: $F(2, 325) = 13.98$, $p < .001$
Served with an Organization during the past year? Yes = 213, No = 113
Yes/No by PIL: $F(2, 325) = 20.98$, $p < .001$
Served with a Class during the past year? Yes = 175, No = 151
Yes/No by PIL: $F(2, 325) = 23.77$, $p < .001$
Served just because I wanted to during the past year? Yes = 201, No = 125
Yes/No by PIL: $F(2, 325) = 24.47$, $p < .001$

made, though it is possible to speculate that these students were achieving a similar sense of life purpose regardless of their chosen field of study. The purpose in life scores in this sample were above average for all groups (see Table 2).

The limitations of this study necessitate some caution when considering our results. Our sample was not representative of the college student population in America as a whole, which may mean that our findings lack generalizability for underrepresented groups.

Despite its limitations, this study contributes to our understanding of altruism, service motivation, and life purpose among college students. Future studies might further investigate college students' academic and career motivations with other facets of student development. Comparing life purpose, service motivation and altruism in students across different undergraduate levels (i.e., freshman, sophomore, etc.) may offer insight into the development of these factors in students during their collegiate career. Future research might include students from other institutions to determine if this university's influence on student development is common or unique. Some experiences provided by this university's service-learning programs may lead to positive outcomes for altruism, service motivation, and life meaning. Faculty at this school are encouraged to include service-learning experiences in their courses, possibly creating data that is not reflective of other institutions. Exploring these variables within universities offering varied levels of service-learning and other experiences may offer student development researchers and student health practitioners' insights as to how to effectively foster a collegiate environment that promotes the growth of these particular outcomes, especially purpose in life.

References

Astin, A. W. (1993). *What matters in college? Four critical years revised*. Jossey-Bass.

Batson, C. D., & Powell, A. A. (2003). Altruism and prosocial behavior. In T. Millon & M. J. Lerner (Eds.), *Handbook of psychology, personality and social psychology* (Vol. 5, pp. 463–484). Wiley.

Batthyány, A., & Guttmann, D. (2005). *Empirical research in logotherapy and meaning-oriented psychotherapy: An annotated bibliography*. Zeig, Tucker & Theisen, Inc.

Batthyány, A., & Levinson, J. (Eds.). (2009). *Existential psychotherapy of meaning: Handbook of logotherapy and existential analysis*. Zeig, Tucker, & Theisen, Inc.

Bowman, N., Brandenberger, J., Lapsley, D., Hill, P., & Quaranto, J. (2010). Serving in college, flourishing in adulthood: Does community engagement during the college years predict adult well-being? *Applied Psychology: Health and Well-Being, 2*(1), 14–34. https://doi.org/10.1111/j.1758-0854.2009.01020.x

Clemmons, A. B., & Fields, D. (2011). Values as determinants of the motivation to lead. *Military Psychology, 23*(6), 587–600. https://doi.org/10.1080/08995605.2011.616787

Crumbaugh, J. C., & Henrion, R. (1988). The PIL Test: Administration, interpretation, uses theory and critique. *International Forum for Logotherapy, 11*(2), 76–88.

Crumbaugh, J. C., & Maholick, L. T. (1964). An experimental study in existentialism: The psychometric approach to Frankl's concept of noogenic neurosis. *Journal of Clinical Psychology, 20*(2), 200–207.

Debats, D. L., Drost, J., & Hansen, P. (1995). Experiences of meaning in life: A combined qualitative and quantitative approach. *British Journal of Psychology, 86*(3), 359–375. https://doi.org/10.1111/j.2044-8295.1995.tb02758.x

Duffy, R. D., & Raque-Bogdan, T. L. (2010). The motivation to serve others: Exploring relations to career development. *Journal of Career Assessment, 18*(3), 250–265. https://doi.org/10.1177/1069072710364791

Frankl, V. E. (1959). The spiritual dimension in existential analysis and logotherapy. *Journal of Individual Psychology, 15*(2), 157.

Frankl, V. E. (2006). *Man's search for meaning*. Beacon Press.

Langridge, N. L., Evans, W. F., Dixon, A. D., & Janser, S. K. (2012). *Meaning in life: Is this the greatest ROI of the collegiate experience?* Unpublished manuscript; pilot study for doctoral dissertation at James Madison University.

Logue, C. T., Hutchens, T. A., & Hector, M. A. (2005). Student leadership: A phenomenological exploration of postsecondary experiences. *Journal of College Student Development, 46*(4), 393–408. https://doi.org/10.1353/csd.2005.0039

Moely, B. E., Mercer, S. H., Ilustre, V., Miron, D., & McFarland, M. (2002). Psychometric properties and correlates of the Civic Attitudes and Skills Questionnaire (CASQ): A measure of students' attitudes related to service-learning. *Michigan Journal of Community Service Learning, 8*(2), 15–26.

Moran, C. D. (2001). Purpose in life, student development, and well-being: Recommendations for student affairs practitioners. *NASPA Journal, 38*(3), 269–279. https://doi.org/10.2202/1949-6605.1147

Pascarella, E. T., & Terenzini, P. T. (1991). *How college affects students: Findings and insights from twenty years of research*. Jossey-Bass, Inc.

Pascarella, E. T., Ethington, C. A., & Smart, J. C. (1988). The influence of college on humanitarian/civic involvement values. *The Journal of Higher Education, 59*(4), 412. https://doi.org/10.2307/1981919

Rushton, J. P., Chrisjohn, R. D., & Cynthia Fekken, G. (1981). The altruistic personality and the Self-Report Altruism Scale. *Personality and Individual Differences, 2*(4), 293–302. https://doi.org/10.1016/0191-8869(81)90084-2

Sax, L. J. (2004). Citizenship development and the American college student. *New Directions for Institutional Research, 2004*(122), 65–80. https://doi.org/10.1002/ir.110

Trudeau, K. J., & Devlin, A. S. (1996). College students and community service: Who, with whom, and why? *Journal of Applied Social Psychology, 26*(21), 1867–1888. https://doi.org/10.1111/j.1559-1816.1996.tb00103.x

Wang, Y., Ye, F., Jackson, G., Rodgers, R., & Jones, S. (2005). Development of Student Service-Learning Course Survey (SSLCS) to measure service-learning course outcomes. *IR Applications, 3*.

William F. Evans, PhD, is a professor of psychology at James Madison University. He earned a BA in religion from Wofford College, an MDiv from Duke University, and a PhD in counselor education and supervision from the University of South Carolina. Dr. Evans is a decorated United States Air Force Colonel (retired) and serves on the International Advisory Board for the Viktor Frankl Institute in Vienna, Austria.

Lindsey Umstead, PhD, is a licensed professional counselor at Three Birds Counseling in Greensboro, North Carolina. She earned her BA in psychology from James Madison University. She earned an MA in counseling, with a specialization in college counseling and student development, and a PhD in counseling from the University of North Carolina, Greensboro.

Cynthia M. Evans, PhD, is an adjunct professor of psychology at Liberty University, teaching at both the undergraduate and graduate levels. She earned her BA in communication studies from The Ohio State University. She earned an MA in counseling and a PhD in professional counseling from Liberty University.

Re-Examining Altruism, Service Motivation, and Life Purpose Among Undergraduate and Graduate Students

William F. Evans and Cynthia M. Evans

The purpose of this study was to explore the relationships between measures of students' self-reported altruism, motivation to serve, and purpose in life. The participants were 583 undergraduate and graduate students from a large, mid-Atlantic university, representing many different majors and professional training programs. An online survey was utilized to assess scores on the three measures and gather demographic data. Four main hypotheses were made for this study: (1) There would be significant positive correlations between all measures, (2) there would be clear differences on all three measures between students who have served compared with those who have not served, (3) there would be a measurable difference between males and females on all measures, and (4) scores for all measures would increase with age. All four hypotheses were either fully or partially supported by the data. Robert Greenleaf (1970, 1977), a well-known author on servant leadership, often wrote that the greatest leaders experienced service to others first; he believed service to be a critical component in the development of leaders, specifically, and human beings, generally. As Sipe and Frick (2015) noted, "true leadership emerges from one whose primary motivation is a deep desire to serve" (p. 36). Greenleaf (1970) also wrote, "The first and most important choice a leader makes is the choice to serve, without which one's capacity to lead is severely limited" (p. 7). Spears (2000) agreed with the importance of service experiences for leadership and personal development.

W. F. Evans (✉)
James Madison University, Harrisonburg, VA, USA
e-mail: evanswf@jmu.cdu

C. M. Evans
Liberty University, Lynchburg, VA, USA
e-mail: cmevans2@liberty.edu

C. L. McLafferty, Jr., J. I. Levinson (eds.), *Logotherapy and Existential Analysis*, Logotherapy and Existential Analysis: Proceedings of the Viktor Frankl Institute Vienna 2, https://doi.org/10.1007/978-3-031-48922-8_19

Sipe and Frick (2015) added: "Greenleaf also articulated two fundamental dimensions of leadership. The first, and best known, is the desire to serve. The second is the desire to serve something beyond or greater than oneself—what he called a 'higher purpose'" (p. 30). This second dimension of leadership, according to Greenleaf, is what Viktor Frankl (Frankl, 2000, 2006) called *self-transcendence*, which Frankl believed to be a clear antecedent to purpose in life.

The collegiate environment allows both undergraduate and graduate students to explore and enhance identity development, interests, skills, and abilities. Potentially, these opportunities place students in a position to discover their purpose in life as they are establishing their sense of identity. Moran (2001) suggested that attaining a sense of life purpose is vital to identity development among college students. The collegiate experience is a popular focus of research when examining purpose in life (Johnson, 2006; Molasso, 2006). Although varying in mission and vision statements, many colleges and universities aspire to help students lead productive and meaningful lives (Johnson, 2006; Langridge et al., 2012). The primary focus of the current research is to seek a better understanding of those experiences in collegiate life that may influence students to attain a greater sense of purpose.

In addition to potentially cultivating a sense of purpose, collegiate life may also be linked with a student's development of altruism. Altruism has been defined as "the motivation to increase another person's welfare" (Batson & Powell, 2003, p. 463). According to Rushton et al. (1981), "some people are consistently more generous, helping, and kind than others" (p. 296). The choices that undergraduate and graduate students make, whether it be selecting their major or professional programs, picking the organizations they will devote their time to, or deciding which extracurricular activities they will involve themselves in, could all potentially develop a sense of altruism. The development of altruism among college students is also a focus of this research project.

Moreover, one's motivation to serve could also be developed within a collegiate environment. Just as with purpose in life and altruism, decisions made by undergraduate and graduate students may well illustrate their values and the motivation behind their behavior. An abundance of research exists on the topic of service engagement, with investigators studying several features of service, including types of service, the benefits of engagement, persistence of commitment, and factors influencing participation (Bowman et al., 2010; Trudeau & Devlin, 1996). Investigators have developed various measures of service motivation to determine individual attitudes and outcomes of service engagement (Moely et al., 2002; Wang et al., 2005).

The purpose of this study was to explore the relationships between students' self-reported altruism, motivation to serve, and purpose in life. Other variables of interest included gender and academic level in collegiate life. Four hypotheses were proposed: (a) There would be significant positive correlations between all measures, (b) there would be clear differences on all three measures between students who have served compared with those who have not served, (c) there would be a measurable difference between males and females on all measures, and (d) scores for all measures would increase with age. An online survey was used to administer measures of altruism, motivation to serve, and purpose in life.

Method

Participants

Participants were undergraduate and graduate students from a large, comprehensive American university (79% female, n = 461; 21% male, n = 122). These students were recruited through a mass e-mail that was sent to a total of 20,583 students from all majors with good academic standing. The e-mail invitation included a link to each questionnaire related to the measures of interest, discussed below. The survey remained active for 3 weeks.

Of the 714 students who started the survey, 583 students (17% freshmen, n = 97; 21% sophomores, n = 120; 25% juniors, n = 148; 21% seniors, n = 125; 3% fifth-year seniors, n = 20; 13% graduate students, n = 73) completed all the items, thus constituting our final sample size.

Our sample included 5.7% Black/African American, 5.2% Hispanic, 6.7% Asian, 0.7% American Indian/Alaskan Native, 79.8% white (non-Hispanic), 0.3% Hawaiian/Pacific Islander, 1.6% multiracial identity. At the time of data collection, the population of the institution consisted of 4.4% Black/African American, 5.7% Hispanic, 4.4% Asian, 0.2% American Indian/Alaska Native, 77.8% white (non-Hispanic), 0.1% Hawaiian/ Pacific Islanders, and 7.4% two or more races or another racial identity. Ethnic demographics of the sample were relatively representative of the institution's population, especially for Black/African American and Hispanic responders.

Materials

Participants completed a questionnaire related to their sense of purpose in life, motivation to serve, and self-report altruism, followed by a set of 17 demographic questions. Life meaning was measured using the Purpose in Life scale (PIL; Crumbaugh & Maholick, 1964). Service motivation was measured using the Civic Action and Social Justice subscales of the Motivation to Serve (MTS) instrument used by Langridge et al. (2012). The Self-Report Altruism scale (SRA; Rushton et al., 1981) measured the level of altruism among participants.

Purpose in Life The PIL is an attitude test that evaluates participants' perceptions of life meaning in terms of the degree they experience "purpose in life" (Crumbaugh & Henrion, 1988, p. 77). Only the quantitative psychometric scale was utilized in the current study, containing 20 statements rated on a 7-point Likert-type scale. Scores range from 20, indicating a low level of meaning, to 140, indicating a high level of meaning and life purpose (Halama, 2009). The reliability coefficient for the PIL was found to be .92 by the original researchers. Our study found an alpha level of .89 for the PIL.

Motivation to Serve Langridge et al. (2012) integrated two well-established measures of MTS related to service learning in a study measuring service motivation and life purpose. Seven items from the Civic Action subscale were included from Moely et al. (2002) to evaluate students' intentions to become involved in community service in the future. Seven items from the Social Justice subscale from Wang et al. (2005) were also used to measure students' attitudes towards helping and changing society. These combined scales were used in this study to assess the level of students' motivation to serve. All items were rated on a Likert-type scale. Moely et al. (2002) found the reliability coefficient for the Civic Action subscale to be .86 and .88 for two separate samples. Wang et al. (2005) reported alpha levels for the Social Justice subscale to be .82. For our sample, we found an alpha level of .92 for the combined MTS score.

Self-Report Altruism The SRA scale is a measure containing 20 items on a Likert-type scale created by Rushton et al. (1981). Regarding the internal consistency of the instrument, the authors reported an alpha of .89. For our sample, we found an alpha level of .88 for SRA.

Procedure

An online survey link containing all three instruments and a series of 17 demographic questions was sent via email to all students in good academic standing at a large university. Students' responses were voluntary. Participants provided informed consent approved by the Institutional Review Board before taking the survey and viewed a debriefing statement following the questionnaire. Data entry was performed using [Excel, software]. All analyses were conducted using SPSS v. 28.0.

Results

Hypothesis 1, which claimed that there would be a significant positive correlation between PIL, SRA, and MTS scores, was analyzed using bivariate correlations to determine whether there were positive relationships between the scores on all three measures: PIL, SRA, and MTS. It was found that there were significant positive correlations between PIL and SRA ($r = .268$, $p < .001$), between PIL and MTS ($r = .388$, $p < .001$), and between SRA and MTS ($r = .432$, $p < .001$). Thus, hypothesis 1 was supported by this data.

Purpose in Life Scores Independent samples two-tailed *t*-tests were performed to compare purpose in life (PIL) between those who served and those who did not during the academic year. Significant differences in scores on the PIL were found: between those who served as a class requirement ($M = 106.30$, SD = 14.15) and those who did not ($M = 102.87$, SD = 16.48); $t(554) = 2.33$, $p = .02$; between those who served with an organization ($M = 105.66$, SD = 15.25) and those who did not ($M = 101.30$, SD = 16.47); $t(554) = 3.20$, $p = .001$; and those who served simply because they wanted to ($M = 106.18$, SD = 14.76) and those who did not serve at all ($M = 101.31$, SD = 16.73); $t(554) = 3.65$, $p < .001$.

Self-Report Altruism Scores Independent samples two-tailed t-tests were performed to compare SRA scores between those who served during the academic year and those who did not. No significant difference was found for SRA scores between those who served as a class requirement ($M = 35.08$, SD = 8.94) and those who did not ($M = 33.80$, SD = 10.25); $t(616) = 1.47$, $p = .142$ (two-tailed). However, there was a significant difference in altruism between those who served with an organization ($M = 35.54$, SD = 9.22) and those who did not ($M = 32.17$, SD = 10.51); $t(616) = 4.20$, $p < .001$. A significant difference was also discovered when comparing altruism between those who served during the academic year simply because they wanted to ($M = 36.46$, SD = 9.78) with those who did not serve at all ($M = 31.68$, SD = 9.43); $t(616) = 6.16$, $p < .001$.

Motivation to Serve Scores Independent samples t-tests (two-tailed) were performed to compare motivation to serve (MTS) between those who served and those who did not serve during the academic year. There was a significant difference in motivation to serve between those who served as a class requirement ($M = 71.39$, SD = 8.62) and those who did not ($M = 66.65$, SD = 12.19); $t(561) = 4.55$, $p < .001$. A significant difference was found between those who served with an organization ($M = 70.53$, SD = 11.04) and those who did not serve with an organization ($M = 64.43$, SD = 11.11); $t(561) = 6.43$, $p < .001$. A significant difference was also discovered between those who served simply because they wanted to ($M = 71.38$, SD = 9.72) with those who did not serve at all ($M = 64.34$, SD = 12.10); $t(561) = 7.64$, $p < .001$. Thus, hypothesis 2 was mostly supported by the data.

Males vs. Females Hypothesis 3, which expected that there would be a difference between males and females among all variables, was analyzed with two-tailed independent samples t-test for all three measures: Significant differences were not found with PIL scores between males ($M = 102.31$, SD = 16.21) and females ($M = 104.52$, SD = 15.62); $t(551) = 1.35$, $p = .178$; nor with SRA scores between males ($M = 34.91$, SD = 9.98) and females ($M = 33.95$, SD = 9.89); $t(613) = .985$, $p = .325$; there was, however, a significant difference between MTS scores of males ($M = 62.76$, SD = 13.38) and females ($M = 69.57$, SD 10.39); $t(558) = 5.92$, $p < .001$. Thus, hypothesis 3 was only partially supported by the data.

Differences in Age: PIL Scores Hypothesis 4 explored age differences among scores for the three variables, expecting scores to increase with age. Independent samples t-tests (two-tailed) were performed to compare purpose in life (PIL) between those students who identified as first year (freshmen) with: (a) second year (sophomores), (b) third year (juniors), (c) fourth year (seniors), (d) fifth year (seniors

+), and (e) graduate students. The differences between PIL scores were not significant when comparing first-year students (M = 102.88, SD = 17.57): with second-year students (M = 103.45, SD = 15.01); $t(252) = .255$, $p = .799$; with third-year students (M = 103.59, SD = 14.70); $t(283) = .356$, $p = .722$; with fourth-year students (M = 105.47, SD = 14.47); $t(285) = 1.31$, $p = .190$; with fifth-year students (M = 96.72, SD = 20.45); $t(186) = 1.39$, $p = .166$; and with graduate students (M = 107.53, SD = 15.57); $t(213) = 1.61$, $p = .108$. Thus, hypothesis 4 was not supported for PIL when comparing first-year students with all other student groups.

Utilizing independent samples two-tailed t-tests with PIL scores when comparing second-year students with third, fourth, fifth, and graduate student groups, no significant differences were found in any of these comparisons between second-year students (M = 103.45, SD = 15.01) and: third-year students (M = 103.59, SD = 14.70); $t(197) = .065$, $p = .948$; fourth-year students (M = 105.47, SD = 14.47); $t(199) = .960$, $p = .338$; fifth-year students (M = 96.72, SD = 20.45); $t(100) = 1.61$, $p = .110$; and graduate students (M = 107.53, SD = 15.57); $t(127) = 1.45$, $p = .149$. Thus, hypothesis 4 was not supported for PIL when comparing second-year students with all other student groups.

Independent samples t-tests (two-tailed) were conducted to compare PIL scores between third-year students in their fourth and fifth years as well as graduate student groups. No significant differences were found comparing third-year students (M = 103.59, SD = 14.70): with fourth-year students (M = 105.47, SD = 14.47); $t(230) = .981$, $p = .328$; fifth-year students (M = 96.72, SD = 20.45); $t(131) = 1.74$, $p = .084$; or graduate students (M = 107.53, SD = 15.57); $t(158) = 1.50$, $p = .136$. Therefore, hypothesis 4 was not supported for PIL when comparing third-year students with all other student groups.

Independent samples t-tests (two-tailed) were performed to compare PIL scores of fourth-year students with those of fifth-year and graduate student groups. A significant difference was found with PIL scores between fourth-year students (M = 105.47, SD = 14.47) and fifth-year students (M = 96.72, SD = 20.45); $t(133) = 2.25$, $p = .026$, but not as expected: Fourth-year students scored higher than fifth-year students. No significant difference was found between fourth-year students (M = 105.47, SD = 14.47) and graduate students (M = 107.53, SD = 15.57); $t(160) = .796$, $p = .427$. Therefore, hypothesis 4 was not supported for PIL when comparing fourth-year students with all other student groups. Finally, in an independent samples two-tailed t-test comparing PIL scores between fifth-year students (M = 96.72, SD = 20.45) and graduate students (M = 107.53, SD = 15.57), the result was significant: $t(61) = 2.27$, $p = .027$.

Thus, hypothesis 4 was only supported when comparing the PIL between fifth-year students and graduate students and was contradicted when PIL scores were compared between fourth- and fifth-year groups.

Hypothesis 4 was also tested through one-way, between-subjects ANOVA for both self-report altruism (SRA) and motivation to serve (MTS) between all student groups, with no significant differences found between groups on either SRA F(6,

661) = 1.82, $p = .092$, or MTS $F(6, 556) = 1.89$, $p = .080$. Therefore, hypothesis 4 was not supported for either SRA or MTS between any groups of students.

Discussion

The findings of this study provide insights into the relationships between purpose in life, altruism, and motivation to serve. Four hypotheses were made for this study. The data supported the first hypothesis, as significant positive correlations between the three primary variables were found. Interestingly, most students at this university seem to engage in some form of service, whether they were motivated to serve for a class, with an organization, or simply because they wanted to. Without stating causality, it appears that students who have higher scores on measures of altruism and motivation to serve also score high in purpose in life.

The second hypothesis of the study explored the relationship between acts of service and the three primary measures. We found that there is a significant relationship between service activities of students and higher PIL, MTS, and SRA scores. This pattern was present regardless of the reason for doing the service, whether for a class, for an organization, or simply because one wanted to serve. Thus, acts of service appear to be related to higher levels of altruism, motivation to serve, and most importantly, to a greater sense of purpose in life.

The third hypothesis for this study stated that there would be a difference between males and females on all three variables. The results partially supported this hypothesis. Specifically, women did score significantly higher on motivation to serve. It could be that women are socialized to display more affection and care; thus, they are more motivated to serve.

The final hypothesis analyzed the relationship between level in school and the three primary variables. The results may be best understood by exploring the relationship between time and maturity. It was expected that older students would display a higher sense of altruism and motivation to serve as well as increasing levels of purpose in life. However, no significant differences were found between scores on the SRA and MTS measures at each grade level, nor for nearly all of the grade-level comparisons with PIL scores. The two exceptions were of interest: Both fourth-year and graduate students' PIL scores were significantly higher than those of fifth-year students.

Though our expectation was that older and more mature students would be more likely to have a greater purpose in life, it was not generally supported by our results. That fourth-year *and* graduate students scored significantly higher than the fifth-year seniors may point to the nonstandard nature of students who take longer to graduate—perhaps they were struggling academically, or establishing a clear sense of identity and life purpose had proven difficult for them within the academic setting. Though the differences of fifth-year PIL scores were not significant compared to first-, second-, and third-year student scores, they were nonetheless the lowest of all the groups on the PIL. Further research is needed to explore this finding.

These results are consistent with the possibility that service experiences are an avenue to finding greater purpose in life though further studies are needed to demonstrate causality. This could be a compelling reason for universities to promote more service-learning experiences for their students, both inside and outside the classroom environment.

We conclude with the words of Robert Greenleaf (1970), who wrote: "the servant-leader *is* servant first.... It begins with the natural feeling that one wants to serve, to serve *first*. Then conscious choice brings one to aspire to lead" (p. 7, italics in original). He added that, for the effectiveness of servant leadership:

> the best test... is: Do those served grow as persons; do they, *while being served*, become healthier, wiser, freer, more autonomous, more likely themselves to become servants? *And*, what is the effect on the least privileged in society; will they benefit, or, at least, not be further deprived? (p. 7, italics in original)

It is our sincere belief that serving to promote positive social and global change is the most needed style of leadership for our planet. We also conclude from this study that serving is a potential pathway to higher purpose in life. This idea is consistent with Viktor Frankl's belief, robustly supported in empirical research (Batthyány & Guttmann, 2005; Evans, 2016), that self-transcendence leads to greater meaning in life (Frankl, 2000, 2006).

References

Batson, C. D., & Powell, A. A. (2003). Altruism and prosocial behavior. In T. Millon & M. J. Lerner (Eds.), *Handbook of psychology, personality and social psychology* (Vol. 5, pp. 463–484). Wiley.

Batthyány, A., & Guttmann, D. (2005). *Empirical research in logotherapy and meaning-oriented psychotherapy: An annotated bibliography*. Zeig, Tucker & Theisen.

Bowman, N., Brandenberger, J., Lapsley, D., Hill, P., & Quaranto, J. (2010). Serving in college, flourishing in adulthood: Does community engagement during the college years predict adult well-being? *Applied Psychology: Health and Well-Being, 2*(1), 14–34. https://doi.org/10.1111/j.1758-0854.2009.01020.x

Crumbaugh, J. C., & Henrion, R. (1988). The PIL Test: Administration, interpretation, uses theory and critique. *International Forum for Logotherapy, 11*(2), 76–88.

Crumbaugh, J. C., & Maholick, L. T. (1964). An experimental study in existentialism: The psychometric approach to Frankl's concept of noogenic neurosis. *Journal of Clinical Psychology, 20*(2), 200–207.

Evans, W. F. (2016). The world still cries for meaning: Are we still listening? In *Logotherapy and existential analysis: Proceedings of the Viktor Frankl Institute Vienna* (pp. 291–301). Springer International Publishing.

Frankl, V. E. (2000). *Man's search for ultimate meaning*. Perseus.

Frankl, V. E. (2006). *Man's search for meaning*. Beacon Press.

Greenleaf, R. K. (1970). *The servant as leader*. The Robert Greenleaf Center for Servant Leadership.

Greenleaf, R. K. (1977). *Servant leadership*. Paulist Press, Inc.

Halama, P. (2009). Research instruments for investigating meaning of life and other logotherapeutics constructs. In A. Batthyany & J. Levinson (Eds.), *Existential psychotherapy of meaning: Handbook of logotherapy and existential analysis* (pp. 415–444). Zeig, Tucker &Theisen.

Johnson, D. (2006). Finding wholeness: Students' search for meaning and purpose in college. *Journal of College and Character, 7*(1). https://doi.org/10.2202/1940-1639.1503

Langridge, N. L., Evans, W. F., Dixon, A. D., & Janser, S. K. (2012). *Meaning in life: Is this the greatest ROI of the collegiate experience?* [Unpublished manuscript; pilot study for doctoral dissertation at James Madison University.]

Moely, B. E., Mercer, S. H., Ilustre, V., Miron, D., & McFarland, M. (2002). Psychometric properties and correlates of the Civic Attitudes and Skills Questionnaire (CASQ): A measure of students' attitudes related to service-learning. *Michigan Journal of Community Service Learning, 8*(2), 15–26.

Molasso, W. R. (2006). Exploring Frankl's purpose in life with college students. *Journal of College and Character, 7*(1). https://doi.org/10.2202/1940-1639.1502

Moran, C. D. (2001). Purpose in life, student development, and well-being: Recommendations for student affairs practitioners. *NASPA Journal, 38*(3), 269–279. https://doi.org/10.2202/1949-6605.1147

Rushton, J. P., Chrisjohn, R. D., & Cynthia Fekken, G. (1981). The altruistic personality and the Self-Report Altruism Scale. *Personality and Individual Differences, 2*(4), 293–302. https://doi.org/10.1016/0191-8869(81)90084-2

Sipe, J. W., & Frick, D. M. (2015). *Seven pillars of servant leadership: Practicing the wisdom of leading by serving*. Paulist Press.

Spears, L. C. (2000). Character and servant leadership: Ten characteristics of effective, caring leaders. *Concepts and Connection, 8*(3), 1–6.

Trudeau, K. J., & Devlin, A. S. (1996). College students and community service: Who, with whom, and why? *Journal of Applied Social Psychology, 26*(21), 1867–1888. https://doi.org/10.1111/j.1559-1816.1996.tb00103.x

Wang, Y., Ye, F., Jackson, G., Rodgers, R., & Jones, S. (2005). Development of Student Service-Learning Course Survey (SSLCS) to measure service-learning course outcomes. *IR Applications, 3*, 1.

William F. Evans, PhD, is a professor of psychology at James Madison University. He earned a BA in religion from Wofford College, an MDiv from Duke University, and a PhD in counselor education and supervision from the University of South Carolina. Evans is a decorated United States Air Force Colonel (retired) and serves on the International Advisory Board for the Viktor Frankl Institute in Vienna, Austria.

Cynthia M. Evans, PhD, is an adjunct professor of psychology at Liberty University, teaching at both the undergraduate and graduate levels. She earned her BA in communication studies from The Ohio State University. She earned an MA in counseling and a PhD in professional counseling from Liberty University.

Part V
Practical Applications of Logotherapy: Education, Youth, and the Workplace

It's a Bird! It's a Plane! It's a Logotherapist! Using Superheroes in Viktor Frankl's Logotherapy

Jared Bishop

In my office there is a sign which reads, "Always be yourself, unless you can be Batman. Then always be Batman." Every person who comes into this office with me, so far, has commented on this sign, usually with laughter and agreement. People are drawn to superheroes, like Batman. In the past year, millions of dollars have been spent by people of all ages flocking to movie theaters to see films with leading characters such as Doctor Strange, Batman, and Thor. TV and streaming services are also capitalizing on the public's interest in superheroes with TV shows like WandaVision, SheHulk, and the Umbrella Academy. Superheroes have become the mythology of modern times (Rubin, 2011). People follow their stories through movies, TV shows, and comic books. Even the most casual follower of popular culture knows the basics of Superman's origin story or can identify popular costumed heroes.

Psychotherapists have a long history of incorporating mythology and stories into therapy (Goodwin, 2015). Superheroes, as modern mythology, have a place in therapeutic settings and can be used to facilitate logotherapeutic intervention and communicate the concepts of logotherapy to our clients.

Superhero Elements

Since the introduction of Superman in 1938, superheroes have become more complex and diverse, yet from the beginning there have been common themes. All superheroes have an origin story which describes how they became the hero they are and acquired their powers. Although each hero's story has unique details, there tend

J. Bishop (✉)
Viktor Frankl Institute of Logotherapy, Stamford, TX, USA

Jane Pauley Community Health Center, Indianapolis, IN, USA

C. L. McLafferty, Jr., J. I. Levinson (eds.), *Logotherapy and Existential Analysis*, Logotherapy and Existential Analysis: Proceedings of the Viktor Frankl Institute Vienna 2, https://doi.org/10.1007/978-3-031-48922-8_20

to be common elements. Many heroes were orphaned, abandoned, or otherwise disconnected from their family of origin. Nearly all experienced violence early in their lives. Superman (Donner, 1978) was separated from his alien parents as an infant. Batman (Reeves, 2022) witnessed the murder of his parents. Spiderman (Watts, 2021) was raised by his aunt and uncle. Magneto (Singer, 2000), similar to Viktor Frankl, lost his family in Nazi concentration camps. Some superheroes are born with innate super abilities, such as Superman or the X-Men (Singer, 2000). Others, such as Spiderman or the Green Lantern (Campbell, 2011), acquire their powers through scientific experimentation gone awry or other fantastic means. A few heroes, including Batman and Iron Man (Favreau, 2008), do not have any superhuman abilities. Regardless, each superhero experiences an event that changes their life and prompts them to respond by creating a superhero identity.

Most superheroes have to navigate the complications of a dual identity. They are both their mundane, everyday, selves as well as masked, powerful, crime fighters. A secret identity allows the hero to conceal their vulnerabilities or, in the case of some, to rise above their weaknesses. Daredevil is an excellent example of this. By day, Matt Murdock is an attorney who was blinded in an accident, but by night he uses his "radar sense" to overcome his disability.

In addition to super powers or incredible abilities, each superhero also has a fatal flaw. Despite all of Superman's amazing abilities, he becomes weak and helpless when he encounters kryptonite. Other fatal weaknesses include Green Lantern's (Campbell, 2011) weakness when exposed to the color yellow and The Hulk's (Lee, 2003) uncontrollable rage. All superheroes have a rogues' gallery of evildoers from whom they must save their community, nation, or planet. In order to do this, most superheroes also have a loyal and helpful sidekick. Additionally, many are part of super teams or families, such as the Guardians of the Galaxy (James, 2014), the Avengers (Russo & Russo, 2019), the X-Men (Singer, 2000), or the Justice League (Snyder, 2017). Most importantly, all heroes are guided by a mission. They have a purpose for putting on a costume and fighting crime.

Superheroes and Logotherapy

These common elements of the superhero story align with the principles of Viktor Frankl's (1988/1969), who built his theory of logotherapy on the assumptions that every person has the freedom to make their own life decisions (*freedom of will*), are motivated to seek meaning in life (*will to meaning*), and are able to discover meaning and purpose through creative values, experiential values, and attitudinal values (*meaning in life*). A lack of meaning results in an *existential vacuum*, which may be characterized by the elements of the mass neurotic triad: depression, aggression, and addiction (Frankl, 2000). Frankl stressed that the will to meaning is the primary motivator of humanity, over Freud's *will to pleasure* and Adler's *will to power* (Frankl, 1988/1969).

The central role of meaning in life is clearly present in superhero narratives. More than a desire to be happy or powerful, most superheroes are pulled to action as a quest for meaning. Batman and Spiderman seek to find meaning in the tragic deaths of their parental figures. Wolverine is motivated by a need to understand his past and find meaning in the traumatic scientific experimentation that was conducted on him. Even the character arc for Iron Man reflects a quest for meaning. From the beginning, Iron Man is presented as egotistical and self-absorbed; however, Iron Man's actions are motivated to improve the world, rather than solely seek pleasure or power. This motivation to transcend himself increases, to the point that he sacrifices himself to save the universe in his final battle, truly finding a unique purpose in life. Not only for Iron Man, but for all superheroes, the personal sacrifice and dedication required often results in the loss of power, prestige, and luxury. Therefore, by seeking meaning, superheroes tend to act in ways that undermine a sense of pleasure or power, despite this being well within their grasp. Bruce Wayne, for example, is a billionaire, who could easily spend all of his time living a hedonistic lifestyle, but instead he devotes much of his time, energy, and resources to his life purpose of protecting Gotham. Professor Charles Xavier's vast telepathic abilities are continually sought after by villains due to their potential for world domination through mind control. Instead, he uses his power to provide education, mentorship, and connection among mutants. Often it is the villains in the superhero narrative whose actions are motivated by self-absorbed needs for pleasure and power. They are also examples of the harmful effects of the existential vacuum.

For most superheroes, their actions are powerful examples of self-transcendence. Rather than focusing their power, abilities, and resources on themselves, they seek to protect and improve the lives of others. Many superheroes are also poignant examples of logotherapy's principles of freedom and responsibility. Very few superheroes had ideal childhoods; as noted, nearly all superheroes are shaped by tragic pasts; however, few would refer to them as victims. Rather than succumb to these blows of fate, story after story tells of how individual characters made the *choice* to determine their own attitudes and responses to life events. Superheroes serve as examples of the *defiant power of the human spirit* and fictional embodiments of humanity's capacity for "resisting and braving even the worst conditions" (Frankl, 1988/1969, p. 16). Superheroes activate attitudinal values by their response to tragedy, abuse, and oppression. As the superhero universe has expanded, so have the traumas experienced by these heroes. They engage creative values through their heroic actions to protect others and uphold justice. Heroes also respond to experiential values, through their connections with sidekicks, other superheroes, family members, and friends.

Superheroes, Logotherapy, and Teens

Logotherapy has strong historical ties to the period of adolescent development. After all, we are reminded that the seeds of logotherapy began to sprout when Viktor Frankl was about 13 years old. As Helen Roberts (1980) recounted the story, Frankl's biology teacher responded to a question about the meaning of life by saying "[It is] a process of combustion, an oxidation process" (p. 19). This was apparently an unsatisfying answer to young Frankl. If logotherapy was tested in concentration camps, it appears to have been born from a search for identity in adolescence, which was not satisfied by reductionistic, nihilistic ideas. Roberts also noted that some of the first applications of logotherapy occurred in Frankl's work in establishing youth guidance centers in Vienna in 1928. Therefore, it is unsurprising that logotherapy touches on the core themes of adolescence: freedom and responsibility, the development of values, and the discovery of meaning and purpose in life.

Adolescence is a period of change. It is not only characterized by the physical changes of puberty, but also changes in relationships, family dynamics, and one's understanding of oneself. The development of identity is one of the key tasks of our teenage years. Erik Erikson (1980) argued that the formation of a healthy identity, while a central task of adolescence, is also the culmination of childhood experiences, as well as a response to hopes for the future. In other words, the core task of adolescence is to identify the values that we will live our lives by and begin the process of discovering the ultimate meaning of our lives.

For many youths, this period is made even more complicated through the experience of relational trauma, particularly complex trauma. Complex trauma refers to exposure to multiple, often chronic traumas from an early age (Wamser-Nanney & Vandenberg, 2013). These children and teenagers have been battered and bruised from their earliest days for offenses as simple as crying too much. Their basic needs have often gone unmet, so that they have had to fend for themselves in a dangerous world in order to survive. The opportunities and experiences that children need to develop into healthy adults have been distorted or taken from them. These are also young individuals without much consistency in their lives. Not only are their families unstable and unpredictable, but they are often thrown into a system of being bounced around from foster family to foster family.

In a follow-up to the Kaiser-Permanente Adverse Childhood Experiences (ACES; CDC, 2019) study, the Centers for Disease Control and Prevention found that 60.9% of their sample had experienced at least one ACE (Merrick et al., 2019). These researchers also found that an individual did not typically experience only one type of adverse childhood experience, such as childhood abuse or household dysfunction. Of those who had experienced at least one ACE, 61.6% had experienced multiple ACEs. They concluded that a greater number of adverse childhood experiences were related to a more complex trauma response and a greater impact on that person's life.

As researchers have explored the effects of complex trauma, they have found that the experience interferes with typical development, including a child's ability to develop a secure attachment, a child's opportunities to interact with the world in a safe manner thereby developing a sense of agency, and a child's sense of identity (Blaustein & Kinniburgh, 2010). These issues continue to compound into adolescence. As children mature into teenagers, they are faced with the developmental task of figuring out who they are against a background of abuse, neglect, and limited opportunity. Many times these youth are burdened with pain, guilt, and death, Frankl's (1984) tragic triad.

Here is the environment in which identity is formed, as adolescents answer the question of "Who am I?" Our sense of identity rests upon balancing tension between "I am" and "I ought"—our current realistic understanding of who we are in the moment and our potential for the future (Frankl, 1988/1969). Frankl pointed out that potential is guided by meaning and values. As Frankl wrote, "The meaning of meaning is to set the pace of being" (p. 51).

This task is complicated even in the best circumstances, but for youth with a history of complex trauma, the search for identity has been warped. Independence, a typical feature of healthy adolescence, has been distorted. Youths in these circumstances have often gravitated to the extremes—complete dependence on others to care for them or complete independence without desire for human connection (Van der Kolk, 2015). Both of these extremes come with a great fear of relationships with others.

Our identity is built upon the messages that we receive from others. The messages youth in the context of complex trauma have received have not generally been positive. Words such as "burden," "mistake," "incapable," "stupid," "unworthy," and "unimportant" are typical words I have heard expressed. These have all shaped an identity that is painful. Avenues that other youth use to discover meaning have not been easily accessible to them. For typically developing children, their creative acts have been praised and encouraged, which has resulted in further successes. For the youth who have experienced complex trauma, their creative contributions are often ignored, at best, and denigrated, at worst. The joy of creating and giving to life has been taken from them.

For children experiencing a typical, healthy development, there have been positive, warm, and encouraging experiences of love and closeness with individuals who care about them. For youth who have experienced complex trauma, their relationships have been empty of such love or have been tainted by inconsistent care. Relationships have become painful and something to be guarded against in the case of absent caregivers. In the case of inconsistent caregivers, youth now desperately cling to shallow and/or abusive relationships. The meaning of experiential values has been distorted for them.

Chronic maltreatment also makes it difficult for these youth to find meaning in suffering that has been all they have ever known. It should come as no surprise that as childhood exposure to trauma increases so do incidents of depression, aggression, and addiction. These are individuals who are trapped in the existential vacuum from an early age. It is within this context that logotherapy is vitally needed as a component in treatment.

Therapies such as trauma-focused cognitive behavior therapy or eye movement desensitization and reprocessing for trauma disorders (Dorsey et al., 2017), or behavior therapy and parent training for conduct problems (Eyberg et al., 2008), have shown effectiveness in treating these psychiatric presentations in adolescence; however, none of these therapy modalities tap into the noëtic dimension. While symptoms do need to be addressed, if they are occurring as a reaction to those experiencing an existential vacuum, it is also necessary to address this underlying problem. Logotherapy may be used in conjunction with other therapy modalities to effectively address issues related to trauma and conduct.

Beyond the use of logotherapy with youth with severe mental health presentations, the use of superheroes in therapy has been described with clients of all ages, but it may be especially salient with teenage clients (Rubin, 2011). Not only are superheroes a topic of interest for most teenagers, many superhero storylines deal with topics that are relatable to them. Superheroes struggle with concepts such as morality, justice, balancing power and vulnerability, and managing conflict. Rubin noted that, like their heroes, many teens are also working through these concepts. Superheroes, like teens, are tackling issues such as autonomy, identity, and relationships. Issues faced by superheroes, not surprisingly, often mirror the developmental tasks of adolescence. In therapy, this can provide practitioners with a window for broaching topics salient to their experience as adolescents.

Overview of the Four Stages of Logotherapy with Youth

The practice of logotherapy with youths follows the same four stages described by Fabry (2013/1968). Schulenberg (2002) later interpreted these stages into guidelines for therapy with youth with behavioral problems. First, there must be *self-distancing from symptoms*. As part of this first stage, the development of rapport is essential. As therapists we provide an opportunity for our clients to learn that they are more than their symptoms. So many of the labels that have been thrown at youth clients over the years have "stuck" and been accepted as part of who they are. Over years of work with adolescents, I can think of many clients who were initially resistant to therapy or medication because their anger, isolation, and aggression were a core part of how they viewed themselves; therapy was initially viewed as an attack on their identity. Over time, the clinician needs to work to develop a sense of identity separate from the symptoms. This is not accomplished through persuasion (Schulenberg, 2002), but through Socratic dialogue. As Lukas (1979) pointed out, we accomplish this by leading the youth "to see themselves from outside as observers, and not from inside their traps, as victims" (p. 97).

The second step is the *modulation of attitudes* (Lukas, 2020). Rice (2000) described a process in which the therapist guides the client to examine their current cognitions and the effect those cognitions have on behaviors and attitudes. This is followed by developing a decision-making process, which emphasizes the adolescent's freedom to choose for themselves and strengthening their ability to accept consequences, which emphasizes responsibility for the choices they make. Our clients—even the most damaged—have the power to heal themselves. This is the defiant power of the human spirit that we must tap in to. We guide our clients to new perspectives about themselves, their identity, and their past traumas.

The third stage is *symptom reduction*. Here we address specific symptoms that have not abated in the first two steps. Any lingering conduct problems should be addressed in a manner that maintains the individual's dignity as a human being and builds on previous work in changing attitudes and discovering avenues of meaning.

Finally, we *orient toward meaning*. Our attention is turned toward the future, so that individuals will be able to generalize their new thoughts, behaviors, and attitudes to new problems in their lives.

Superhero Therapeutic Techniques

Now that we have established that superheroes embody many logotherapeutic principals and reviewed the stages of logotherapeutic counseling, let us consider how superheroes can be used in therapy. The use of superheroes in therapy requires several prerequisites of the therapist (Rubin, 2011). Therapists using superheroes must be imaginative and fun-loving. They should be open and flexible to the needs of the client. Also vital to the effective use of superheroes in therapy, they need to have an interest in superheroes. However, there is no need to have encyclopedic knowledge of every issue of *The Batman* (Reeves, 2022) or be able to immediately identify the most minor superhero. When a client identifies a hero with whom the clinician is unfamiliar, acknowledgment of the lack of familiarity often allows the client to share a special interest and to deepen rapport with the clinician. Afterwards, additional information about the particular hero can be sought out. A fuller understanding of an unfamiliar hero only requires a small amount of research and interest. This may involve reading their character's Wikipedia page, watching a movie featuring the character, or perhaps reading a few comics. Therapists using superheroes should also value and respect superheroes. In the 1954 Kefauver hearings, the US Senate (1954) sought to determine whether superhero stories were detrimental to youth. Some mental health professionals argued that the violence of these comics and, what these experts perceived as emblems of homosexuality and fascism (Wertham, 1954), made them harmful to adolescents. Other experts found value in the stories of these superheroes as metaphors for teenagers and as ways to expressing and dealing with trauma, conflict, and upheaval in their lives. As time has progressed, the former group of professionals has grown smaller; however, clinicians who view superheroes with suspicion may find that their use in therapy is not appropriate for them.

Finally, using superheroes in therapy is significantly helped by having access to superhero paraphernalia. Some therapists have written about how their entire office is decorated in superhero themes, with posters, insignia, and toys covering their workspace. For myself, I have the one sign mentioned at the beginning of this chapter. Having something superhero-related in your office provides an opening and can aid in rapport building. For superhero fans, seeing something hero related in their new counselor's office may be a comforting sign and a point of connection, even before the first words are spoken. Even though a therapist and client may have never met before, it may create an immediate bond through a shared interest. When a client comments on my Batman sign, it is an opening to ask about their favorite superhero, ask what super powers they wish they possessed, and their level of interest in superheroes. Obviously, not every client has an interest in superheroes. For this reason, I generally wait until the client mentions superheroes and determine their level of interest before incorporating them into the session.

In therapy, superheroes work very effectively for many clients as a metaphor (Rubin, 2007). Parallels can be drawn from the client's situation to situations faced by superheroes. Particularly thanks to the social awareness of comic book creators, it is very likely that there is a superhero out there who has faced a similar situation to the one the client is encountering. Batman deals with grief and loss; Superman, with being adopted and living as an outsider; the Hulk, with uncontrollable rage; Spiderman, with sexual abuse as a child; Daredevil (Johnson, 2003) and Professor X, with physical disabilities; X-Men, with discrimination. The role of metaphor is nearly endless. Regarding the principles of logotherapy, many superhero stories embody these principles and serve as useful metaphors for communicating these ideas to clients.

To this end, Robertie and colleagues (2007) describe the "What If" technique, which I have modified to incorporate the principles of logotherapy. In this technique, clients and therapists engage in a discussion of what would have happened if the character had made a different choice. For example, Spiderman, through a series of events, lets loose the Green Goblin, who later murdered his Aunt May. Spiderman has many choices he could have made in response to this event, reflecting his freedom of will: He could have used his powers to exact revenge, he could have become despondent, or he could have drowned his sorrows in a bottle of alcohol. Instead, he chose to use his powers to embody his aunt's mantra: "With great power comes great responsibility." Spiderman's choice reflects his choice of meaning, while overcoming depression, senseless violence, and addiction. Following the "What If" technique, the discussion can be guided to the examination of these ideas in the life of the client. By discussing events through the lens of the superhero narrative, the client is allowed to self-distance from their own situation. It also serves as a point of connection with another person (albeit fictional) who has faced a similar life challenge. Superheroes are particularly effective as metaphors for efficacy and competence, conflict resolution (both internal and external), the freedom of will, and a common person accomplishing uncommon things (Rubin, 2011).

If your knowledge of specific superhero conflicts is limited, or, as is often the case, your superhero knowledge is different from your client's, a technique described by Nelson (2007) may be useful. The "What Would Superman Do?" technique challenges the client to place their favorite superhero in their own situation and explore how the character would respond to the real-life challenges facing the client. This is also a simple question that can be taught to clients as they work through difficult decisions outside of the counseling office. Despite their hero's fantastic abilities, it is their values that shape their response. A word of caution is in order regarding antiheroes, or superhuman characters that are morally ambiguous (e.g., Deadpool or characters for the Umbrella Academy): If your client identifies with an antihero, this technique would likely not be beneficial; however, antiheroes can provide a wealth of material for discussions on morality and decision making.

Because superheroes tend to live by a code of ethics, they can provide a powerful context for value-exploration activities. Superheroes can be used to bookend a discussion of personal values. The client and therapist begin by discussing the character of superheroes. For example, "Would Clark Kent respond to a situation differently from Superman?" As the discussion unfolds, it should become clear that, although the super alter-ego may be more likely to act in a superhuman fashion, Clark Kent and Superman are one individual with the same values. The therapist then guides the client into a discussion about how the superhero developed these values. Often, these values have strong significance to the superhero because of their past experiences. The client and therapist then transition to focusing on the client's values using a values-clarification activity, such as the one developed by Joseph Fabry (2021/1988) or the Personal Values Card Sort (Miller et al., 2001). These activities ask clients to compare commonly held values in order to determine their most important values. The client and therapist can then explore how past events have shaped these values. To end the values-clarification experience, the therapist returns to the superhero, emphasizing that superheroes make conscious choices to live lives consistent with their values, which is sometimes challenging. For example, due to Batman's value of human life, he never kills his enemies, which often makes his mission more challenging and puts him at greater risk. The client and therapist can then reflect on how the client's own actions going forward can reflect their life values.

Eisenberg, Welter, and Hutzell (cited in Welter, 1995) developed the Movie Experience as a tool for logotherapists to guide clients as they examine the "degree of meaning in their lives up to the present" (p. 65). This technique can be modified for the superhero fan. I generally begin by exploring the life of a favorite superhero, to serve as a model. Together, we discuss the chosen superhero's background, their supernatural aids, and the symbols associated with them. We then discuss challenges faced by the superhero, both internal and external. The client discusses the superhero's sidekicks and supports, as well as their nemesis. Finally, we identify a theme that unifies the superhero's experience and a life purpose. The client is then asked to imagine their life as a superhero movie. What role do they play? Are they the superhero, the sidekick, the villain, or just a bystander? What is their origin story and how do they acquire their superpowers? What powers and supports do they have? What symbols represent their super identity? The therapist and client discuss villains and internal challenges faced. Finally, the therapist guides the client into looking back over their life for a unifying theme and life purpose. This can be similarly done with second part of the Movie Experience. Superhero stories can also be enacted using role play, sand tray, or art.

The options for using superheroes in therapy are nearly limitless. Expressions from superheroes can become mantras for clients or link them back to their superhero metaphor. Examples include Spiderman's (Watts, 2021) theme "With great power, there must also come great responsibility," Hulk's (Lee, 2003) warning "You wouldn't like me when I'm angry," and Green Lantern's (Campbell, 2011) oath, "In brightest day, in blackest night, no evil shall escape my sight." Additionally, client discussions of how they would use superpowers and how they might backfire can be highly engaging and meaningful. Similarly, clients and therapists can discuss superhero weaknesses, and how they can be overcome or transformed into meaningful actions.

In therapeutic work using superheroes, clients may use this discussion to avoid focusing on real-life problems or become so involved in the fantastic elements of the story that they cannot see how this relates to their own life. Throughout the use of superheroes, therapists should emphasize the "everyday hero" qualities that are just as "super" as the hero's superhuman powers. These qualities, rather than their powers, are what makes them heroes rather than villains. The qualities of everyday heroes include: showing up, being responsible, helping others, standing up for what is right, telling the truth, asking for help, caring for self and others, battling monsters, and coping with challenges (Rubin, 2011). These are things that all clients can do! Be sure to praise them for their actual feats of "everyday heroism."

Conclusion

Novelist Ursula Le Guin (1979) wrote:

> The great fantasies, myths, and tales are indeed like dreams: They speak from the unconscious to the unconscious, in the language of the unconscious-symbol and archetype.... They short-circuit verbal reasoning, and go straight to the thoughts that lie too deep to utter. (p. 62)

This may represent superheroes' true greater power: They give us a tool to interact meaningfully with our clients at a deeper level. The values and missions of superheroes can serve as metaphors and examples of the principles of logotherapy acted out. The possibilities for logotherapeutic healing using superheroes are limitless.

References

Blaustein, M., & Kinniburgh, K. (2010). *Treating traumatic stress in children and adolescents: How to foster resilience through attachment, self-regulation, and competency*. Guilford Press.

Campbell, M. (Director). (2011). *Green Lantern* [motion picture]. United States: Warner Bros.

CDC. (2019). *Preventing adverse childhood experiences: Leveraging the best available evidence*. US Department of Health and Human Services. CDC Retrieved from https://www.cdc.gov/violenceprevention/pdf/preventingACES-508.pdf

Donner, R. (Director). (1978). *Superman* [motion picture]. United States: Dovemead Ltd.

Dorsey, S., McLaughlin, K. A., Kerns, S. E., Harrison, J. P., Lambert, H. K., Briggs, E. C., et al. (2017). Evidence base update for psychosocial treatments for children and adolescents exposed

to traumatic events. *Journal of Clinical Child & Adolescent Psychology, 46*(3), 303–330. https://doi.org/10.1080/15374416.2016.1220309
Erikson, E. H. (1980). *Identity and the life cycle*. Norton.
Eyberg, S. M., Nelson, M. M., & Boggs, S. R. (2008). Evidence-based psychosocial treatments for children and adolescents with disruptive behavior. *Journal of Clinical Child & Adolescent Psychology, 37*(1), 215–237. https://doi.org/10.1080/15374410701820117
Fabry, J. B. (2013/1968). *The pursuit of meaning: Viktor Frankl, logotherapy, and life*. Purpose Research. (Original work published 1968)
Fabry, J. B. (2021/1988). *Guideposts to meaning: Discovering what really matters* (2nd ed.). Purpose Research. (Original work published 1988)
Favreau, J. (Director). (2008). *Iron Man* [motion picture]. United States: Marvel Studios.
Frankl, V. E. (1984). *Man's search for meaning* (3rd ed.). Pocket Books. (Original work published 1946)
Frankl, V. E. (1988/1969). *The will to meaning: Foundations and applications of logotherapy*. Meridian.
Frankl, V. E. (2000). *Man's search for ultimate meaning*. Perseus. (Original work published *Der Unbewusste Gott*, 1948 and English translation, *The Unconscious God*, 1975)
Goodwin, C. J. (2015). *A history of modern psychology*. Wiley.
James, G. (Director). (2014). *Guardians of the Galaxy* [motion picture]. United States: Marvel Studios.
Johnson, M. (Director). (2003). *Daredevil* [motion picture]. United States: Marvel Studios.
Le Guin, U. K. (1979). *The language of the night: Essays on fantasy and science fiction* (2nd ed.). G.P. Putnam's Sons.
Lee, A. (Director). (2003). *The Hulk* [motion picture]. United States: Universal Pictures.
Lukas, E. (1979). The four steps of logotherapy. In J. B. Fabry, R. P. Bulka, & W. S. Sahakian (Eds.), *Logotherapy in action* (pp. 95–103). Jason Aronson.
Lukas, E. (2020). *Meaningful living: Introduction to logotherapy theory and practice*. J. B. Fabry, Trans (2nd ed.). Purpose Research.
Merrick, M. T., Ford, D. C., Ports, K. A., Guinn, A. S., Chen, J., Klevens, J., et al. (2019). Vital signs: Estimated proportion of adult health problems attributable to adverse childhood experiences and implications for prevention—25 States, 2015–2017. *Morbidity and Mortality Weekly Report, 68*(44), 999–1005.
Miller, W., C'de Baca, J., Matthews, D., & Wilbourne, P. (2001). *Personal values card sort*. University of New Mexico. Retrieved from http://www.motivationalinterviewing.org/sites/default/files/valuescardsort_0.pdf
Nelson, C. A. (2007). What would Superman do? In L. C. Rubin (Ed.), *Using superheroes in counseling and play therapy* (pp. 49–67). Springer.
Reeves, M. (Director). (2022). *The Batman* [motion picture]. United States: Warner Brothers.
Rice, G. E. (2000). An optimistic stance toward disruptive behavior. *International Forum for Logotherapy, 23*, 30–39.
Robertie, K., Weidenbenner, R., Barrett, L., & Poole, R. (2007). A super milieu: Using superheroes in the residential treatment of adolescents with sexual behavior problems. In L. C. Rubin (Ed.), *Using superheroes in counseling and play therapy* (pp. 143–168). Springer.
Roberts, H. (1980). Logotherapy's contribution to youth. *International Forum for Logotherapy, 3*(1), 19–21.
Rubin, L. C. (2007). Introduction: Look, up in the sky! An introduction to the use of superheroes in psychotherapy. In L. C. Rubin (Ed.), *Using superheroes in counseling and play therapy*. Springer.
Rubin, L. C. (2011). *Superheroes in play therapy and counseling*. Paper presented at the South Carolina Association for Play Therapy.
Russo, A., & Russo, J. (Directors). (2019). *Avengers: Endgame* [motion picture]. United States: Marvel Studios.

Schulenberg, S. E. (2002). Logotherapy and conduct disorder. *International Forum for Logotherapy, 25*(1), 52–59.
Singer, B. (Director). (2000). *X-Men* [motion picture]. United States: Twentieth-Century Fox.
Snyder, Z. (Director). (2017). *Justice League* [motion picture]. United States: Warner Brothers Pictures.
U.S. Senate. (1954). *Juvenile Delinquency (comic books). US Congressional Senate hearings before the subcommittee to investigate Juvenile Delinquency. Committee on the Judiciary, United States Senate, eighty-third congress, second session pursuant to Senate resolution, 190. Investigations of Juvenile Delinquency in the United States*. US Government Printing Office.
Van der Kolk, B. (2015). *The body keeps the score: Brain, mind, and body in the healing of trauma*. Penguin Books.
Wamser-Nanney, R., & Vandenberg, B. R. (2013). Empirical support for the definition of a complex trauma event in children and adolescents. *Journal of Traumatic Stress, 26*(6), 671–678.
Watts, J. (Director). (2021). *Spider-Man: No way home* [motion picture]. United States: Columbia Pictures.
Welter, P. (1995). *Franklian psychology and attitudinal change*. Viktor Frankl Insititue of Logotherapy.
Wertham, F. (1954). *Seduction of the innocent*. Rinehart.

Jared Bishop, is a licensed psychologist in East Central Indiana where he is the Director of Behavioral Health Training at the Jane Pauley Community Health Center. He earned a Bachelor of Arts degree in Psychology and a Master of Education degree in Counseling and Human Development from Hardin-Simmons University. Dr. Bishop graduated from Ball State University with a Doctor of Philosophy Degree in Educational (School) Psychology and completed his doctoral internship at the Onarga Academy site of the Illinois School Psychology Internship Consortium. He has been active in the Viktor Frankl Institute of Logotherapy since 2009. He has experience providing counseling and psychological assessments in various settings, including community mental health, school districts, and residential treatment facilities. Dr. Bishop's clinical interests include sand-tray therapy, meaning-centered therapy, eye movement desensitization and reprocessing (EMDR), and complex trauma. Dr. Bishop serves as the Vice President of the International Board of Directors for the Viktor Frankl Institute of Logotherapy.

Logotherapy: Educating Students to Search for Meaning

Cynthia Wimberly

The search for meaning and purpose is a quest as old as the history of mankind. Our earliest stories tell of heroic journeys in which the beast must be slain, the evildoer overcome, and the good for all must win. We root for the underdogs, those individuals who must discover their roles through the struggles and unfair events fate has ordained. And as old as this story is, it is also the newest story reflected in the box office hits of the season, the Star Wars stories, superheroes, and heroines, Frozen, Harry Potter, and so on. We struggle, we mourn, we celebrate, we cry, we fear, we live… in the understanding that these epic adventures reflect that deep yearning of living a life with meaning that transcends our personal journeys.

Perhaps hidden in this search by living life vicariously through movies, video games, and technology is the very real fear of living a life without meaning. Today's youth face a different landscape from previous generations. Names reflecting the struggle for the young generation range from the E-Generation, the Scapegoat Generation, the Ambitious Generation, and the iGeneration. By reducing them down to a generic commodity, society has moved from Generation Y to Generation X to the current Generation Z.

Generation Z, those born between 1995 and 2015, number nearly 74 million in the USA. This group is characterized by heavy use of technology, including mobile devices and the internet. They live in a world with instant access and instant connection. On average, they spend three hours on these devices daily (Kasasa, 2019). Riehm et al. (2019) concluded that those adolescents who spend more than three hours per day involved in social media may be at a higher risk for mental health problems.

This generation has never known a world without war, social media, and smartphones. Not content to simply watch from the sidelines, this generation: (a) is much

C. Wimberly (✉)
Viktor Frankl Institute of Logotherapy, Stamford, TX, USA

C. L. McLafferty, Jr., J. I. Levinson (eds.), *Logotherapy and Existential Analysis*, Logotherapy and Existential Analysis: Proceedings of the Viktor Frankl Institute Vienna 2, https://doi.org/10.1007/978-3-031-48922-8_21

more involved in social causes while at the same time slowing their transition into adulthood, (b) is much more tolerant and inclusive while suffering from a fragility that causes a need for "trigger warnings" and "safe spaces," and (c) is much more open to others while spending an inordinate amount of time experiencing relationships only though technology (Haidt & Lukianoff, 2018).

How do nations, societies, communities, and parents tackle this challenge of rearing the next generation to find meaning? How do we teach the individual to accept responsibility for making decisions and for being accountable for the consequences while ensuring they remain true to the unique meaning of the moment? How do we honor the uniqueness and value of the individual while demanding a meaningful, purposeful, and socially responsible treatment of others? How do we help our younger generation find their way?

Perhaps the first step is in acknowledging the right of our young people to ask the hard questions. But instead of offering them an answer, perhaps the correct response is to admit their motivation to ask these questions is hard-wired into their being and to encourage them to develop the skills to find their answers.

The *Oxford Learner's Dictionaries* ("Education," 2019) defines *education* as "the process of receiving or giving systematic instruction, especially at a school or university." Historically, the role of education has included the concept of preparation for a vocation. Vocation ("Vocation," 2019) is defined "as a strong calling, impulse or inclination to follow a particular activity or career; a function to which one is called" and transcends the idea of finding a job. The definition of education could then be the process of receiving or giving systematic instruction, in which the individual learns to listen to a strong inclination to follow a particular calling. The emphasis then is on the process, not the end product—on the way of life, not the acquisition of a job. The role of education is then to teach students how to search out the "right" answer to life's questions, not simply to regurgitate knowledge on a standardized test. As Frankl (2000) explained:

> A doctor cannot give meaning to his patients, nor can a professor give meaning to his students.... What he may give, however, is an example, the existential example of his personal commitment to the search for truth. The answer to the question of what is the meaning of life can be posited only out of one's whole being—one's own life is the answer to the questions of the meaning of life (p. 46).

Logotherapy, developed by Viktor Frankl (1986) prior to World War II, provides a template for this type of educational experience. He coined the term *logotherapy*, derived from the Greek word *Logos*, which denotes *meaning*. The logotherapist calls for the finding of unique meanings in all circumstances of life. In addition to the body (soma) and the mind (psyche), Frankl added the unique human dimension of spirit (*noös*), which is defined as separate from any religious connotation of the word *spiritual*. Frankl noted that meaning is rooted in this noëtic, spiritual dimension, which is unique in his theoretical three-dimensional framework of a human being.

Frankl (1986) explained that it is in the noëtic dimension that the search for meaning originates, that the human kingdom is different from the plant and animal kingdoms. Fabry (1988/2021) quoted Frankl as saying that the human spirit is our instrument for finding meaning. Meaning is the reality of one's life. This spiritual dimension contains such faculties as freedom of choice, intentionality, creative and artistic interest, and religious and ethical sensitivity. The human conscience is found in this dimension; it also includes an understanding of values and love, as well as the capacity to be awed by experiences, intuition, and inspiration (Frankl, 1988/1969).

In addition, the American Counseling Association (ACA) in 1995 and the American School Counseling Association in 2004 recognized the importance of addressing the spiritual component. Both organizations, like Frankl, defined spirituality by differentiating it from the concept of religion. The American Counseling Association definition of spirituality is:

> A capacity and tendency that is innate and unique to all persons. [It] moves the individual toward knowledge, love, meaning, hope, transcendence, connectedness, and compassion. Spirituality includes one's capacity for creativity, growth, and the development of a value system. Spirituality encompasses the religious, spiritual, and transpersonal. (MacDonald, 2004, p. 294)

Traditionally, educators have felt comfortable addressing the physical and academic needs of the student. However, without incorporating the spiritual dimension, a student is left with a standardized approach to education. By ignoring the uniquely human quality, the spirit or noös, the student obtains knowledge without direction. This lack of direction or meaninglessness creates a void that Frankl (1969/1988) labeled the *existential vacuum* (pp. 83–98), which is reinforced by an educational system that avoids challenging students with values.

To be clear, the school system is doing a superlative job of preparing students for college. For example, a study done in 2017 shows that 47% of students graduated with an "A" average from high school (Hurwitz & Lee, 2018). Perfect ACT scores have doubled since 2015 (Sparling & Horn, 2019). However, in conjunction with these studies, the rates of serious depression, anxiety, and substance use have risen, especially among the more affluent teenagers who are expected to do well (Roy, 2019).

A student experiencing an existential vacuum is living in a world in which there are no guideposts, no values, and no traditions that provide a firm foundation for the future. It is a world in which it is difficult to identify goals for the day, much less for a life after graduation. It is a world of isolation, of loneliness. For young people experiencing this vacuum, they may conform and follow the crowd or abdicate their choices and simply do what they are told. Both conformism and totalitarianism are symptoms of an existential vacuum. Students who are experiencing this will often manifest feeling bored, apathetic, or uncaring and this can escalate into feelings of aggression, depression, and addictions (Frankl, 1969/1988).

Today, this existential vacuum translates into statistics showing the lack of meaning and purpose in students' lives. Miron et al. (2019) reported that the rate of US adolescents and young adults dying of suicide is at the highest level since 2000. In 2017, it was reported on the *PBS News Hour* that there were 47% more suicides among young people aged 15–24 years of age (Frazee, 2019, June 18). In addition, more children ages 10–14 are likely to die of suicide than in an automobile accident. Suicide is the culmination of the ultimate feelings of hopelessness (Kominiak, 2019).

In addition to suicide, additional challenges face students today. The opioid epidemic is the latest and perhaps most deadly addiction young people have faced. The National Institute on Drug Abuse (2019) reported that as of January 2019 more than 130 people in the US were dying daily of an opioid overdose. The National Alliance on Mental Illness (n.d.) reported that 17% of children and youth, aged 6–17 years, experience a mental health disorder. According to the U.S. Department of Health and Human Services (n.d.), between 25% and 33% of students have been bullied at school with this extending to off-campus bullying, often through cyberbullying. Perhaps the most extreme form of aggression aimed at trying to inappropriately fill the existential vacuum plays out in school shootings. In addition, there have been 1924 school shooting incidents since 1970 with 246 reports in 2021, though this number includes brandishing a firearm or shooting at a school (U. S. Department of the Navy, 2022).

To combat the existential vacuum, a student must discover meaning. Frankl (1984) defined *the will to meaning* as the primary human motivation and explained that meaning can be approached as a search for the meaning of the moment or in the ultimate meaning of life. The tension that is created between *what is* and the striving toward *what should be* is healthy. Meaning gives an individual a unique purpose in life and provides the three pillars of logotherapy: (1) Meaning exists under all circumstances, (2) All persons have the innate desire (motivation) to find meaning in all circumstances, and (3) All persons have the capacity to find meaning by changing the situation or one's attitude. Labeled as the *meaning triangle,* Frankl (1969/1988) identified three ways to discover meaning: (1) through a deed (work, activity, actualization of *creative values*); (2) through experiences (art, nature, beauty, truth, love—*experiential values*); or (3) through a change of attitude (towards life experiences that cannot be changed—*attitudinal values*).

In the philosophy of logotherapy, a student's motivation for living is to find meaning. It is in the noëtic—spiritual—dimension of our being, that each individual asks the questions that provide the desire to focus life in a purposeful manner. Life always has the potential for meaning, and the educator's task is to guide students in finding their own abilities to discover it. Within this framework, educators encourage students to search for answers. "What is the meaning of life?" may be an ultimate question, but more importantly it is possible to ask: "What is the meaning of this moment and how do I choose to respond to it?" (Fabry, 1968/2013; Frankl, 1969/1988).

Frankl (1969/1988) identified key concepts that have been labeled guideposts and/or the medicine chest of logotherapy. These resources of the human spirit must be utilized in order to find meaning. They include self-discovery, choice, uniqueness, responsibility, self-transcendence, will to meaning, task orientation, conscience, self-distancing, and humor. Each of these resources can be applied to the three areas mentioned in the meaning triangle—creativity, experiencing values, and attitude—through implementation of Socratic dialogue. Socratic dialogue is the most common interaction to help students find meaning by reflecting back to the individual. This is used to draw forth knowledge that is intuitively known. The educator throughout the process is listening for logohooks, logoanchors, and logohints (Fabry, 1968/2013).

Applications of Logotherapy in Education

In the discussion that follows, specific ways will be explored in which I have incorporated these topics into the education system. These interventions are based on a research study done with at-risk students (Wimberly, 2006).

Using concepts of logotherapy, the following outline was developed to work with students in classroom settings, group sessions, and individual meetings. The purpose of the discussion is to create an environment where students are able to identify, discover, and make use of meaning and meaning potentials. Since these interactions are directed at all students, the level of emotional risk has to be kept at a minimum. In the school setting it is vital to not open up issues when there is not the time and space to process them. Since confidentiality cannot be guaranteed, the level of risk must be minimized. The professional judgment of the educator is vital in recognizing if issues beyond the school environment exist; appropriate resources have to be available as needed (Wimberly, 2006).

The following topics and accompanying activities were developed to assist students in a search for meaning and were organized for my research study (Wimberly, 2006). These themes center around the meaning triangle. In addition, the majority of the books listed are under the category of children's books; however, it has been my experience that adolescents and adults learn from them, enjoy being read to, and resonate with the message being shared. At the same time, both written and nonwritten options are given for most activities so all students may participate. The foundation of all of these interactions is based on respect, positive regard, and a closeness with scientific detachment. The topics are:

Logotherapeutic Guideposts

1. What is in a name?	Uniqueness
2. What is important to me?	Self-discovery
3. Where do I want to go from here?	Choice
4. How do I get there from here?	Task Orientation/Goals
5. What stands in my way?	Responsibility
6. What choices do I have?	Conscience/Responsibleness
7. How do I fit into the rest of the world?	Self-transcendence
8. Celebration—Show me your stuff	Self-worth

Uniqueness

The first area to be addressed is uniqueness since it is difficult to move a student forward until the concept of being unique is understood and accepted. Many individuals find it difficult to recognize any situations where they cannot be easily replaced. If students feel they are replaceable, then not only is there no meaning or purpose in their life, but also there is no reason to search for it (Wimberly, 2006).

During the first meeting, the three-dimensional concept of the human being (soma, psyche, and noös or spirit) is discussed. Students seem to grasp the concept easily. A clear definition of the spiritual dimension is given to ensure there are no religious connotations. A vital component to this discussion is the introduction of the idea of conscience. My experience has been that the majority of the students at all grade levels have an intuitive understanding of the concept of right and wrong. Students also tend to be comfortable with the concept that the spirit is what defines them as a human as compared to other living things. Without these concepts, educators are reducing students to objects (Wimberly, 2006).

Viktor Frankl quoted William Irwin Thompson to emphasize this point: "Humans are not objects that exist as table and chairs; they live, and if their lives are reduced to the mere existence of chairs or tables, they commit suicide" (cited in Frankl, 1969/1988, pp. 85–86).

A nonthreatening activity that can open the conversation to each person's uniqueness is to explore the history of how a student's name is selected and the emotions the name invokes for the students. Do they like their names? Are they named after someone? Do they like who they are named after? Does their name carry a family responsibility with it? Does it connect with a culture or tradition? Is the name a blessing or a curse? Because of the myriad of different possibilities of what constitutes a family, this can be modified to a nickname, initials, etc. Depending on the age of the student, different art activities can be incorporated with this discussion (Fabry, 1988/2021).

The key to this exercise is having the student share with others both verbally and creatively. Each student receives a blank folder to decorate, a blank piece of cardstock to create a nameplate, and art supplies and magazines. The students are instructed to decorate the folder and nameplate to reflect their uniqueness in 10 different areas. These areas include activities, experiences, and relationships. It is often helpful, if not necessary, for educators to have a resource to guide students to explore this area. Sadly, many will not have 10 items to list. (Wimberly, 2006).

Uniqueness exercise: Meaning triangle

Creative. Decorating nameplate and folder, list 10 ways you are unique;
Experiential. Sharing uniqueness, interview family members or friends;
Attitudinal. During the course of the activity, if it seems that a student has nothing positive about the name or nickname or if it carries a burden, then explore ways to reframe or rewrite the thought process;
Reading. *It's OK To Be Different* by Todd Parr (2011).

In my experience, this first step has had notable results in creating an environment of cooperation and connection. Having done this activity with children, adolescents, and adults, the rise in the energy level in the room and the connections that are being made as stories are shared is immediately noticeable. It has provided insight into what students view as important and unique about themselves and has laid the foundation for future group work.

Self-Discovery

Once students begin to grasp their uniqueness, then the next step is for them to understand the self. Self-discovery is key to finding meaning but, in order to do so, façades must be removed and the true person at the core must be found. Just as each person is unique in mental and spiritual attributes, the conscience of each person that can speak for the noös is also unique. Although there are many different value exercises available to introduce and determine what is important to a student, the method used here is storytelling and games (Wimberly, 2006).

Students are given a certain amount of play money to bid on or purchase important items. These items include money, friends, love, intelligence, health, hero status, physical attractiveness, athletic ability, family, fame, leadership, education, reputation, respect, and one blank for them to determine. Guidelines are put in place so that students have to make some choices and not simply put a small amount of money on each area. Since there is a limited amount of money, they have to determine what is most valuable and needed. Students then process and share their reasons for purchasing key items and not others (Wimberly, 2006).

Through the discussion, students identify what is important to them; in this process, underlying values emerge. Students are then asked to write a story titled, "What would you risk it all for?" Using these themes, students write a story or create a video or picture in which the aliens, monsters, bad guys (their determination) are attacking. Students are given a limited amount of time to save the top five items chosen. The story is to explain why these items were chosen. It is assumed that "living things" (family and pets) will automatically be protected. When their life depends on it, will the items stay the same between the purchase and the story? Educators must guard against imposing personal values on the students' exploration. However, depending on the age, Socratic dialogue is utilized to process value identification and to challenge unhealthy choices (Fabry, 1968/2013; Wimberly, 2006).

Self-discovery exercise: Meaning triangle

Creative. Determining how to safeguard key items in return for being willing to lose others, writing and illustrating story—Mountain Top Exercise, if time permits;
Experiential. Sharing stories, videos, and pictures;
Attitudinal. The options taken in selections since no one can possess all items;
Reading. Individual student stories.

Choice

The third guidepost to be explored is choice. By progressing from "I matter and am unique" to "this is what is important to me"—because of who I am at my core—students can then be challenged as to the choices they make. (The reverse of this is if I don't matter and I don't know who I am, then I simply react instead of act.) In addition, this concept along with the next three, task orientation/goals, responsibility, and conscience/responsibleness, build on each other and work in tandem in decision making. Although listed by steps, in practice these areas blend together during implementation and discussion (Wimberly, 2006).

Choice exercise Students are given a 15-inch piece of machine, adding paper or strips of paper cut into 2-inch widths. The following instructions are then given:

Write your birth date and place it on one end of the tape.
How old will you live to be?
Write that number on the other end of the tape.
Fold the paper in half and write the "halfway" age.
Fill in key dates in life until the present.
Now place key dates for your future and what you will be doing along your lifeline.
Finally, select one important future date on your lifeline and describe in detail what that future event entails.

Students then create a collage of that event and share it with the class. These topics often include a special job, a university, marriage, or moving to a new area. Key to this discussion is the choices that must be made before that goal can be reached. The idea of locus of control is introduced in an age-appropriate manner, as well as the idea that not making a choice is itself a choice (Wimberly, 2006).

Information concerning the Meaning Triangle will be combined with the next steps. Although making a conscious decision, a choice, to reach a certain goal is the first step; it is only a first step. This next activity builds into the following steps.

Task Orientation and Goals

The logical next step from realizing they do have choices is to also accept that with the ability to make choices comes the necessity of identifying the tasks that need to be met to support the choices. During this time the difference between a dream and a goal is discussed. The explanation given is "a goal was a dream with shoes on." It was movement and planning, not just thinking or daydreaming (Wimberly, 2006).

Exercise: SMART goals This is goal setting and one of the methods used with students was the SMART goal setting process; SMART goals are Specific, Measurable, Attainable, Realistic, and Time-limited.

In this step, students identify a short-term goal, one within the current school year, and address the five areas listed to work toward that goal. The majority of these topics tend to center around grades, attendance, and extracurricular involvement. Then they are to brainstorm the five areas to meet their future, long-term goals chosen in the last unit. Students are allowed to work in pairs or small groups to brainstorm options (Wimberly, 2006).

With the realization that task orientation is based on individual choices, the concept of responsibility emerges. Each choice brings consequences and a student must learn to accept the responsibility for those choices. Much discussion centers around the fact that doing nothing is a choice with consequences. By accepting responsibility, a person is then free to confront the obstacles that prevent the achievement of identified tasks.

Exercise: Overcoming obstacles Students brainstorm a list of challenges that stand in their way. Often these include the very items identified earlier as creating an existential vacuum: bullying, poverty, addictions, anger, low grades, feelings of hopelessness, and lack of being listened to or empowered. They then select one of these obstacles and research how they can confront this challenge (Wimberly, 2006).

Vitally important in this exercise is the concept of locus of control. Although internal/external locus of control has already been introduced, this deepens the conversation. What items are under students' control and can be changed? Students can then identify the items not within their control and discuss ways to change their attitude. They quickly grasp that the only thing they can control is the self. However, this knowledge does not easily translate into a change in behavior. I have students copy onto their folder, "Draw a circle around my feet. What is within the circle I can control?" If there is room to do this, have them actually draw a circle around their feet (Wimberly, 2006).

Responsibility and Conscience

Building on the previous lesson, students examine the role of their conscience in responding. The five-step approach to problem solving of Elisabeth Lukas (2000, 2015) is used. Through this approach, students are synthesizing the previous steps and reviewing ways to apply them to solve the problem. I have used this approach frequently in individual counseling sessions and published a case study in *The International Forum for Logotherapy* (Wimberly, 2010).

Exercise: The five-step approach of Lukas (2000, 2015) involves the following:

1. *Name the problem.* Vital to this step is to be able to identify the problem in a sentence or less. This step involves self-distancing and dereflection.
2. *What scope of free action is available?* Areas of control are discussed and those not within the student's control are removed from the plan. During this

discussion, the educator can explain the difference between being a victim and being an overcomer. The healthy core of the human spirit is emphasized to provide strengths to overcome being a victim.

3. *What options do I have?* Action steps are discussed as well as attitudes. Attitudes impact all areas but specifically those outside a student's control that are limiting future courses of action. Students should be encouraged to brainstorm all options, whether they seem probable or not and to create a list that identifies consequences. This step also allows discussion around the belief that between all stimulus-response, there is an option to act instead of react. Again, "acting" can be defined as not taking any action.
4. *What option is most meaningful?* Values from the second unit are incorporated in the discussion as to options. The student must be willing to accept the consequences of the choices selected. Once an individual has meaning or purpose in life, choices can be made based on personal values and can carry the weight of the responsibility of that option.
5. *The option I want to put into action is...* The concept that once a choice is implemented all the previous choices disappear is discussed. However, with the new choice, a new set of options emerge. An "act as if" exercise is used to practice their choices by dividing them into small groups to role play.

Conscience and responsibleness exercise: Meaning triangle (Activities are interchangeable in the previous four steps as the educator sees best.)

Creative. Imagining their future, creating a collage, evaluating and analyzing new ways to meet the chosen goal, the movie experience, act as if, role-playing.

Experiential. Sharing collage, goals, and plans to meet their goals, group interaction with fingercuffs, group activities (research, organizing, preparation, presenting).

Attitudinal. Discussion of items that are outside students' control and how they will be addressed, e.g., fingertraps or fingercuffs are shared and students are allowed to brainstorm how to free their fingers. (The "trick" to free your fingers is that the student must think differently and "give in"—not by struggling, but by a change in attitude.)

Reading. *What Do You Do with A Chance?* by Kobi Yamada (2021); *Oh, The Places You Will Go!* by Dr. Seuss (1990).

The key to each of these decision-making processes (choice, task orientation/goals, responsibility, conscience/responsibleness) is the understanding that in the noëtic dimension, human beings are meant to struggle and question. This existential tension creates growth. This is in opposition to the homeostasis principle of finding rest or balance that may be obtainable in the physical and psychological realm. Within the noëtic dimension, there is always meant to be a positive, healthy tension—a need to grow (Frankl, 1969/1988).

Self-Transcendence

Finally, the concept of self-transcendence is introduced. It is only when the students recognize the rights and response-abilities they have toward others that the above concepts can lead to meaning. Meaning is what is meant for the good of others, for society, for something greater than the self. Depending on the school setting, this step may be a discussion focused on concepts and events. However, a much more powerful way to teach about self-transcendence is by *doing*. When possible, students need to get outside their classroom. This may be as simple as reading to other students or as involved as volunteering time at a nonprofit or raising money and supplies for others in need (Wimberly, 2006).

The concept of homeostasis has already been introduced, but at this step the idea must be challenged most strongly. Educators must be willing to allow the tension to exist as the students encounter a conflict between *what is* and *what ought to be*. As Frankl (1969/1988) stated, "What man needs first of all is that tension which is created by direction" (p. 48). It is the movement beyond self to right a wrong that resonates with the student individually and in which meaning is recognized (Wimberly, 2006).

Regardless of the activity, the students must discuss, process, and share. Frankl (1984) wrote:

> For success, like happiness, cannot be pursued; it must ensue, and it only does so as the unintended side-effect of one's personal dedication to a cause greater than oneself or as the by-product of one's surrender to a person other than oneself. Happiness must happen, and the same holds for success: you have to let it happen by not caring about it. (pp. xiv-xv)

In light of this idea, it is beneficial to discuss the emotions felt during this challenge of trying to right a wrong. Students should be assured that the struggle for finding answers to a wrong is appropriate and a healthy response of the defiant power of human spirit: the noös (Wimberly, 2006).

Self-transcendence exercise: Meaning triangle

Creative. Energy stick conductor (see https://www.amazon.com/s?k=B08998PKXN [–Ed.]). This stick conducts energy; when students grasp hands and close the circuit by the student on each end grasping the end of the stick, a light is produced. It is a physical way of showing we are all intertwined. Our actions impact others and helping others has a ripple effect.

Experiential. Act as if.... If I were ruler for a day, role play, discuss consequences.

Attitudinal. It is vital to summarize the previous learnings in this area. What meaning has been discovered, what areas of freedom to change exist, and what attitude must be adjusted for those areas that are changeable to continue the movement toward meaning.

Readings. *The Rainbow Fish* by Marcus Pfister (1992); *The Giving Tree* by Shel Silverstein (1964).

Reflections on Applications of Logotherapy in the Classroom

Interestingly, the results of my study (Wimberly, 2006), which was done with at-risk students, found that the students who received a logotherapeutic intervention scored statistically higher for meaning in life as scored on the Purpose in Life Test (Crumbaugh & Maholick, 1964) than the control group who did not receive the intervention. Students also showed positive growth toward an internal locus of control as measured by the Nowicki Strickland Locus of Control (Nowicki & Strickland, 1973). Although this study was done in 2005 and has not been replicated, the same interactions have been used with positive changes in student's attitudes and behaviors as reported in the schools. In addition, although this study was done on a specific population of students (i.e., at risk), the search for meaning is universal to all students and these activities have been productive with students, prekindergarten through university graduate level, and with adults in various settings. Activities must be modified to fit the population and the educator must process all interactions through Socratic dialogue as needed. And finally, it is important to celebrate the growth of each student in their personal journey; a celebration of recognizing the value of self and realizing the search for meaning is an individual, moment by moment responsibility. It is the purpose of living.

Educators (teachers and counselors) can make a difference in teaching students how to find meaning. Meaning cannot be given, but an environment can be created to allow students the freedom to examine choices, make mistakes, and learn skills to make responsible decisions in a safe environment. Although this example utilizes activities outside the standard curriculum, all of these concepts could be implemented into coursework in any subject.

Samuel Johnson (1869/1759), an eighteenth-century English author, wrote, "Integrity without knowledge is weak and useless, and knowledge without integrity is dangerous and dreadful" (p. 158). Fabry (1968/2013) noted that "the mission of education is not merely to pass on knowledge but to help refine their individual conscience, so they become able to understand the meaning requirement of the specific moment" (p. 97). The choice between students with straight As and a perfect ACT score but with no access to the noëtic or the conscience should be an easy one. Perhaps then, there is a better option for professionals in the educational system than simply high-stakes testing and grades. Instead, we can be working toward equipping students with the tools needed to become better human beings. Educators can provide the tools that will enable a student to become a total person, one that has the potential to reach the highest standards of a successful life.

In conclusion, Frankl (1969/1988) stated:

> The foremost task of education, instead of being satisfied with transmitting traditions and knowledge, is to refine that capacity which allows man to find unique meanings. Today education cannot afford to proceed along the lines of tradition but must elicit the ability to make independent and authentic decisions. (p. 64)

The results of this study and my personal experience show that educators have the ability to positively impact students' abilities to search for meaning and to live their lives with meaning. Education can be a method to equip Generation Z with tools to respond to life and all of the challenges it brings by discovering meaning.

References

"Education." (2019). Oxford learner's dictionaries online. In *Oxford learner's dictionaries online*: https://www.oxfordlearnersdictionaries.com/us/definition/american_english/education

"Vocation." (2019). *Oxford learner's dictionaries online*. Retrieved from https://www.oxfordlearnersdictionaries.com/us/definition/english/vocation

Crumbaugh, J. C., & Maholick, L. T. (1964). An experimental study in existentialism: The psychometric approach to Frankl's concept of noogenic neurosis. *Journal of Clinical Psychology, 20*(2), 200–207.

Fabry, J. B. (2013). *The pursuit of meaning: Viktor Frankl, logotherapy, and life*. Purpose Research. (Original work published 1968)

Fabry, J. B. (2021). *Guideposts to meaning: Discovering what really matters* (2nd ed.). Purpose Research. (Original work published 1988)

Frankl, V. E. (1984). *Man's search for meaning* (3rd ed.). Pocket Books. (Original work published 1946)

Frankl, V. E. (1986). *The doctor and the soul*. (R. Winston & C. Winston, Trans.). Alfred A. Knopf. (Original work published in 1946 as *Ärztliche Seelsorge*)

Frankl, V. E. (1988). *The will to meaning: Foundations and applications of logotherapy*. Meridian. (Original work published 1969)

Frankl, V. E. (2000). *Man's search for ultimate meaning*. Perseus. (Original work published *Der Unbewusste Gott*, 1948 and English translation, *The Unconscious God*, 1975)

Frazee, G. (2019, June 18). PBS News Hour. *Suicide among teens and young adults reaches highest level since 2000.* Retrieved from https://www.pbs.org/newshour/nation/suicide-among-teens-and-young-adults-reaches-highest-level-since-2000

Haidt, J., & Lukianoff, G. (2018). *The coddling of the American mind: How good intentions and bad ideas are setting up a generation for failure*. Penguin UK.

Hurwitz, M., & Lee, J. (2018). Grade inflation and the role of standardized testing. In *Measuring success: Testing, grades, and the future of college admissions* (pp. 64–93).

Johnson, S. (1869/1759). *Rasselas, Prince of Abyssinia*. Sampson, Low, Son, and Marston. (Original work published 1759)

Kasasa. (2019). *Boomers, Gen X, Gen Y, Gen Z, and Gen A explained*. Retrieved from https://www.kasasa.com/articles/generations/gen-x-gen-y-gen-z

Kominiak, T. (2019). *Top stories of 2019: K-12 schools face a rise in student suicide*. Retrieved from https://www.k12insight.com/news/k-12-schools-face-rise-student-suicide/

Lukas, E. (2000). *Logotherapy textbook: Meaning-centered psychotherapy*. (T. Brugger, Trans.). Liberty Press. (Original work published *Lehrbuch der Logotherapie*)

Lukas, E. (2015). *The therapist and the soul: From fate to freedom*. Purpose Research.

MacDonald, D. (2004). Collaborating with students' spirituality. *Professional School Counseling, 7*, 293–300.

Miron, O., Yu, K.-H., Wilf-Miron, R., & Kohane, I. S. (2019). Suicide rates among adolescents and young adults in the United States, 2000-2017. *JAMA, 321*(23), 2362–2364. https://doi.org/10.1001/jama.2019.5054

National Alliance on Mental Illness. (n.d.). *Mental health by the numbers*. Retrieved from https://www.nami.org/mhstats

National Institute on Drug Abuse. (2019). *Drug overdose death rates*. Retrieved from https://www.drugabuse.gov/drugs-abuse/opioids/opioid-overdose-crisis

Nowicki, S., & Strickland, B. R. (1973). A locus of control scale for children. *Journal of Consulting and Clinical Psychology, 40*(1), 148.

Parr, T. (2011). *It's okay to be different*. Little, Brown Books for Young Readers.

Pfister, M. (1992). *The rainbow fish*. Simon and Schuster.

Riehm, K. E., Feder, K. A., Tormohlen, K. N., Crum, R. M., Young, A. S., Green, K. M., et al. (2019). Associations between time spent using social media and internalizing and externalizing problems among US youth. *JAMA Psychiatry, 76*(12), 1266–1273. https://doi.org/10.1001/jamapsychiatry.2019.2325

Roy, P. (2019). *The real cost of a meaningless education*. Retrieved from https://pamroyblog.com/the-real-cost-of-a-meaningless-education

Seuss, D., & Richardson, M. (1990). *Oh, the places you'll go!* Random House.

Silverstein, S., & Fu, W. (1964). *The giving tree*. HarperCollins.

Sparling, H. K., & Horn, D. (2019). ACT test: The number of perfect scores is soaring everywhere, as expensive test prep booms. *USA Today*. Retrieved from https://www.usatoday.com/story/news/education/2019/05/01/act-sat-scholarships-college-admissions-scandal-scores-test-prep/3640007002/

U. S. Department of the Navy. (2022). *51 years of data: K-12 school shooting statistics everyone should know*. Retrieved from https://www.campussafetymagazine.com/safety/k-12-school-shooting-statistics-everyone-should-know/

U.S. Department of Health and Human Services. (n.d.). *Facts about bullying*. Retrieved from https://www.stopbullying.gov/resources/facts#stats

Wimberly, C. L. (2006). *Impact of logotherapy on at-risk African American elementary students*. (Unpublished doctoral dissertation, Texas Tech University). Retrieved from https://ttu-ir.tdl.org/handle/2346/1297

Wimberly, C. L. (2010). Intervention with an at-risk student. *The International Forum for Logotherapy, 33*(1), 10–17.

Yamada, K. (2021). *What do you do with a chance?* Compendium.

Cynthia Wimberly, received her PhD in counselor education from Texas Tech University. She has over 40 years' experience in education and counseling, working as a school counselor at all levels. She retired from the University of Texas Rio Grande Valley in 2018, where she served as Chair of the Department of Counseling. Currently, she works at the Noah Project, a shelter for individuals experiencing domestic violence, in Abilene, Texas, where she is director of primary prevention and coordinator of the Batering Intervention and Prevention Program. Wimberly serves as president of the Viktor Frankl Institute of Logotherapy (US). Her areas of research include school counseling, at-risk students, domestic violence, and the application of logotherapy in each of these areas.

New Work: How Important Is the Orientation of Meaning? Reflections on the Basis of Frankl's Dimensional Ontology

Bernd Ahrendt

The term *new work* is currently the subject of much debate, as it is nothing less than a concept of work that does not exhaust people but one that is intended to give them energy and strength (Bergmann, 2017, p. 11). It is about a new view of the relationship between the human being and work and thus about the expectation that the current challenges facing many companies can be successfully mastered. If you want to understand the core of new work, you have to deal with both the question of meaning in general as well as the question of meaning in the context of work.

In order to approach the phenomenon of new work and its concept of meaning, the following section first looks at an increasingly dynamic work environment commonly known as VUCA before deriving the need for a humanization of work and considering it on the basis of Frankl's dimensional ontology. From this, considerations on a human-oriented level as well as on an organizational level of companies are derived, which point out the meaning as a core element of new work. It is clear that orientation of meaning is the foundation on which many of the current issues are built.

New Work and VUCA

Many companies live in an increasingly dynamic environment, which is characterized by the acronym *VUCA* (Mack & Khare, 2016), which stands for: *volatility* (increasing speed and dynamics of change); *uncertainty* (decreasing degree of predictability and events); *complexity* (increasing number of connections, dependencies, and possibilities for action that make a topic inscrutable); and *ambiguity*

B. Ahrendt (✉)
FOM University of Applied Sciences, Hanover, Germany
e-mail: bernd.ahrendt@fom.de

C. L. McLafferty, Jr., J. I. Levinson (eds.), *Logotherapy and Existential Analysis*, Logotherapy and Existential Analysis: Proceedings of the Viktor Frankl Institute Vienna 2, https://doi.org/10.1007/978-3-031-48922-8_22

(ambiguous facts, meaning that general conditions and prerequisites can be interpreted in several ways).

Thus, VUCA represents the dynamic milieu in which companies are involved: An environment that is characterized by both evolutionary and disruptive developments and therefore constantly poses new challenges that must be addressed. The answers are both evolutionary and disruptive, which in turn influence the dynamics as effects on the respective market, so that direct and indirect effects will be difficult to manage. The VUCA model therefore requires company leadership to be able to continuously make changes in order to remain sustainable in the market. This model places high demands on every company and thus on its employees, who have to find the appropriate answers.

It is ultimately the employees who must shape this constant change; the importance of human resources in general, and the individual in particular, are increasing for the company. Often it used to be the case that individuals or a small group of people were able to steer the company decisively on the basis of well-founded decisions. However, the application of new work principles requires a fundamentally different approach: Instead of specific persons, it is now up to everyone in the company to identify trends in environmental development at an early stage, so that they can be addressed at that point in the company where they are needed. It is not every person in a company that must react to VUCA stressors; rather, response is required only from the affected parts, which leads to the following internal requirements:

1. At the organizational level, dealing with VUCA issues requires a significantly higher degree of flexibility. However, such flexibility is only possible if the company succeeds in developing a corresponding ability to shape itself, that is not be planned centrally, but can only be implemented decentrally.
2. On a human-oriented level, active interaction with VUCA-related situations requires employees who can "think in VUCA." Thus, behind a successful approach to VUCA is the demand for committed people, who are willing to think for and to stand up for the company. These individuals are capable of helping to shape the necessary entrepreneurial self-determination, which in turn requires a corresponding individual willingness to shape one's own self.

Employee commitment (i.e., extra-productive, voluntary behavior that has a positive effect on the company and is not directly covered by the formal incentive system) is becoming a central intangible resource for companies (Nerdinger et al., 2019, p. 492). This type of commitment cannot be demanded by the company; in order to be able to use this resource, leadership of a company must create appropriate framework conditions in which people are willing to get involved. Thus, the corporate culture is of great importance. This illustrates why new work has become so popular, on the one hand, and why its implementation is nontrivial in nature, on the other, because it is about the core of a company: the VUCA-compatible design of corporate culture. VUCA demands an entrepreneurial, decentralized self-creation potential, which is to be found above all in the people of the company with their self-creation potential. By implementing new work, this potential for self-determination in people can be used for the company.

Corporate culture is a common basic understanding that allows people in their entrepreneurial environment to work together and achieve the company's goals. This culture expresses the way in which a company conducts its business (Homma & Bauschke, 2015, p. 2) and arises through the interaction of people in the company. It is the result of various aspects, such as the company's history, the structures and processes created, and the joint realization of the goals set. All members are both cultural bearers and cultural imprinters (Sackmann, 2002, p. 259). In this respect, corporate culture is also something that itself is subject to constant change and can therefore be changed.

Many studies show a positive correlation between corporate culture and success (Sackmann, 2002, Table 5.1). Sackmann also reported a positive correlation between corporate culture and employee commitment (p. 147).

Anyone who wants to use new work should establish a culture within the company that exerts a pulling effect on people and invites them to participate in a committed way. New work is therefore about humanizing companies.

New Work from the Perspective of Frankl's Dimensional Ontology

A humanization in the sense of new work—that is, what someone would like to do "really, really" (Bergmann, 2017, p. 10)—refers to the basic needs of the individual and the ways in which these needs are connected with the demand for meaning. Grawe (2000, pp. 383–420) described four equally entitled basic needs in the context of his contingency theory:

- Orientation and control: The need to develop and maintain an individual model of reality. The human being has the need to understand and control reality, to gain an appropriate overview of situations and to receive feedback on his behavior.
- Pleasure gain and avoidance on unpleasure: The need for behavior adapted to the environment. It includes the fundamental tendency for a person to bring about pleasant experience and to avoid painful ones.
- Binding: The need to develop a stable relationship with a caregiver who provides security. Every human being has this need and experiences it at an early age.
- Self-esteem: The need to be accepted by others and to feel competent and valuable.

People want to be able to think positively about themselves. Accordingly, they have a fundamental need to increase their self-esteem and to avoid injuries.

All four basic needs influence each other and are networked accordingly. They refer to the dimensions of the human body and psyche (also called the psychophysical dimensions), which strive to satisfy as many needs as possible in these dimensions in order to remain both physically and psychologically healthy. Accordingly, preference will be given above all to those possibilities which serve this satisfaction, while those which jeopardize satisfaction will be fended off or avoided as far as possible (Peters & Ghadiri, 2011, p. 188).

New work thus focuses on the basic needs of people. But not only that. As Kurz (2011, pp. 33–38) made clear, these basic needs are based on a striving for meaning. However, this orientation of meaning goes beyond the dimensions of body and psyche and can only be explained with another dimension. In this respect, the dimensional ontology of Viktor Frankl (2015) can be taken up here, which recognized the spiritual (noëtic) as the third dimension alongside the body and the psyche (p. 55ff). In Frankl's ontology the human being *is* a spiritual person ("geistige Person," p. 331) who strives to fulfill meaning in the world. And this spiritual person *has* a body and a psyche. While in the physical and psychological dimensions human beings might want to implement personal development in their lives that is seen as appropriate, the noëtic, spiritual dimension goes beyond that. It is not a matter of direct view of oneself and a subjective view of one's own development, but of a meaning that can be realized in the world. Only and precisely this dimension points to life in its entirety. It is oriented towards something or someone other than the self (Frankl, 2015, p. 54) and is in this sense self-transcendent (Frankl, 1966). According to Frankl, this meaning (from the Greek "*Logos*") is something objective. Thus, meaning cannot be constructed by a human being, but meaning is always there. In this respect, it can be found subjectively by humans, but not invented or self-created (Berschneider, 2018, p. 104).

These considerations are of great importance because it is precisely this noëtic, spiritual dimension that is specifically human in the individual: It is that which strives for meaning in people and allows them to develop in the dimensions of body and psyche. On the one hand, personality development is therefore only a consequence of the orientation towards logos. And it is the person who has to decide whether to implement the meaning possibilities that are available. At the same time, however, the spiritual dimension needs the psychophysical dimension to become effective in the world. In this respect, it is always a matter of striving for the fulfillment of meaning as well as of paying attention to the satisfaction of basic needs.[1]

Human-Oriented Conclusions for New Work Based on the Dimensional Ontology

Understanding new work means recognizing all human dimensions, which include the idea that people aspire to a meaning in life that is oriented to the world. For this, they need a good basis so that they can become effective as spiritual beings. The meaning of the moment can serve as the decisive standard for the human being here, which in this way becomes the "pacemaker of being" ("Schrittmacher des Seins," Frankl, 2015, p. 114). Thus, the human being's engagement is directed toward the intended. In other words: It is only through the fulfillment of meaning

[1] Maslow (1966) agreed with Frankl that self-realization can only be realized in a self-transcendent form; he described self-realization in this sense as a "meta-need" (p. 108).

that a person succeeds in striving for personal development and a successful life in which he feels joy.

Such an observation makes it possible to recognize the human being in its entirety, consisting of body, psyche, *and* spirit. A humanization of the corporate culture must therefore encompass all three dimensions.

A system of motivation based on this idea includes the satisfaction of basic needs and accordingly encompasses both extrinsic and intrinsic aspects of motivation on the physical and psychological dimensions (Fig. 1) as well as the human orientation to meaning in the spiritual dimension. The term *logofocal* (Lukas, 2014, p. 282) will be used to refer to motivation involving the spiritual dimension, in contrast with extrinsic/intrinsic motivation of the psychophysical dimensions (see also Ahrendt et al., 2023, Chaps. 3 and 4). This refers to motivation that recognizes the *will to meaning* (Frankl, 1986, p. 27) as the primary motivation.

With regard to the psychophysical dimension, employees—also in comparison to their colleagues—would like to have

- an appropriate employment contract, which takes into account duration and remuneration (orientation/control and self-esteem);
- a trusting cooperation with executives and colleagues which makes them feel comfortable (orientation/control, pleasure/unpleasure, and binding);
- an experience of social resonance (Berschneider, 2018, pp. 111–112) (pleasure/unpleasure, binding, and self-esteem);
- preparation for changes and the ability to flow with them (orientation/control and pleasure/unpleasure);
- an understanding of decisions (orientation/control); and
- a contextual leadership at eye level (orientation/control and self-esteem).

Design of a motivational system is essentially about the aspects of fairness and personality development. This design has to take place on the basis of an orientation to meaning, which forms the foundation of this approach.

Managers at a company that want to have committed employees must show each individual what meaning the company in general—and the work in particular—serves (thus, a logofocal motivation). To this end, leadership must ensure that each person's striving for meaning is not frustrated and that the possibilities for the individual to realize meaning are expanded.

Fig. 1 Relationship between motivation and Frankl's dimensions of the person

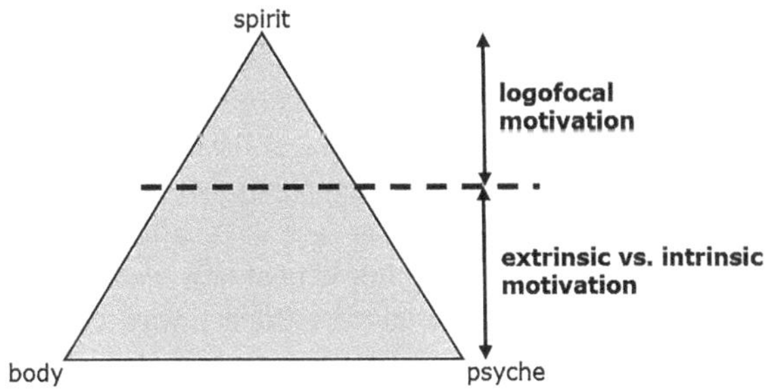

Such a view poses great challenges for any company's leaders, as it involves very subjective views of meaning. Some individuals are mainly influenced by material incentives and do not know the spiritual dimension or are not interested in it. Conversely, others may emphasize the spiritual dimension; a material reward (though reasonable!) is of secondary importance to them. (For more detailed explanations on logofocal leadership, see Ahrendt et al., 2023, Chap. 8.)

Whatever values a person is currently orienting towards, those who implement new work start with an orientation to meaning and demand that the person is willing and able to develop or expand a corresponding *competence of meaning* ("Sinnkompetenz", Berschneider, 2003, p. 52–54).

Organizational Conclusions for New Work Based on the Dimensional Ontology

The company is a system that is geared to the company's objective and thus to the fulfillment of tasks. It is characterized by the aspect of economic profitability and always includes the perspectives of efficiency (exploitation) and effectiveness (exploration) (see Welpe et al., 2018, pp. 31–36). New work considers this aspect, but complements it, however, with the previously mentioned aspects of fairness and personality development by including the realization that the company is oriented towards meaning. This can be demonstrated to employees by examples such as: what living conditions are improved and for whom, what positive values are eventuated for customers and employees, or how the company's product results in a social and/or ecological benefit. In order to implement new work, the company as a whole pursues a meaning in order to give people a space on this basis to find their meaning in their work. Thus, new work is based on an orientation toward meaning of the company, which is to be shaped under the aspects of profitability, fairness, and personality development (see Fig. 2).

This arrangement refers to both indirect and direct human resources management. In order to implement an orientation to meaning, a vision, a mission, and values statement must be developed for the company, which should be carried out in participatory manner with a view to better implementation (fairness; profitability). Instruments must be developed that enable people to develop their competence of meaning, while new employees should already have a corresponding competence of meaning in order to be able to make a value adjustment between the company and the individual (personality development, profitability). It should be noted that meaning cannot be arranged by a manager/executive, but can only be found by employees themselves within the framework of the corporate culture.

New work requires an organizational and human-oriented corporate culture. Large companies in particular face the challenge of having to transform their existing culture if they want to implement new work. This does not succeed in a revolutionary way, but only in an evolutionary way, because new work—as has become clear—cannot be prescribed. The people in the company must want, and be able, to participate in this transformation.

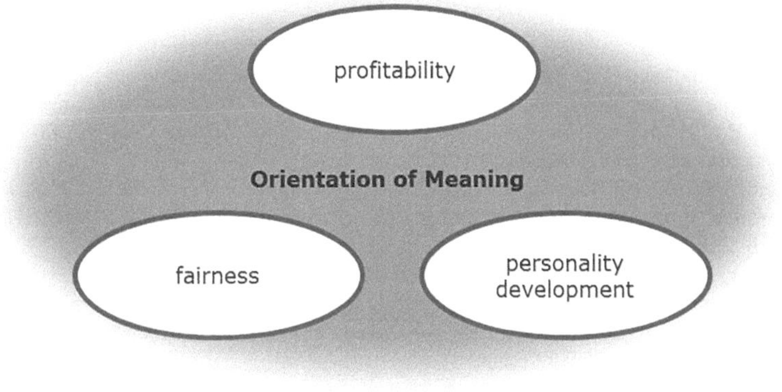

Fig. 2 Corporate orientation of meaning and its aspects

To this end, they must partly question their previous extrinsic and intrinsic motivational aspects and rediscover what requires time and courage. In the context of such a transformation, managers/executives are of particular importance, because they serve both as role models and pioneers. They have to exemplify the logofocal motivation and develop it directly with their employees. They have to face the different aspects of fairness and take them into account.

Since this transformation can only be shaped by people, every company (or in large companies every department) will need time, so that different speeds within a company can be expected (see Voigt, 2018).

Conclusion

At new work, orientation of meaning is of great importance for successful action in a VUCA environment. Meaning forms the foundation on which the other aspects are built and together form the cornerstones of an appropriate corporate culture. Major upheavals in companies without a meaningful foundation will only be successful to a limited extent. With new work, it is possible for employees to become involved in their company by drawing energy and strength from their work and finding adequate answers to the VUCA environment whenever needed. In this sense, new work gives companies organizational resilience.

And something else becomes clear: The currently intensively discussed keywords such as "agile company," "digital transformation," "self-organization," "self management" are partial aspects that are based on the fundamental orientation towards a company's orientation of meaning. In this respect, they are never equal to this orientation, but always subordinate. This should also be taken into account in new work.

References

Ahrendt, B., Nikolaus, R. S., & Zilinski, J. (2023). *Das organisationale Ikigai. Theoretische Grundlagen für die Transformation zu einer purpose-driven Organisation*. Springer Gabler.

Bergmann, F. (2017). *Neue Arbeit, neue Kultur* [In English: *New work new culture: Work we want and a culture that strengthens us* (2019)]. Arbor Verlag.

Berschneider, W. (2018). Personalmarketing aus logotherapeutischer Sicht: Führung mit Sinn und Werten. In B. Ahrendt & S. Wöhrmann (Eds.), *Personalmarketing in 3D—Die vielfältige Disziplin* (pp. 99–116). Thurm Verlag.

Berschneider, W. (2003). *Sinnzentrierte Unternehmensführung: Was Viktor E. Frankl den Führungskräften der Wirtschaft zu sagen hat*. Orthaus Verlag.

Frankl, V. E. (2015). *Ärztliche Seelsorge. Grundlagen der Logotherapie und Existenzanalyse* (6th ed.). Deutscher Taschenbuch Verlag.

Frankl, V. E. (1966). Self-transcendence as a human phenomenon. *Journal of Humanistic Psychology, 6*(2), 97–106.

Frankl VE (1986) Die Psychotherapie in der Praxis. Eine kasuistische Einführung für Ärzte. R. Piper GmbH & Co. KG.

Grawe, K. (2000). *Psychologische Therapie* (2nd corrected ed.). Hogrefe.

Homma, N., & Bauschke, R. (2015). *Unternehmenskultur und Führung. Den Wandel gestalten – Methoden, Prozesse, Tools* (2nd ed.). Springer Gabler Verlag. https://doi.org/10.1007/978-3-8349-4758-1

Kurz, W. (2011). Sinn und Lebensqualität. Das Sinnbedürfnis in Relation zu den Grundbedürfnissen. In O. Zsok (Ed.), *"Du kannst dem Sinn nicht ausweichen." Existenz als Herausforderung für den Einzelnen und für die Gesellschaft. Vorträge und Seminare zum 25-jährigen Bestehen des Süddeutschen Instituts für Logotherapie und Existenzanalyse gAG. Jubiläumskongress am April 1–2, 2011 in Fürstenfeldbruck* (pp. 25–38). Süddeutsches Institut für Logotherapie.

Lukas, E. (2014). *Lehrbuch der Logotherapie: Menschenbild und Methoden* (4th ed.). Profil Verlag.

Mack, O., & Khare, A. (2016). Perspective on a VUCA world. In O. Mack, A. Khare, A. Krämer, & T. Burgartz (Eds.), *Managing in a VUCA world* (pp. 3–19). Springer. https://doi.org/10.1007/978-3-319-16889-0_1

Maslow, A. H. (1966). Comments on Dr. Frankl's paper. *Journal of Humanistic Psychology, 6*(2), 107–112.

Nerdinger, F. W., Blickle, G., & Schaper, N. (2019). *Arbeits-und Organisationspsychologie* (4th ed.). Springer.

Peters, T., & Ghadiri, A. (2011). *Neuroleadership—Grundlagen, Konzepte, Beispiele: Erkenntnisse der Neurowissenschaften für die Mitarbeiterführung* (2nd ed.). Springer. https://doi.org/10.1007/978-3-658-02165-8

Sackmann, S. A. (2002). *Unternehmenskultur: Erkennen—Entwickeln—Verändern: Erfolgreich durch kulturbewusstes Management* (2nd ed.). Springer. https://doi.org/10.1007/978-3-658-18634-0

Voigt, T. (2018, July 26). Interview by Bernd Ahrendt. [Online transcript]. Interview mit Thomas Voigt über die bewusste Veränderung einer Unternehmenskultur. https://wissenschafts-thurm.de/bewusste-veraenderung-der-unternehmenskultur-ein-interview-mit-schokolade/

Welpe, I. M., Brosi, P., & Schwarzmüller, T. (2018). *Digital work design. Die Big Five für Arbeit, Führung und Organisation im digitalen Zeitalter*. Campus Verlag.

Bernd Ahrendt, Professor of General Business Administration, in particular Human Resources Management, teaches and researches at the FOM University of Economics & Management in Hanover and works as a meaning-centered coach. Research priorities include meaning-centered mindset, purpose-driven organizations, competence management.

Meaning-Centered Job Crafting: A Way to (Re-)Discover Meaning at Work

Sabine Indinger

Given the important role of work in the lives of human beings (Frankl, 1973; Kovacs, 1986), finding meaning at work is of great importance to many people to live fulfilled lives. Finding meaning at work is an individual task and presents freedom and responsibility for the person (Frankl, 1973; Pattakos, 2019; Pichler, 2019). It cannot be delegated to organizations or managers in a "done-for-you" way. At the same time, the individual search for meaning and the will to find meaning at work seem to have steadily increased over the past few decades (Burger et al., 2013); Pattakos (2018) spoke of the search for meaning as a "megatrend of the new millennium."

As a result of the weakening of religious and spiritual systems, the question of the meaning of work has become inevitable. It has been argued that the role of work goes beyond providing one with a paycheck but also relates to aspects such as personal development, identity, self-esteem, and ultimately meaning in life (Burger et al., 2013, p. 3).

Meaningful work becomes more crucial when the world of organizations and business is rapidly changing, requiring individuals to take on more responsibility for their careers and job descriptions and designing and navigating the course of their work lives. Organizations, companies, and managers will be less able and willing to do this for employees. Providing traditional work contracts becomes increasingly fluid and varied (Bridges, 1996; Burger et al., 2013; Slim, 2013; Wrzesniewski et al., 2010). Therefore, many people will no longer find stable, full-time

With kind reprint permission, adapted from *The International Forum for Logotherapy* (originally published in Vol. 45, No. 2).

S. Indinger (✉)
Ferdinand Porsche Fernfachhochschule/University of Applied Sciences,
Wiener Neustadt, Austria
e-mail: sabine@indinger.at

C. L. McLafferty, Jr., J. I. Levinson (eds.), *Logotherapy and Existential Analysis*, Logotherapy and Existential Analysis: Proceedings of the Viktor Frankl Institute Vienna 2, https://doi.org/10.1007/978-3-031-48922-8_23

employment. Employees frequently change their work–life and employment environments and hold multiple (part-time) positions. Increasingly, people are working as freelancers, on temporary projects, often with multiple temporary contracts for different organizations, in virtual teams and remote locations, and increasingly need more immediate guidance of job descriptions and direct managerial supervision (Dundon, 2019).

Berg et al. (2013a) stated that the "idea of employees working from a fixed job description is becoming less common" (p. 83). These circumstances require a continual definition and redefinition, evaluation, and re-evaluation of the tasks employees are performing and their understanding of their role within an organization—independent of the specific form of work contract or relationship they have with this organization. When considering the increasing commonality of agile, project-based work within organizations and work relations (Kotrba & Miarka, 2015), new projects and steps, milestones, and phases within projects become necessary for (re-)defining and (re-)designing jobs, concrete tasks, and relationships. Employees under these circumstances cannot wait for the organization or their managers to define the exact scope and boundaries of their jobs and roles within the organization and projects—and the organization then relies on employees to be capable of ongoing, adaptive, and evolutionary processes independently (Berg et al., 2013a; Burger et al., 2013; Wrzesniewski & Dutton, 2001).

An additional topic has increased in relevance over the past few decades: Employees are increasingly expecting more from their work than financial rewards and promotions (Rampton, 2017). Individuals often seek occupations that will provide fulfillment of core personal values, meaning and purpose (Wrzesniewski et al., 2003), self-expression, and opportunities to help others. People within diverse work contexts are looking for a job and a calling (Berg et al., 2010; Wrzesniewski et al., 2003). Conversely, the inability to pursue a calling may undermine psychological well-being by producing frustration, disappointment, or regret, ultimately hindering job performance (Berg et al., 2010).

Organizations confronted with a workforce experiencing increased work dissatisfaction and delayed retirement age are experiencing employees who are staying longer in jobs they might not enjoy (Berg et al., 2013a). At the same time, many Generations X and Y members believe that they can "be anything they want to be" and thus have solid expectations for the meaningfulness they would like to derive from their careers (Bresman & Rao, 2017).

Job Crafting as a Starting Point

Such challenges in the workforce and organizations present the question: "How do individuals find or rediscover meaning at work under these circumstances?" Berg et al. (2013a) pointed to *job crafting* as a way for people to deal with these changes and challenges at the workplace. Wrzesniewski and Dutton (2001) defined the term: "We use the term *job crafting* to capture the actions employees take to shape, mold, and redefine their jobs" (p. 180). Whether formal or informal, employees use work tasks and interactions as raw materials and building blocks to construct, craft, and tailor their jobs according to their needs, values, and preferences (Berg et al., 2007; Wrzesniewski & Dutton, 2001). Job crafting emphasizes "the proactive behavior that employees use when they feel that changes in their job are necessary" (Petrou et al., 2012, p. 1120).

Wrzesniewski and Dutton (2001, p. 185) presented three ways in which employees can specifically enact job crafting. The first approach involves changing the job's *task boundaries* by changing the number, scope, or type of job tasks done at work (cited in Wrzesniewski et al., 2010). The second form of job crafting entails changing the *relational boundary of the job* by changing how, when, or with whom employees interact within the execution of their jobs. The third method, *cognitive crafting*, occurs when employees change their perceptions of, or attitudes toward, their jobs, their tasks, and relationships, as well as how they think about the purpose of certain aspects of their job or reframe the job (Berg et al., 2013a, p. 82).

"Job crafting is neither inherently good nor bad for organizations" (Wrzesniewski & Dutton, 2001, p. 195)—or the individual employee, which means that "even when the crafting is beneficial for the individual job crafter, it still may be harmful to the overall organization" (Berg et al., 2007, p. 7)—and vice versa. Wrzesniewski et al. (2010) even sent out a warning to potential job crafters: "Not all job crafting is beneficial. It can be stressful if, as a result, you take on too much or alter tasks without understanding your manager's goals" (p. 117). Their findings are more descriptive than normative, stating a fact of organizational reality, whether employees or managers acknowledge it, like it, or even actively support or hinder it. Job crafting as a phenomenon is not surprising either since we invariably bring our uniqueness to each job and thus perform tasks individually. Job crafting is a proactive activity by the employee (Wrzesniewski et al., 2010; Wrzesniewski & Dutton, 2001) and does not necessarily infer the process to be conscious. The positive potential of job crafting involves the acknowledgement of the extent to which the individual actively seeks to realize meaning potentials within or beyond the formally or informally defined job boundaries and the extent to which they experience themselves as playing an active role in shaping their job. Only then is it possible for the employee to actively and creatively (re-)discover and actualize meaning, as "conscious awareness is required for the recognition of meaning" (Marshall & Marshall, 2012, p. 41).

With increased expectations of what work offers the employee (i.e., providing a source of income *and* meaning) against the modern-day work life presenting changes, challenges, chances, disruptions, and possibilities, it might not come as a surprise that phenomena like burnout syndrome (Riethof & Bob, 2019) or what Frankl called *existential frustration* and the *existential vacuum* (Frankl, 1969/1988, 1973, 2006, 2010) are increasing. Pichler (2019) put the topic in its historical and highly topical context when he observed:

> Eighty years ago, Frankl drew attention to the connection between the actualization of personal meaning and effects on health. Today, his work has been confirmed by a number of scientific studies. The German health insurance fund AOK dedicated a 600-page study

report to the importance of meaning at work; Viktor Frankl was cited on the first page (Badura et al., 2018).

With the steady increase of burnout syndrome (cf Badura et al., 2018), a consequence of existential frustration in life, at work, and in work life (Riethof & Bob, 2019), a kind of meaning-centered job crafting might be a promising route to counter this development.

Riethof and Bob (2019) looked at LTEA in the context of burnout syndrome and concluded that "very few studies have explored the connection of burnout with loss of meaning in one's work and life. Recent findings suggest burnout syndrome is a form of existential vacuum described by Viktor Frankl" (p. 1). Existential frustration is a "lack of fulfillment of the will to meaning" (Frankl, 2010, p. 61) and a "sense of meaninglessness and emptiness" (Frankl, 1969/1988, p. 83). It has the potential to motivate, inspire, and empower healthy, stable, meaning-seeking employees to "craft their jobs," affording them a chance to realize meanings (Frankl, 1967, 1978, 2010). Some individuals struggle existentially and cannot find a way out of it independently.

Today, organizations and C-suites of corporations have heard the "unheard cry for meaning" (Frankl, 1978). In 2017, the World Economic Forum prominently broadcast a roundtable discussion on "Creating Profit Through Purpose" (World Economic Forum, 2017). Early in 2019, Larry Fink (2019), the CEO of Blackrock, a leading investment company, urged companies to balance profit with purpose in his annual letter to CEOs. Later that year, 181 CEOs at the Business Roundtable committed to leading their companies for the benefit of all stakeholders by issuing an open letter titled "Statement on the Purpose of a Corporation," prioritizing people over profits (Business Roundtable, 2019; Gartenberg & Serafeim, 2019). Organizations (and their C-suites, HR departments, and line managers) are determined to provide meaning for the employee (and to the stakeholders, to the markets they serve, and to the world).

Meaning-Centered Job Crafting as the Answer

I contend that meaning-centered job crafting, i.e., conscious job crafting activities that are firmly rooted in logotherapy and existential analysis (LTEA), is sorely needed in the workplaces of the twenty-first century. In short, finding meaning is the highest responsibility (and the greatest freedom) of each individual.

Researchers and scholars (cf Bailey & Madden, 2016; Bailey et al., 2017) have argued over the varying degrees to which management and organizations may be able and ethically allowed to "manage meaningfulness" (Bailey & Madden, 2016, p. 60). Bailey et al. (2017) found that when organizations try to define and impose a universal sense of meaning in the workplace as a top-down initiative, workers end up doing what Bailey et al. (2017) call "existential labor." A false sense of meaning presents as aligning with directives, or the sense of what is meaningful to them alters to meet the requirements. Such approaches are unsustainable and lead to exhaustion, stifled expression, burnout, leading eventually to a sense of depersonalization and demotivation, alienation, dissatisfaction, and intent to quit (Bailey & Madden, 2016, p. 29; Hakner, 2017). Bailey et al. (2017) also stated that "employees may also, of course, discern their work to be meaningful independently of any active efforts on the part of the employer to manage their experience" (p. 16).

By postulating that meaning is the primary source of motivation for the human being (Frankl, 1969/1988, 1973, 2006), LTEA is not only uniquely qualified but also compelled to play an essential role in the workplace of the twenty-first century. At the same time, LTEA postulates that meaning is always present and, therefore, cannot (and need not) be created but can only be discovered and found (Frankl, 1969/1988). If we assume that meaning is central to the twenty-first-century world, meaning is not a management miracle weapon whose proper application requires providing "meaning-creating trainings" for all managers.

On the contrary, a consistent LTEA-based approach means putting meaning discovery and meaning actualization back where it belongs: into the realm of freedom and responsibility of the individual, whether the individual confronts the question of meaning as a leader/manager or as an employee. The person will always encounter the question as an individual human being.

Conscience, Orientation to Meaning, and Meaning-Centered Job Crafting

Berg et al. (2013b) explained that "Research suggests that many individuals can and do engage in job crafting, but many people have unrealized opportunities to *beneficially* [emphasis added] craft their jobs." (p. 3). While job crafting offers excellent opportunities for rediscovering meaning in the workplace by changing the task or the relational and/or cognitive (attitudinal) boundaries of a person's formal job, there are also risks involved. The authors noted that the final result might differ from the individual employee's intentions and the organization's needs.

Job crafting needs to become a conscious effort, a planned activity directed towards meaning (*Logos*). Incorporating the principles of LTEA is thus needed to develop a job-crafting approach that is beneficial and meaningful for the employee as the job crafter and for managers and the organization as a whole.

According to Lukas (2006–2008; from personal notes taken during lectures and logotherapy training in Kremsmünster, Austria), "meaningful" in the context of LTEA means that a given situation:

- has the potential to be beneficial for all involved or has the probability of positive outcomes for the largest number of all involved;
- neither overburdens the person nor limits challenges for the person (e.g., is perceived as boring); and, as a possibility, lies within the realm of the person's freedom and responsibility;

- resonates with a person's true nature, in the sense of Pattakos and Dundon (2017): "Meaning is what resonates with my core essence, my true nature" (p. 9);
- has within it the optimum (i.e., the best possible) solution, option, alternative, answer to the question life is asking the person at this moment in this situation; and
- allows the person to choose to the best of their ability, knowledge, and conscience, "half-sure and whole-hearted" (Gordon Allport, as cited in Frankl, 1969/1988, p. 66).

Opening to the Noëtic Dimension

LTEA adds the noëtic dimension, which helps people to (re-)discover meaning under all circumstances, even the worst, and overcome existential frustration, ideally before they burn out. Practitioners of LTEA do not discuss *creating meaning* but *finding and discovering meaning* (Frankl, 1969/1988, 1973, 2006). We can see this in meaning-centered job crafting, as it presupposes that there is meaning to be found under all circumstances at the workplace. As Frankl (1973) stated:

> The job at which one works is not what counts, but rather the manner in which one does the work. It does not lie with the occupation, but always with us, whether those elements of the personal and the specific which constitute the uniqueness of our existence are expressed in the work and thus make life meaningful....
>
> People's natural relationship to their employment as the area for possible actualization of creative values and self-fulfillment is often distorted by prevailing conditions of work. (p. 118, 120)

These conditions underscore the call for meaning-centered job crafting.

From this perspective, those who practice LTEA offer a different approach towards meaning that turns the focus of the individual towards questions such as, "What is asked from me specifically at my workplace?" or "What question is life asking me specifically, individually, and uniquely in this situation, in this (work) place, in this moment?" rather than: "What is the job doing for me?" "What is the organization giving me?" Such questions offer a healthy way to manage expectations towards work and organizations.

Frankl stated that "meaning is fulfilled by realizing values" (as cited in Sárkány, 2016, p. 77). Frankl (1969/1988, 2006) proposed three different ways for discovering meaning in life: (a) by creating a work or doing a deed (*creative values*: what we give to the world), (b) by experiencing something or encountering someone (*experiential values*: what we take from the world; encounters with other human beings), and (c) by the attitude we take toward unavoidable suffering (*attitudinal values*: the stance we take toward the conditions that we must face).

The three forms of job crafting (crafting tasks, relationships, and cognitions as noted above) echo the three avenues to meaning LTEA noted by Frankl. What LTEA adds is the noëtic dimension, e.g., realizing attitudinal values rather than making cognitive changes. Adding the noëtic dimension to the job crafting approach transforms it into a uniquely humane approach that relates to the true nature and core essence of human beings.

Noëtic Dimension Opens the LTEA "Medicine Chest"

Adding the noëtic dimension also opens what Fabry (1988/2021) called "the medicine chest of logotherapy" (p. 6), making it available for meaning-centered job crafting activities to be applied by the individual meaning seeker and those who support and guide them along the way. Human resources to be found in the medicine chest of LTEA are as follows:

- The will to meaning is the source of motivation and inspiration for the search for meaning.
  - *The concept of noö-dynamics*: Frankl called noö-dynamics "a tension between existence and essence or being and meaning.... [Meaning] must always be one step ahead of being—only then can meaning fulfill its own meaning, namely, to be a pacemaker of Being" (as cited in Marshall & Marshall, 2012, p. 54).
  - *Task orientation* based on the demand character of life: "The conviction that one has a task before him has enormous psychotherapeutic and psychohygienic value.... Nothing is more likely to help a person overcome or endure objective difficulties or subjective troubles than the consciousness of having a task in life" (Frankl, 1973, p. 54).
- Freedom of will is the ability to choose.
  - *Freedom of will* is the ability (and response-ability) to choose "to take a stand on whatever conditions might confront them" (Frankl, 1969/1988, p. 16). Frankl (1973) also called it "freedom of decision" (p. 86), not as freedom *from* conditions, but as the freedom *to choose* how a given situation (e.g., intended or involuntary actions of others, a pleasant encounter, a blow of fate, a new idea, etc.) is regarded, what meaning is possible, or if the meaning is at all found in the circumstances of life (Frankl, 1967)—thus, each person decides what their life will be by the choices made moment to moment.
  - *Self-transcendence* is "the essence of existence" (Frankl, 1969/1988, p. 50). Self- transcendence is a uniquely human capacity and "denotes the fact that being human always points, and is directed, to something or someone other than oneself" (Frankl, 1982, p. 345). This illustrates that human beings are able and willing to reach beyond their egocentricity (Frankl, 2004, p. 4).
  - *Self-distancing* is the uniquely human capacity to detach from a situation or oneself, allowing the person to choose an attitude toward the situation or self: "In *self-distancing*, the spiritual 'you' steps away from the physical 'you'.... You have, as Frankl expressed it, 'the defiant power of the human spirit,' a vital resource of your inner medicine chest" (Fabry, 1988/2021, pp. 7–8).

- Conscience is the "meaning-organ."
  - *Conscience* guides and supports the person trying to discover what is meaningful and what the meaning of the moment is: "Conscience could be defined as the intuitive capacity of man to find out the meaning of a situation" (Frankl, 1969/1988, p. 63).
  - Fabry (1988/2021) painted a vivid picture of conscience as a "compass needle that points in the direction of the meaning of the moment" (p. 6). While the meaning organ can guide the person, Frankl (1975) noted that individuals need to follow where the compass needle leads them in discovering, rediscovering, and reclaiming meaning, e.g., at work "within the thousand meanings of the thousand demands and commandments hidden in the ten thousand situations with which life is confronting [them]" (p. 120). "Apart from being intuitive, conscience is creative.... Conscience also has the power to discover unique meanings that contradict accepted values" (Frankl, 1969/1988, p. 63). In this respect, meaning-centered job crafting humorously becomes: "job (description) meets conscience."

The medicine chest of LTEA *expands* the currently available tools, exercises, interventions, and instruments that originate in positive psychology, solution-focused therapy (De Shazer, 1988; Jackson & McKergow, 2007; Kotrba & Miarka, 2015), coaching practice, organizational psychology, work/labor/occupational psychology, and other schools of psychotherapy by "elevating" them to the noëtic dimension. It also excludes the application of some instruments, exercises, tools, and strategies.

Conclusion

Finding, discovering, and rediscovering meaning at work through meaning-centered job crafting could help people stay healthy, sane, and well in the workplace, even when the world of work, with its tasks and requirements, is subject to constant change and challenge for the individual.

Meaning-centered job crafting is a preventive and curative approach for human beings and their work lives. It is preventive, as it prevents the experience of a lack or loss of meaning if applied from the very beginning (before people even start to experience a lack or loss of meaning at work). It can also have curative effects, albeit not in a clinical sense, as it supports people to (re-)discover meaning at their workplaces, jobs, and occupations.

Meaning-centered (i.e., logotherapeutic) job crafting is highly relevant for the twenty-first century because it empowers individuals to craft their jobs meaningfully so that they can work in a humane way, one which is personally satisfying on an existential, noëtic level. What is even more important is that it prevents existential frustration and thus also helps to prevent burnout syndrome, which is an increasingly prevalent problem in the world of work (Riethof & Bob, 2019).

Meaning-centered logotherapeutic job crafting strives to provide individuals with the knowledge, ability, tools, instruments, and processes to craft their jobs responsibly, i.e., humanely. This ability to define the boundaries of one's job and work life becomes a critical life competence for humanity in the twenty-first century—and beyond.

References

Badura, B., Ducki, A., Schröder, H., Klose, J., & Meyer, M. (2018). *Fehlzeiten-Report 2018: Sinn erleben-Arbeit und Gesundheit*. Springer-Verlag.

Bailey, C., & Madden, A. (2016). What makes work meaningful—or meaningless. *MIT Sloan Management Review, 57*, 53. https://sloanreview.mit.edu/article/what-makes-work-meaningful-or-meaningless/

Bailey, C., Madden, A., Alfes, K., Shantz, A., & Soane, E. (2017). The mismanaged soul: Existential labor and the erosion of meaningful work. *Human Resource Management Review, 27*(3), 416–430. https://doi.org/10.1016/j.hrmr.2016.11.001

Berg, J. M., Dutton, J. E., & Wrzesniewski, A. (2007). *What is job crafting and why does it matter?* https://positiveorgs.bus.umich.edu/wp-content/uploads/What-is-Job-Crafting-and-Why-Does-it-Matter1.pdf

Berg, J. M., Wrzesniewski, A., & Dutton, J. E. (2010). Perceiving and responding to challenges in job crafting at different ranks: When proactivity requires adaptivity. *Journal of Organizational Behavior, 31*(2–3), 158–186. https://doi.org/10.1002/job.645

Berg, J. M., Dutton, J. E., & Wrzesniewski, A. (2013a). Job crafting and meaningful work. In B. J. Dik, Z. S. Byrne, & M. F. Steger (Eds.), *Purpose and meaning in the workplace* (pp. 81–104). American Psychological Association.

Berg, J. M., Dutton, J. E., Wrzesniewski, A., & Baker, W. E. (2013b). *Job crafting exercise*. University of Michigan Ross School of Business.

Bresman, H., & Rao, V. D. (2017). A survey of 19 countries shows how generations X, Y, and Z are—and aren't—different. *Harvard Business Review, 25*, 1–8. https://hbr.org/2017/08/a-survey-of-19-countries-shows-how-generations-x-y-and-z-are-and-arent-different

Bridges, W. (1996). *Jobshift: How to prosper in a workplace without jobs*. Addison Wesley.

Burger, D. H., Crous, F., & Roodt, G. (2013). Exploring a model for finding meaning in the changing world of work (Part 3: Meaning as framing context). *SA Journal of Industrial Psychology, 39*(2). https://doi.org/10.4102/sajip.v39i2.1022

Business Roundtable. (2019). *Business roundtable redefines the purpose of a corporation to promote 'an economy that serves all Americans.'* www.businessroundtable.org/business-roundtable-redefines-the-purpose-of-a-corporation-to-promote-an-economy-that-serves-all-americans

De Shazer, S. (1988). *Clues: Investigating solutions in brief therapy*. WW Norton & Co.

Dundon, E. (2019). Causes of the lack of meaning at work: Understanding why there is a crisis of meaning in the workplace. *Psychology Today Online*. https://www.psychologytoday.com/us/blog/the-search-for-meaning-after-age-50/201911/causes-of-the-lack-of-meaning-at-work

Fabry, J. B. (1988/2021). *Guideposts to meaning: Discovering what really matters* (2nd ed.). Purpose Research. (Original work published 1988)

Fink, L. (2019). *Larry Fink's annual letter to CEOs*. https://www.blackrock.com/corporate/investor-relations/larry-fink-ceo-letter

Frankl, V. E. (1967). *Psychotherapy and existentialism*. Washington Square Press.

Frankl, V. E. (1969/1988). *The will to meaning: Foundations and applications of logotherapy*. Meridian.

Frankl, V. E. (1973). *The doctor and the soul*. (R. Winston & C. Winston, Trans.). Penguin Books. (Original work published 1946 as *Ärztliche Seelsorge*; Franz Deuticke)
Frankl, V. E. (1975). *Anthropologische grundlagen der psychotherapie*. Huber.
Frankl, V. E. (1978). *The unheard cry for meaning: Psychotherapy and humanism*. Simon and Schuster.
Frankl, V. E. (1982). Opening address to the First World Congress, 1980: Logotherapy on its way to degurufication. In S. A. Wawrytko (Ed.), *First World Congress of Logotherapy* (pp. 340–351). Institute of Logotherapy.
Frankl, V. E. (2004). *On the theory and therapy of mental disorders: An introduction to logotherapy and existential analysis*. (J. DuBois, Trans.). Brunner-Routledge. (Original work published *Theorie und Therapie der Neurosen Einfuhrung in die Logotherapie und Existenzanalys*)
Frankl, V. E. (2006). *Man's search for meaning*. Beacon Press. (Original work published 1946)
Frankl, V. E. (2010). In A. Batthyany & A. Tallon (Eds.), *The feeling of meaninglessness: A challenge to psychotherapy and philosophy*. Marquette University Press.
Gartenberg, C., & Serafeim, G. (2019). 181 top CEOs have realized companies need a purpose beyond profit. *Harvard Business Review, 20*, 2019. https://hbr.org/2019/08/181-top-ceos-have-realized-companies-need-a-purpose-beyond-profit
Hakner, J. (2017). *Imposing "meaningful work" leads to staff burnout*. https://www.sussex.ac.uk/broadcast/read/38643
Jackson, P. Z., & McKergow, M. (2007). *The solutions focus: Making coaching and change SIMPLE* (2nd ed.). Nicholas Brealey.
Kotrba, V., & Miarka, R. (2015). *Agile Teams lösungsfokussiert coachen*. dpunkt.verlag.
Kovacs, G. (1986). Phenomenology of work and self-transcendence. *The Journal of Value Inquiry, 20*(3), 195–207. https://doi.org/10.1007/bf00148299
Marshall, M., & Marshall, E. (2012). *Logotherapy revisited: Review of the tenets of Viktor E. Frankl's logotherapy*. Ottawa Institute of Logotherapy.
Pattakos, A. (2018). Why put meaning first? *Psychology Today Online*. https://www.psychologytoday.com/us/blog/the-meaningful-life/201812/why-put-meaning-first
Pattakos, A. (2019). MEANINGology: A cure for todays modern day crisis of meaning. *Working on purpose*. https://www.voiceamerica.com/episode/116003/meaningology-a-cure-for-todays-modern-day-crisis-of-meaning
Pattakos, A., & Dundon, E. (2017). *Prisoners of our thoughts: Viktor Frankl's principles for discovering meaning in life and work* (Kindle ed.). Berrett-Koehler Publishers.
Petrou, P., Demerouti, E., Peeters, M. C. W., Schaufeli, W. B., & Hetland, J. (2012). Crafting a job on a daily basis: Contextual correlates and the link to work engagement. *Journal of Organizational Behavior, 33*(8), 1120–1141. https://doi.org/10.1002/job.1783
Pichler, H. (2019). Is your leadership meaningful? Website of the international platform for *Meaning at Work*. Retrieved from https://meaning-at-work.com/is-your-leadership-meaningful/
Rampton, J. (2017). *Different motivations for different generations of workers: Boomers, Gen X, Millennials, and Gen Z: An honest day's pay for an honest day's work isn't always the case*. https://www.inc.com/john-rampton/different-motivations-for-different-generations-of-workers-boomers-gen-x-millennials-gen-z.html
Riethof, N., & Bob, P. (2019). Burnout syndrome and logotherapy: Logotherapy as useful conceptual framework for explanation and prevention of burnout. *Frontiers in Psychiatry, 10*, 382–382. https://doi.org/10.3389/fpsyt.2019.00382
Sárkány, P. (2016). *Meaning-centred existential analysis: Philosophy as psychotherapy in the work of Viktor E. Frankl*. Könighausen & Neumann.
Slim, P. (2013). *Body of work: Finding the thread that ties your story together*. Portfolio/Penguin.
World Economic Forum. (2017). *Creating profit through purpose*. https://www.youtube.com/watch?v=a5duxtCh3DU
Wrzesniewski, A., & Dutton, J. E. (2001). Crafting a job: Revisioning employees as active crafters of their work. *Academy of Management Review, 26*(2), 179–201. https://doi.org/10.5465/amr.2001.4378011

Wrzesniewski, A., Dutton, J. E., & Debebe, G. (2003). Interpersonal sensemaking and the meaning of work. *Research in Organizational Behavior, 25*, 93–135. https://doi.org/10.1016/s0191-3085(03)25003-6

Wrzesniewski, A., Berg, J. M., & Dutton, J. E. (2010). Turn the job you have into the job you want. *Harvard Business Review, 88*(6), 114–117.

Sabine Indinger (Master of Organisational Psychology), completed her studies of logotherapy with Elisabeth Lukas in 2008 and received an Academic Associate Credential in Logotherapy (Viktor Frankl Institute of Logotherapy USA) in 2009. Since 2011 she has been a Life Member of the Viktor Frankl Institute of Logotherapy (USA). She completed her Diplomate in 2020 and was accredited by the Viktor Frankl Institute Vienna in 2020. She works as an HR executive and as an HR & business consultant, coach and trainer/educator, finding ways to apply Viktor Frankl's Logotherapy to the workplace.

Nominal Socratic Dialogue or Finding the Basic ID: An Existential Analytical Tool for Finding Meaning

Willem Maas

It was Viktor Frankl's lecture on the "Arguments for a Tragic Optimism" (in English, see Frankl, 1984, pp. 137–154) that enabled me to find and construct the Nominal Socratic Dialogue (NSD) tool (Maas, 1989, 1999, 2013). The phrase "*omnia mea mecum porto*" ("All that is mine I carry with me"; attributed to Bias von Pirene, a Greek philosopher, cited in Polak, 1949, p. 1) is the point where the dialogue begins. As a therapist I know that, although our clients may have forgotten it or are not yet aware of it, it implies an inner dialogue of the client, one that requires Socratic dialogue on the part of the therapist.

The NSD helps therapists to deal with unconscious values of the client, and helps the client to find their own value hierarchy in order to reintegrate it into a personalized, situational meaning statement. This empowers the individual to reintegrate as a person into social exchange. "Nominal" refers to nouns, which represent important as well as essential issues that are part of their attitude towards their situation in life.

The first public application of the NSD took place during a training event for individuals who were chosen to rise from middle management to a higher echelon of a large telecommunications company in the Netherlands in 1989. I was invited by one of my students at the Netherlands Institute for Logotherapy and Existential Analysis to present the tool to his trainees.

There were about 20 adult males in the room who were focused on advancing themselves in their respective careers; they could be considered high-flying top performers. I was invited to deliver a short presentation on logotherapy in a setting in which one would normally not include any sort of psychological self-assessment. These individuals knew who they were and what they wanted; they were independently driven, proud to be elected to rise to new responsibilities.

W. Maas (✉)
Netherlands Institute for Logotherapy, Wijk bij Duurstede, Netherlands

C. L. McLafferty, Jr., J. I. Levinson (eds.), *Logotherapy and Existential Analysis*, Logotherapy and Existential Analysis: Proceedings of the Viktor Frankl Institute Vienna 2, https://doi.org/10.1007/978-3-031-48922-8_24

Most of the participants said that the idea of values was too far removed from their day-to-day working situation; it was of no practical value for the business decisions they had to make. I agreed with them, but insisted, even in voicing their opinions, they were expressing a kind of personal "business mission statement." This statement, underlying their actual behavior in situations in which their leadership would be requested, would possibly be an important tool to help them better understand the people they might be managing in the near future.

That got their attention, and one of them asked if I could present any evidence for my thesis. I replied that I could. They were curious as to how I would present the evidence. Because I did not know any of these participants, nor anything about their background (not even their names), I was able to present the exercise.

I invited them to take a blank piece of paper and write down six items, six nouns of importance, using free association. Paper, pencil, and eraser were provided.

There were some common expectations as to what they would write, because some nouns would be almost universal as well as socially expected: These might include spouse, kids, home, car, health... whatever else first came to mind. I instructed them to leave these out; even when these were taken away, they still had to live their own lives. Anyone familiar with logotherapy will have recognized the context of my remarks; however, these participants were not familiar with the concentration camp experience that Frankl (1984) described in *Man's Search for Meaning*. They were in unfamiliar territory.

After 10 minutes, all of them had managed to put down six words. I then asked them to pick out and mark the three most important ones, each with a plus sign: **+**. From these three, I asked them to indicate the most important one, and to mark that one with a double plus sign: **++**. Three nouns were left unmarked. I suggested that it might be possible to see these as potential sources or causes of trouble, discomfort, or danger. Only one was troublesome for sure; participants were instructed to mark it with the minus sign: **–**. Finally, because the remaining two nouns could not readily be assigned a position in their lives, they were instructed to mark them with a question mark: **?**. Though the participants were unsure of the purpose of the exercise, all completed the task.

I then asked them to draw a hexagram, a compound of two equilateral triangles, such as the Star of David, on their piece of paper. In fact, I instructed them to orient their triangles as a Star of David for the purposes of this exercise. Because we can possibly visualize that each of us is a star, I asked them to put a large *P* for "person" in the center of the star.

Now I asked them to copy their nouns onto the points of the star; the noun with the double pluses **++** at the top of the star, and the two nouns with the plus sign **+** at the bottom points of the upward-pointing triangle. The noun given the minus sign **–** was to be placed at the bottom point of the star, and the two nouns with questions marks were to go at the remaining points at the outer top (see Fig. 1).

What we now have, I explained, is not just a hierarchy of items, which are called *values*, but also a picture of the interactive, dynamic, relationship of these values, being put into their right place and order.

Fig. 1 Placing the nouns on the star

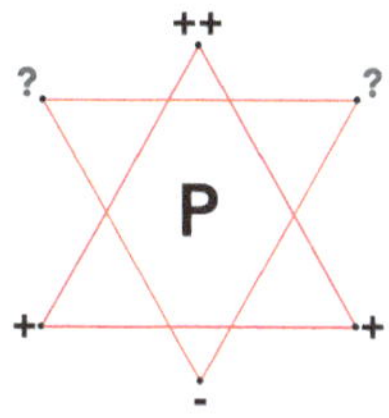

The final step was to start writing a statement, beginning with the word "I" representing the *P* (person) and use the items from the star, beginning at the top, integrating each item in clockwise order until the last item was integrated, and then add a full stop. I told them it might not be an easy task; however, I was confident that each of them would succeed in the exercise.

It took about quarter of an hour for all participants to complete their statements. After they had finished, I asked the person finishing last to read out his statement. With tears in his eyes and a choking voice, he read his statement:

> I was given a second chance in order to change my situation, becoming the best possible person I could be, knowing that I cannot be perfect but I am confident that I will be able to return the trust which the company has put in me.

He was a robust man; he had started his career digging trenches for cables and had been working hard to advance his position; today, he was receiving the training which would help him rise on the ladder from overseer in the trenches to a position of leadership over 100 people. In this exercise, he retrieved his actual, *basic existential ID*. He formulated his challenge as a human person in connection with the burden his actual life represented. He found his individual arguments for a tragic (that is, a realistic) optimism, trying to be the best possible person he thought he could become. He had never realized all these insights about himself and his life was within him.

We might expect an average group of individuals to talk about superficial topics, such as social situations, current events, the economy, or politics. This group had not been used to discussing their feelings, let alone their existence.

All participants read their statements, though some of the narratives did not flow very well. The use of pencil and eraser allows participants to change or reposition their previously stated value hierarchy in order to turn it into a self-explanatory mission statement. I was able to explain the why and the how of the exercise, showing that in each line arguments for a so-called tragic optimism were integrated in an individual, and very personal, way.

Frankl (1984) spoke about the *optimistic triad* (pp. 137–154); he also explained the *tragic triad* of pain, suffering, and death (Frankl, 1969/1988, p. 73). The tragic triad relates to reality, it points "down to earth." Every person will be confronted with suffering, loss, and guilt. I explained that suffering is not necessarily an illness or a matter of fate or bad luck. Suffering, or its equivalent, as each of us knows, implies our own unconditional involvement. It is the time in which a person finds a challenge, which equals a freedom for some burden to be carried, which equals personal responsibility. I told the participants:

Such a mission statement can be found in the heart and mind of every single person, denoting for whom or for what that person is actually contributing in life in a dignified, meaningful way. It is like a basic existential ID. The statement makes sense, because it is the very personal explanation of the cause or purpose of being in a situation like ours here today.

If you really want to know what kind of a person is in front of you, you may remember your mission statement and act upon it. If you do, you will find the other person in an actual phase of their own personal mission in life. It will help you to assist those who are suffering from burnout to find another job or to recognize talents that will help you to successfully manage your part of the business. It may even assist you in finding external help for people who need a different orientation although they think they cannot afford to.

What Is The Background of this Exercise?

Anyone familiar with logotherapy knows that I was speaking about the unconditional "Yes" towards life (Frankl, 2020), i.e., the moment that situational meaning occurs and is put into action. The noun marked with ++ represents this unconditional "Yes."

Values are like telecommunication, they are essential—as this exercise demonstrates. The NSD is designed as an existential–analytical tool, not to interfere, but to observe without judging, and to assist personal growth towards the freedom one is able to be responsible for.

In working with clients, we ask and observe, we postpone our conclusions, waiting for them to explain to us for whom or what the presented problem has appeared. In explaining the exercise, I avoid using the words "love, hope, and faith" and "suffering, transience, and guilt." The reason for that may sound simple: These almost universally known nouns would fill out the thoughts of the person taking the NSD and block the free association on what really matters. Had I mentioned them, as in Frankl's lecture, almost everyone would have used those, and all of their narratives would have sounded alike, instead of unique for each person.

When a client comes in for therapy, we know there is a problem. Even if we are familiar with their individual situation, we do not know what else is being brought into our room. We need a fast entry, a certain amount of dereflection in order to enable the person to speak for themselves, not just to express the psyche and its everlasting series of problems. We need to find out where and how our client is able to defy their situation. In short, we need to find out what the intention of the spiritual person is.

The mission statement that results from the NSD exercise is explaining the existential dignity to its own creator (Frankl, 2007a, pp. 70–71). It "uncovers," so to speak, what is hidden behind the façade of individual psychological and social conformity.

It is, however, possible that the statement doesn't smoothly flow, or that it contains issues that do not fit in with the other issues. For example: "I love life although it sometimes is so hard to keep up hope, especially during times of loss and failure, but I am confident that I can overcome my sorrow and repay my debts."

During the exercise, participants may decide to exchange **+** or **?** marked values, and try again to write down in one sentence the mission statement. The pencil and eraser are, in fact, symbols of our conscience; they are there to provide the freedom to change what is truly important in our lives, even though this is only a sketch. Because our time has not been used up, we still are in the process until we have completed our lives.

If no statement seems possible, we then have an entrance to ask questions about the mentioned order of importance, as decided in the second step of the exercise. We do not want to know what someone has or doesn't have. We want to know what givens someone carries as truly important. We also are aware of things we cannot want, such as wanting to want, wanting to will, wanting to hope for or experience faith, or wanting to be happy. If such issues do occur in the optimistic triangle, we are aware of incongruency or disharmony which needs to be explored. They could be the causal element in the neurotic problems of the client.

The spiritual person, the *P* author of the individual statement, does not pretend (Frankl, 2007a, p. 71); as we know from medicine, bodies do not lie. We know that logotherapy is a "person-to-person" method (Frankl, 2007b, see also theses 1, 5, 6, 7 in Frankl, 2021), rather than a "therapist-to-problem-or-disorder" type of psychotherapy.

It is the Socratic aspect combined with the notion of the *nominal* (substantives for basic issues). Each item in the star represents an aspect of *logos*—a meaningful, valuable, and valid complex relationship between the person and their situation (Frankl, 1939, p. 707; 1984). The personalized mission statement explains the attitude towards the requirement of the situation (Polak, 1949), which may differ from third-party expectations and social demands.

For many participants, it was a profoundly moving experience; so much so that for the first time in their lives they could describe themselves, explaining what truly matters for each of them. This is obviously what the "existential" is all about: the moments that really move us showing us that we matter and make a difference.

It is the hallmark of what exists in the background of our awareness, the spiritual dimension that is normally unconscious and sometimes appears like a flash of light to encourage us. In a therapy setting, people expect to first and foremost discuss their problems. In the forefront of their mind are things that are required, issues that bother or block them, reactions that must be controlled.

In a logotherapy setting, the initial aim is to foster resilience, and only then search for the meaning of the moment, which is that which is required to be done in order to solve a problem, to overcome despair, and to restart—even when it is "sadder and wiser"—into a meaningful context.

The NSD can be extended into the field of emotions, feelings, and actual options. Each of the six items from the exercise carries emotive (emotion + motive) aspects. They are aspects of individual attitudinal value, supported by experiences, each one of which are supported by creative values. It is therefore possible (and even of great importance) to write the experiential values down, three at each point of the star, building new triangles.

The two triangles with their six points now carry issues that might need to be opened and unpacked. We can explore such issues and differentiate them into how we felt when the issue occurred, finding an emotional harvest. For therapy, it is preferred to focus on the optimistic triangle for obvious reasons. We want our client to find his or her resilience, exploring the defying power of the human spirit rather than deepening the problematic and harsh characteristics of the experienced reality.

Each of our situations—challenging and positive as well as problematic—is integrated within the at least 72 facets of awareness about an individual's dignity and about the meaning waiting to be fulfilled. That may not look like a sheer endless number of possibilities; however, it is the nature of meaning.

Emotional memories are what Frankl (1969/1988) defined as *experiential values*. Such moments support rapid and complete change of mind and matter, confirmed by behavioral and neurobiological research. Positive experiences, feelings, and emotions will open the window towards life itself.

If we start our therapeutic work using the optimistic triad by ways of finding the experiences underpinning the decision (*attitudinal values*, Frankl, 1969/1988), the psycho-neuro-endocrine-immunological organism will reproduce the positive situation. It will enhance the possibilities to change, the resort of our spiritual freedom to live our life response-able.

The exercise provides self-distancing, trailing the actual problem towards challenge, for which the capacity to grow, to interact, and to overcome, called *self-transcendence*, is put into action. The items in the tragic triad keep us, so to speak, with our two feet in our individual "down to earth" reality. It is the actual involvement in life, e.g., to endure and not despair, to overcome and not lose faith. Life will offer us the insight about what we are about to do in order to become the best possible person we can be. The actual problem (the one a client brings into therapy) is included, as part of the individual reality of things that need to be completed, redeemed, and healed.

Logotherapy is a truly realistic therapy; it is not spiritualistic but it deals with the way a person searches for and finds meaning and dignity, even in individual tragedy. Logotherapy is the essential way to "reach" the person who has to decide what they will do next. It is pragmatic, while concentrated on "being within the responsible awareness of acting" ("Sein in der Verantwortung der Tat," Frankl, 2007a, p. 236), in order to deliver the congruent human answer to the requirements of any given situation.

That is why I told the training group that each person carries a "personal mission statement," which is the energy that ensures being a good manager. In terms of a therapeutic goal, the value and meaning awareness allows the client to heal and proceed with life, maybe sadder and wiser, but wholeheartedly and prepared for their individual future.

Another aspect of the NSD-Tool is that the experiential values found actually are substitutes or synonyms of past experiences. Human beings collect experiences that help them to survive and overcome (even if only situationally and temporarily) their natural anxiety. That is why we remember, and recognize experiences as enlarging our freedom or as limiting it. Frankl (1984) quoted Spinoza: "'*Affectus, qui passio est, desinit esse passio simulatque eius claram et distinctam formamus ideam.*' Emotion, which is suffering, ceases to be suffering as soon as we form a clear and precise picture of it" (p. 74).

Early memories of limiting nature are necessary to survive, and we usually find those and their situational substitutes in the tragic triad. Nonetheless, logotherapy is not a therapy delving into the past; rather, it is rather a realistic one exploring the creative options of a person in the here and now (of individual suffering).

The complete, integrated mission statement is therefore the situational *simile,* of the unconscious and unconditional commitment to live life as it develops, from situation to situation, preventing the neurotic provisional state of being in which psyche expects life to serve it; moreover, it includes an unconditional personal commitment towards dignity and meaning in suffering. As Frankl (1984) noted: "Suffering ceases to be suffering at the moment it finds a meaning, such as the moment of a sacrifice" (p. 113).

Suffering therefore is not only social, mental, emotional, or physical suffering, it also denotes the self-transcendent decision to stand in for someone or for something and to dedicate one's life to alleviate suffering. Finding meaning in a given situation arrives only from self-transcending, because meaning itself is transcendent; it exists, may be shared, cannot be taken away or lost, because we cannot "have" meaning. We can only fulfill the call for this special meaning with our own existence as an answer and bring meaning into reality. We are not looking for "meaning of life"; that is Adler's turf, denoting a compensatory activity to face the basic anxiety or frustration of not having (received) enough. Therefore, the NSD procedure helps our clients to experience their very own dimensional differences and to find the energy to understand the challenge of the moment as a possibility to grow as a human being towards dignity. From existence to act, "being within the responsibility of the act" (Frankl, 2018, p. 61). That differs from the reductionist or nihilistic focus on feelings arriving from bad experiences and broken dreams.

The well-known founder of homeopathy, Samuel Hahnemann (1810), is noted for saying that, in order to become a successful healer, it is necessary to exactly replicate his method and intention.

The simplest of solutions are most of the times the ones that are hardest to find. Similar to Frankl's insight and wisdom, I followed his directions. I was just lucky to find the NSD Tool, owing the direction and background to Viktor Frankl.

Final Remarks Related to the Exercise

As noted earlier, it is of vital importance to *not* mention the tragic or optimistic triads to the client at the start of the exercise. If I had, I would have transferred my understanding onto the participants' psyches and, in so doing, would have prepped them to answer to our premeditation (Frankl, 1959). Logotherapists tend to explain to clients their trade secrets because logotherapy is not like popular psychology, and certainly not a psychodynamic psychology. As Frankl noted, we want a causal therapy, not one that is suggestive or autosuggestive (p. 22ff).

The second reason for not mentioning the tragic or optimistic triads is that the instrument is a one-time instrument, an opportunity that is needed in both counseling and therapy.

Still another reason is that, if we told our client about love, hope, faith as well as of suffering, guilt, and transience, the opportunity of a true set of issues from the unconscious will be blocked by the psychological wish to comply. We do not want compliance in a psychological way, because it will only deliver us the answers clients think that their therapist expects them to give. We would have suggested that such an approach would actually tell us about the deepest aspirations of our client, and spoiled the opportunity of the spiritual person to explain in terms of attitudinal values what their life was really about in an existential perspective.

So, we keep quiet, as Socrates did when he asked his uneasy questions to his audience. He knew what he was evoking; his aim was to make his public feel ashamed. That is definitely not our intention. Our intention is to help our client become aware of their essence in life—an essence, if we follow Spinoza (cited in Frankl, 1984), that will not stop striving for realization (which is what personal growth is) in spite of circumstances, conditions, and social structure. The essence is to become aware of being a person and express a meaningful life which positively contributes to the enterprise of humanity itself.

Thus, it is only after the value hierarchy is formed, after the statement beginning with "I" reaches its full stop in allocating all six values as they have been put into the hexagram, that we show our cards and explain the essence of the existential dynamics of this exercise.

The last remark is about the fractal nature of the points of the star. We as therapists are looking for a peak of the very person ($N = 1$) knowing what this person is not aware of, namely, that the number of meaning possibilities is approximately endless ($\approx\infty$). Both behavioral options as well as meaning possibilities are variable; if not, there would be no possibility to mature. There is no "standard human being," and there is no such thing as a universal "meaning of life."

Although it is clear that it is possible to further explore each of the points in psychological terms by asking about the experiences and activities that are associated with each point, it is *not necessary*. It may be helpful in cases that include statements such as "I never received love, so I cannot give it," or "just let me be, I am who I am" to explore a single issue, and show, for example where a paradox has emerged. That is: During the course of a therapy or counseling process, we may get back to one of the issues and find a key question.[1]

[1] Further professional education in the use of the above method is available at the Netherlands Institute of Logotherapy and Existential Analysis. The BasicID exercise is part of the actual training program. For more information, please contact Dr. Pieter Hoekstra at info@viktorfrankl.nl.

References

Frankl, V. E. (1939). Philosophie und Psychotherapie: Zur Grundlegung einer Existenzanalyse [Philosophy and psychotherapy: On the basis of existential analysis]. *Schweizerische Medizinische Wochenschrift, 69*, 707–709.

Frankl, V. E. (1959). *Das Menschenbild der Seelenheilkunde, Kritik des dynamischen Psychologismus* [The image of man in psychiatry: A critique of dynamic psychologism]. Hippokrates Verlag.

Frankl, V. E. (1969/1988). *The will to meaning: Foundations and applications of logotherapy*. Meridian. (Original work published 1969)

Frankl, V. E. (1984). *Man's search for meaning* (3rd ed.). Pocket Books. (Original work published 1946)

Frankl, V. E. (2007a). *Theorie und Therapie der Neurosen* [Theory and therapy of mental disorders]. Reinhardt.

Frankl, V. E. (2007b). *Ärztliche Seelsorge, Grundlagen der Logotherapie und Existenzanalyse [In English, published as The doctor and the soul]. Deutscher Taschenbuch. (Original work published 1946)*

Frankl, V. E. (2018). *Der leidende Mensch: Anthropologische Grundlagen der Psychotherapie* [The suffering person: Anthropological foundations of psychotherapy]. Hogrefe AG.

Frankl, V. E. (2020). *Yes to life: In spite of everything*. Beacon Press.

Frankl, V. E. (2021). *Zehn Thesen über die Person* [10 theses on the person]. In *Der Wille zum Sinn* (pp. 87–94). Hogrefe.

Hahnemann, S. (1810). *Organon der rationellen Heilkunst* [Organon of the art of healing]. Stuttgart Homoion-Verlag.

Maas, W. J. (1989). *Basic ID, training manuals NILEA*. Netherlands Institute for Logotherapy and Existential Analysis.

Maas, W. J. (1999). Value analysis, gateway to the ultimate human dream. *Bulletin voor Logotherapie en Existentiële Analyse, 2*, 11. http://viktorfrankl.nl/Bulletins/Bulletin%20Vol09-2-1999.PDF

Maas, W. J. (2013). *Nieuwsbrief* [Newsbrief]. Nederlands Instituut voor Logotherapie, *2*. https://drive.google.com/file/d/16KVL2u4PTFRSzDBQW3cqD5E0XL8Sy9LK/view

Polak, P. (1949). *Frankl's Existenzanalyse in ihrer Bedeutung für Anthropologie und Psychotherapie* [Frankl's existential analysis in its importance for anthropology and psychotherapy]. Tryolia-Verlag. [Translation available on request from the author.].

Willem Maas, Ph.D. (1948) studied philosophy and theology at the Protestant Theological University in Brussels and specialized in meaning-centered pastoral psychology. In 1989 he founded the Netherlands Institute for Logotherapy, with the personal recommendation of Viktor Frankl. He worked as an international trainer/supervisor in the Netherlands, Malta, and in the United Kingdom. He retired in January, 2023.

Logo-CareerSkills: A Logotherapeutic Intervention for Resilient Career Development in Youth

Memduh Nezih Ozmert

The beginning of the twenty-first century was accompanied with huge problems: environmental issues, economic and financial crises, regional clashes, mass migrations, income inequalities, a pandemic (Covid-19), and technological disruption. These changes, challenges, disasters, and chaos make careers more dynamic, requiring employees to keep up with ever-increasing changes in the job and labor markets. Harari et al. (2020) asserted that automation and artificial intelligence would eliminate millions of jobs.

One of the main consequences of all these challenges is an increase in the mismatch between job listings and the skills of those who are seeking employment. This increase might cause multiple issues stemming from the existential vacuum and collective neuroses, including unemployment neurosis. Frankl (1986) emphasized that the most prominent symptom of unemployment neurosis is not depression, but apathy.

As an effort to contribute to finding a resolution for these challenges, an intervention program titled "Logo-CareerSkills" (LCS) was established to stimulate career competency development and resilience of the work force. LCS is based on the JOBS career competency model (Price et al., 1998) developed at the Michigan Prevention Research Center as a preventive intervention for recently unemployed job seekers. JOBS is a short, group-based program focused on acquiring job skills and strengthening self-efficacy and problem-solving approaches (Vinokur et al., 1995, p. 40). LCS is a modification of the JOBS method in accordance with the philosophy, the anthropological view of the human being, and the tools and techniques of logotherapy.

M. N. Ozmert (✉)
Viktor Frankl Enstitüsü Türkiye, Ataşehir, Istanbul, Turkey

C. L. McLafferty, Jr., J. I. Levinson (eds.), *Logotherapy and Existential Analysis*, Logotherapy and Existential Analysis: Proceedings of the Viktor Frankl Institute Vienna 2, https://doi.org/10.1007/978-3-031-48922-8_25

The advantages of modifying the JOBS method in accordance with logotherapy are:

- This modification contributes to the vision that individuals can dedicate themselves to their call of meaning and become free and responsible under all circumstances.
- It broadens the viewpoint of work, as Viktor Frankl (1986) stated:
  - Work usually represents the area in which the individual's uniqueness stands in relation to society and thus acquires meaning and value. This meaning and value, however, is attached to the person's work as a contribution to society, not to the actual occupation as such (p. 63).
- It addresses the meaninglessness that accompanies unemployment, as noted by Frankl (1946/1986):
  - Fifty years ago, I published a study devoted to a specific type of depression I had diagnosed in cases of young patients suffering from what I called "unemployment neurosis." And I could show that this neurosis really originated in a twofold erroneous identification: being jobless was equated with being useless, and being useless was equated with having a meaningless life (p. 91).
- It adds Frankl's (1986, 1946/1986) concept of the existential vacuum, and its tools and techniques to enable self-distancing and self-transcending capabilities.
- In brief, LCS is an education and coaching intervention program targeted not only to increase the career competencies of individuals but their resilience under all circumstances and situations as well.

Because unemployment—specifically youth unemployment—became a major issue globally as noted in the 2022 statistics on youth unemployment prepared by the Organisation for Economic Cooperation and Development (2022), the LCS program was specifically focused on youth unemployment.

The main objectives of this intervention were:

- to make job seekers aware of their future hopes, their deepest motivations;
- to increase awareness of their strengths, shortcomings, and skills related to their personal careers;
- to enhance their skills to use and develop their social support networks;
- to develop their self-profiling skills, which refers to presenting and communicating their personal knowledge, skills, and abilities to the labor market;
- to assist them in setting goals, planning, and taking action;
- to increase their creativity by developing out-of-the-box thinking abilities; and
- to grow their resilience in the face of difficult conditions and "hitting the wall."

The LCS Intervention

The LCS intervention involves two phases: Phase I was comprised of six workshops, and Phase II was interwoven with Phase I with three personal coaching sessions over a 6-week period, as shown in Fig. 1.

All workshops lasted 4 hours. After every two workshops, a one-on-one coaching session took place. In workshops, active learning methods such as brainstorming, social modeling, and role playing were applied in a socially supportive environment, and homework was assigned. The main objective of the individual coaching sessions was to ensure that the participants understood the material and completed their homework, which are the main deliverables, the outcome of this intervention program.

Phase II was comprised of these three one-on-one coaching sessions, conducted biweekly. All coaches were certified as Academic Associates in Logotherapy by the Viktor Frankl Institute of Logotherapy (USA).

The LCS Training Program

In workshops and coaching, all the layers of the LCS model depicted in Fig. 2 were addressed. As will be shown, the training, feedback, and support were integrated carefully into both phases, which alternated.

Session 1 In the first session, instruments were administered in order to study the success of the program (see study details below), as well as the VIA Character Strength Survey (Peterson & Seligman, 2004; available at www.viacharacter.org), a psychological assessment designed to identify an individual's profile of character strengths. Self-discovery was the main theme of this session, and principles of logotherapy in the form of logo-education were introduced, which included questions such as, "What does it mean to be human?" "What are the attributes of humanness?" The *Workbook to Increase your Meaningful and Purposeful Goals (MPG)* (Hutzell & Jerkins, 2009) was introduced for participants to clarify their value hierarchies.

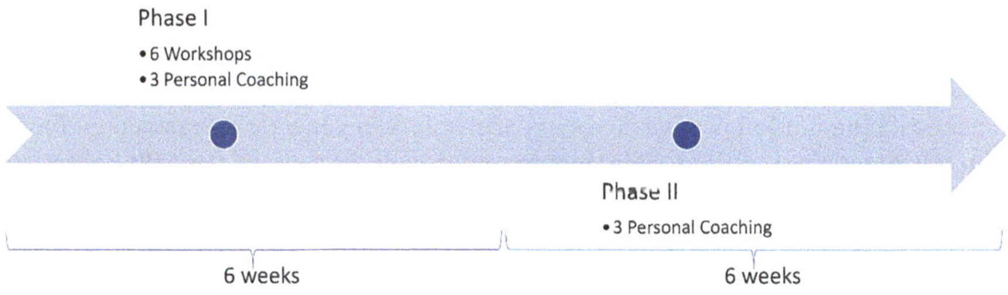

Fig. 1 LCS intervention Phases I and II

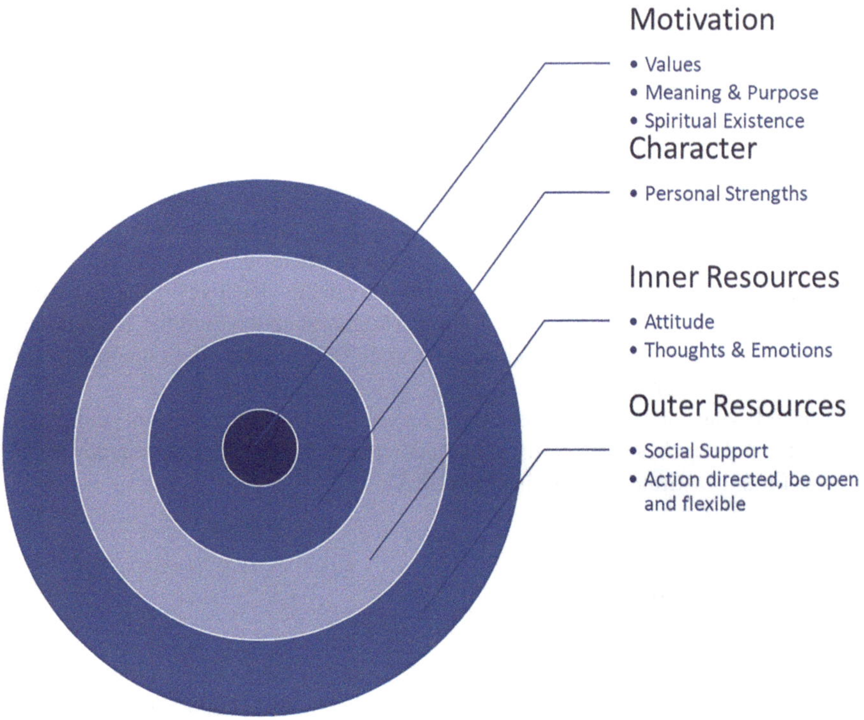

Fig. 2 The LCS Resilient Career Competency development model

Session 2 In the second session, each participant was challenged existentially to discover answers to questions such as: "Do your current career ideals match with your value hierarchy and your character strengths?" "Which roles and responsibilities match with your values and character strengths in the industry in which you intend to work?" Participants were invited to step into a figurative "time machine" to discover their dream jobs and visualize themselves fulfilling this possibility. Through this phenomenological exercise they were encouraged to visualize and describe what they were doing in their ideal job, how they were doing it, for what they were accomplishing this goal, and to understand the essence of who they are.

Personal Coaching 1 After the second session, the first one-on-one coaching took place. Each participant was assigned a coach. The main objective of this initial personal coaching conference was to help participants to generate a personal emblem which is comprised of their value hierarchy through the help of the MPG exercise (Hutzell & Jerkins, 2009), integrating the strengths and weaknesses identified in the VIA Character Strength Survey (Peterson & Seligman, 2004). A visualization experience was used to explore who they are and who they want to become.

Session 3 In the third session, work exploration, establishing an action plan with short-, medium-, and long-term breakdown, and self-profiling were addressed. Participants were asked about their values and skills and ways in which they exhibited these competencies to significant others. They were asked to present themselves as convincingly as possible in a brief "elevator speech."

Session 4 In the fourth session, networking was the central topic. Participants were given guidelines to utilize and expand their professional network. They were requested to enrich their action plans with activities related to expanding their professional networks. Finally, participants were requested to cross-reference each of the tasks in their action plans to their values, which is the final step of the MPG exercise (Hutzell & Jerkins, 2009).

Personal Coaching 2 After completing the fourth session, another one-on-one personal coaching conference took place. The objective was to validate and verify that the participants established their action plans with a breakdown of short-, medium-, and long-term time frames and to discuss cross-referencing all the tasks to their value hierarchy. Their elevator speeches were discussed and, if needed, rerecorded.

Session 5 The theme of the fifth session was how to utilize inner resources. Frankl's (1946/1986) concept of tragic optimism and the logotherapy techniques of paradoxical intention and dereflection were introduced. Participants were invited to experience Frankl's (1986) Copernican twist through the conduct of nominal Socratic dialogue technique (Maas, 2021, p. 25; see also Maas, this volume). The participants were introduced to experience both: (a) paradoxical intention as a technique to learn how to fight with fear and wrong passivity and (b) dereflection to overcome the vicious circles of hyperintention and hyperreflection.

Session 6 The themes of the sixth session were "out of the box" thinking and problem solving. Instead of chasing job vacancies, job creation was considered. Total Quality Management tools and techniques were introduced based on David Allen's (2019) recommendations.

Personal Coaching 3 The third one-on-one personal coaching objectives were to cultivate an attitude of tragic optimism towards life and to learn to use techniques of paradoxical intention and dereflection (Frankl, 1946/1986).

The second phase of the LCS program was based on integration of the bi-weekly personal coaching sessions. The intention was to retain resilience against setbacks. The protocol suggested by Close (2006) was used as a guideline.

In week 12, all participants and their coaches met to review the LCS program, which ended with a certification ceremony. Two instruments were completed by participants at this endpoint in order to assess the program (see below). Analysis of pre- and post- assessments were used for testing the hypotheses noted in the study below and to improve the LCS program.

A Study of the Effectiveness of the LCS Program

The impact of this intervention was assessed with two hypotheses:

- Hypothesis 1: The LCS intervention significantly increased the level of career competencies of the participants.
- Hypotheses 2: The LCS intervention increased participants' level of career resilience.

Selection of Participants

The LCS program was implemented twice (in 2020 and 2022), under close cooperation with a nongovernment organization in Turkey (Değiştiren Adımlar https://degistirenadimlar.org/). This organization was running a Responsible Leadership Program for university students from disadvantaged backgrounds (individuals with socioeconomic disadvantages or disabilities). The criteria to participate in the LCS program was offered to those students who completed the Responsible Leadership Program and having either difficulty finding a job or desiring to change their career. The students had to sign an agreement committing to: (a) attend all workshops, coaching sessions; (b) show their best effort to produce the deliverables in requested quality and duration; (c) to complete and submit the VIA Character Strength Survey, the Career Competencies Questionnaire (CCQ), and the Connor-Davidson Resilience Scale (CD-RISC).

In all, 34 participants attended; each group was comprised of 17 unemployed university graduates coming from different social strata. Since the LCS program was modified prior to the second implementation, only the 2022 group results are reported.

Method

Assessment Measures The hypotheses were tested using several instruments, which were completed before the first workshop session: Career competency was assessed using the Career Competencies Questionnaire (CCQ; Akkermans et al., 2013); Resilience was measured with the Resilience Scale Connor-Davidson Resilience Scale (CD-RISC; Connor & Davidson, 2003).

The data were analyzed using paired sample (pre-post) *t* test using Microsoft® Excel® 2021 MSO (Version 2206 Build 16.0.15330.20246) 32-bit for the statistical analysis.

Results

The results of a paired *t*-test comparing CCQ scores in pre- and post-intervention are depicted in Table 1. The average scores increased significantly and meaningfully (24 points) as a result of the intervention.

The results of a paired *t*-test comparing the Connor-Davidson Resilience Scale (CD-RISC) scores are presented in Table 2. Participants' average scores increased significantly and meaningfully as a result of the intervention.

Discussion

The execution of the LCS program within a nongovernment organization resulted in a significant improvement in measures of career competence and resilience scores in the 17 participants of the 2022 group. For this program to be effective in an ecosystem of fighting with youth unemployment, the following objectives are critical: (a) The effectiveness of this intervention must be evaluated and adjusted on an ongoing basis, with consultancy and quality assessment services acquired from international authorities on logotherapy; and (b) the program will have to become scalable in order to meet the demand leading to challenges of increasing the number of coaches within the predefined quality standards, utilizing information

Table 1 Paired t-test results for Career Competencies Questionnaire scores

CCQ	N	$\bar{X}$	SD	Difference	t value
Pre-intervention	17	72.8	13.1		
Post-intervention	17	96.4	8.1	23.6	9.12[a]

[a]df = 16, $p < 0.001$

Table 2 Paired t-test results for Connor-Davidson Resilience Scale

CD-RISC	N	$\bar{X}$	SD	Difference	t value
Pre-intervention	17	93.4	6.9		
Post-intervention	17	110.2	9.9	16.8	10.1

[a]df = 16, $p < 0.001$

technology, and technological capabilities such as gamification. To accomplish these objectives, we are in the process of writing a grant proposal to be awarded with European funding.

References

Akkermans, J., Brenninkmeijer, V., Huibers, M., & Blonk, R. W. (2013). Competencies for the contemporary career: Development and preliminary validation of the Career Competencies Questionnaire. *Journal of Career Development, 40*(3), 245–267. https://doi.org/10.1177/0894845312467500

Allen, D. (2019). *Getting things done: The art of stress-free productivity*. Piatkus Books.

Close, R. E. (2006). A logodiagnostic interpretation of a case of unemployment neurosis. *Journal of Spirituality in Mental Health, 9*(2), 75–84. https://doi.org/10.1300/J515v09n02_06

Connor, K. M., & Davidson, J. R. (2003). Development of a new resilience scale: The Connor-Davidson resilience scale (CD-RISC). *Depression and Anxiety, 18*(2), 76–82. https://doi.org/10.1002/da.10113

Frankl, V. E. (1946/1986). *Man's search for meaning* (3rd ed.). Washington Square Press/Pocket Books. (Original work published 1946)

Frankl, V. E. (1986). *The doctor and the soul* (R. Winston & C. Winston, Trans, p. 64/153). Alfred A. Knopf. (Original work published in 1946 as *Ärztliche Seelsorge*)

Harari, Y. N., & Rutte, M. (Directors) & Gadiesh, O. (Director). (2020). *How to survive the 21st century: DAVOS 2020*. YouTube. Retrieved from https://www.youtube.com/watch?v=eOsKFOrW5h8&t=3s

Hutzell, R. R., & Jerkins, M. E. (2009). *A workbook to increase your meaningful and purposeful goals (MPGs)* (2nd ed.). Viktor Frankl Institute of Logotherapy Press.

Maas, W. (2021). Existential analysis: The precondition for effective psychotherapeutic help. *The International Forum for Logotherapy, 41*(2), 15–32.

Organisation for Economic Cooperation and Development. (2022). *Youth unemployment rate*. [Website] Retrieved from https://data.oecd.org/unemp/youth-unemployment-rate.htm

Peterson, C., & Seligman, M. E. (2004). *Character strengths and virtues: A handbook and classification* (Vol. 1). American Psychological Association and Oxford University Press.

Price, R. H., Friedland, D. S., Choi, J. N., & Caplan, R. D. (1998). Job-loss and work transitions in a time of global economic change. In X. B. Arriaga & S. Oskamp (Eds.), *Addressing community problems: Psychological research and interventions*. Sage.

Vinokur, A. D., Price, R. H., & Schul, Y. (1995). Impact of the JOBS intervention on unemployed workers varying in risk for depression. *American Journal of Community Psychology, 23*(1), 39–74.

Memduh Nezih Ozmert With a B.Sc. in Statistics and M.Sc. in Management Science and Operational Research from Warwick University, UK, Memduh has more than 30 years of experience in academia, government, and IT industry mainly in people management, consultancy, and program management. In 2016, he established the "Viktor Frankl Enstitüsü Türkiye" which is an accredited member of The International Association of Logotherapy and Existential Analysis. As a Diplomate in Logotherapy and a faculty member of the Viktor Frankl Institute of Logotherapy, he is interested in Edmund Husserl's phenomenology. Ozmert initiated a meaningful living movement in Istanbul and is leading a social volunteering project on Career Resilience with young unemployment based on Viktor Frankl's Logotherapy framework. He sees his mission to contribute to people to become more meaning and purpose oriented and to humanize workplaces and businesses.

Part VI
Theory and Philosophy of Logotherapy

Logotherapy and Mindfulness: An Anthropological Perspective

David Srakar

Psychotherapy as a science and profession has recently shown serious interest in Buddhist meditation techniques, particularly those that cultivate mindfulness (*sati*).[1] In recent decades, there has been a huge development in the field of introducing Buddhist-derived intervention methods into traditional psychotherapeutic settings. One can observe many new therapeutic approaches arising and remodeling or even adapting already existent psychotherapeutic models to incorporate mindfulness as its main therapeutic tool, for example, in mindfulness-based stress reduction, mindfulness-based cognitive therapy, mindfulness-based relationship enhancement, mindfulness-based relapse prevention, mindfulness-based eating awareness training, mindfulness-based cancer recovery, dialectical behavior therapy, as well as acceptance and commitment therapy (McCown, 2013, pp. 23–26).

Based on these recent developments, it can be observed that Indian approaches to mental health are becoming of great interest to current Western psychotherapy (Kristeller & Rikhye, 2008, pp. 507–508).[2] Within this interest and progressive development, the fields of non-Western psychology and cross-cultural psychotherapy are becoming one of the most important current research areas, since the need for appropriate understanding of methods for alleviation of human suffering deriving from

[1] The technical Buddhist terms in Pāli are followed in parentheses, in Roman transliteration. All Pāli terms referred to in the text are transliterated according to the internationally accepted transliteration standards. In the direct in-text citations which do not follow these transliteration rules, appropriate changes are made; these modifications are not specifically noted in the text.

[2] The term "Western" used throughout this work refers to cultures, societies and the body of knowledge founded by and developed from the Western Classical philosophy, such as the Greek philosophers' perspective on the nature of the human being.

D. Srakar (✉)
Private Practice, Ljubljana, Slovenia
e-mail: info@psihoterapija-srakar.si

C. L. McLafferty, Jr., J. I. Levinson (eds.), *Logotherapy and Existential Analysis*, Logotherapy and Existential Analysis: Proceedings of the Viktor Frankl Institute Vienna 2, https://doi.org/10.1007/978-3-031-48922-8_26

non-Western cultural contexts demands a broader and interdisciplinary approach in order to be fully grasped and wisely applied in new contexts, such as clinical psychotherapeutic practice (Berry et al., 2011, p. 425; Chakkarath, 2012, pp. 80–81; Lavelle, 2016, p. 233; Manickam, 2008, p. 501; Virtbauer, 2016, p. 75).

Thus a cross-cultural approach will be used for this work, since the research question focuses on the exploration of the potential introduction of mindfulness (*sati*), as understood and presented in the textual sources of Theravāda Buddhism,[3] (e.g., Anuruddha, trans. 1993; Buddhaghosa, trans. 1999; *Dīgha Nikāya*, trans. 1995; *Majjhima Nikāya*, trans. 1995; *Saṃyutta Nikāya*, trans. 2000) into an anthropological model of one of the existential schools of psychotherapy: Viktor Frankl's (1946/1986) logotherapy and existential analysis.[4] Can logotherapy's dimensional anthropology be enriched through the Theravāda Buddhist concept of the five aggregates (*pañcakkhanda*) in order to provide a solid theoretical framework for exploring potential possibilities of introducing the concept of mindfulness (*sati*) into logotherapy? What are the divergences and confluences between the anthropological models of logotherapy and Theravāda Buddhism? What is mindfulness (*sati*), how is it developed and cultivated according to the Theravāda Buddhism, and where is it situated in the concept of the five aggregates (*pañcakkhanda*)? Can the concept of mindfulness (*sati*) be theoretically introduced into logotherapy's dimensional anthropology?

In the first part of this chapter, an introduction to both anthropological models is given, namely to the dimensional anthropology and to the five aggregates (*pañcakkhanda*). A brief outline of the Frankl's anthropological model and its main components and dynamics is presented, followed by exploration of the Theravāda Buddhist anthropological model of the five aggregates (*pañcakkhanda*), as described in the textual sources of Pāli Canon, particularly in the *Book of Aggregates* (*Khandhavagga*) of *The Connected Discourses of the Buddha* (*Saṃyutta Nikāya*, trans. 2000) and the commentarial work of Buddhaghosa's (trans. 1999) *The Path of Purification* (*Visudhimagga*). The discussion then focuses on the later development of the Buddhist anthropological model as presented in the Abhidhamma portions of the Pāli Canon and summarized in *A comprehensive manual of Abhidhamma* (*Abhidhammattha Sangaha*) of Ācariya Anuruddha (trans. 1993), who perceived the human experience as being constituted of four ultimate realities (*dhamma*s), and situates mindfulness (*sati*) as being a part of one of these ultimate realities (*dhamma*s), namely the mental factors (*cetasika*s).

The second part of this chapter offers a brief description of mindfulness (*sati*) and ways it is cultivated according to the Theravāda Buddhist thought; the last part explores the accommodation of the model of the five aggregates (*pañcakkhanda*)

[3] Interpretations of mindfulness that have evolved in modern Buddhism very frequently refer back to Theravāda sources. Therefore, in discussions of the concept of mindfulness, this article draws from the Theravāda Buddhist canon with the technical terms for mindfulness and the related concepts given in Pāli.

[4] The term *logotherapy* is used throughout this work as an abbreviation of the full name of the psychotherapeutic school known as "logotherapy and existential analysis," as established by Viktor Frankl (1946/1986).

into Frankl's (1969/1988, 1946/1986) dimensional anthropology in order to theoretically situate mindfulness (*sati*) into the logotherapy's anthropological model, without neglecting its ethical characteristics as outlined in the Theravāda Buddhist psychological and ethical system of thought.

The inquiry in this work is inspired by the current lack of emphasis on the ethical dimension of mindfulness (*sati*) and its role in the contemporary psychotherapeutic forms of its application (Monteiro et al., 2015, p. 11). The acknowledgement of ethical dimension as an irreducible characteristic of mindfulness (*sati*), situated at the core of practices for its cultivation, is crucial, and to explore potential ways of actively integrating and enhancing this dimension in the context of psychotherapy is an important next step in the dialogue between contemporary psychotherapy and mindfulness (*sati*), as a component of Buddhist psychology (Brown, 2017, p. 45; Ditrich, 2013, p. 60; Nilsson, 2014, p. 172; Virtbauer, 2012, p. 254). The key assumption of this research is that logotherapy can be enriched by the Buddhist concept of the five aggregates (*pañcakkhanda*) to such a degree that it can theoretically incorporate in its anthropological model the concept of mindfulness (*sati*), without neglecting its ethical foundation emphasized by the Theravāda Buddhist doctrine.

Anthropological Models of Logotherapy and Theravāda Buddhism

The inquiry into the question of what human beings are, what constitutes them, and how to apply this knowledge to enhance both material and experiential living conditions in order to live a less painful life has been the topic of many great thinkers. The conceptual representation of the nature of the human being has been established in many forms throughout human history. Based on these representations, various approaches to relieve human suffering have been (and are still being) developed, among which two such approaches are being considered in this work, namely, logotherapy (Frankl, 1946/1986) and Theravāda Buddhism (e.g., Anuruddha, trans. 1993; Buddhaghosa, trans. 1999; *Dīgha Nikāya*, trans. 1995; *Majjhima Nikāya*, trans. 1995; *Saṃyutta Nikāya*, trans. 2000). Both systems of thought developed their own culturally informed representations of the human being and the ways to approach human suffering. Logotherapy developed an anthropological model called "dimensional anthropology and ontology" (Frankl, 1969/1988, p. 22) while Theravāda Buddhism outlined the model of the five aggregates (*pañcakkhanda*) (*Saṃyutta Nikāya*, trans. 2000, pp. 853–1041, *SN III 1–278*)[5] and later reinterpreted

[5]The in-text references of classical Pāli texts are cited according to the APA guidelines and followed in italics by abbreviation of Pāli source and the quotation system according to the Pāli Text Society transliterated edition of the text. The numbers in the quotations refer to the volume and page of the Pāli edition of the text (e.g., *MN I 21* refers to the *Majjhima Nikāya*, vol 1, page 21). See also Rhys Davids & Stede (1921–1925), Trenckner et al. (1924–1992) and Gethin (2008, pp. xi–xliv).

it in terms of the four ultimate realities (*dhammas*) (Anuruddha, trans. 1993, pp. 23–365 [excluding explanatory guide] *Abhidh-s*). These two models differ from each other in many ways, since they were conceived in two very different cultural and historical contexts.

Dimensional Anthropology

The logotherapeutic model was put forth in the early 1930s by Viennese psychiatrist and philosopher Viktor Frankl (2010) as a response to a highly reductionistic and pandeterministic approach of Western medical and psychological sciences towards understanding the human being and its suffering (Cooper, 2003, pp. 51–53). Frankl (2000) focused his theory on the "*rehumanization of psychotherapy*" (p. 105) and strived to establish an anthropological model that would encompass the contemporary scientific findings in his approach while not neglecting the specifically human dimension of existence, which was often the case in the early twentieth century debates on conceptual formulation of the human being as a machine rather than a living being. The model was developed in a dialogue with various philosophical, psychiatric, and psychotherapeutic movements of that time. Those that most influenced Frankl's (1969/1988, 2000) perspective were Sigmund Freud (the founder of psychoanalysis), Alfred Adler (individual psychology), Edmund Husserl and Max Scheler (phenomenology), Nicolai Hartmann (ontology), Martin Heidegger (existential phenomenology), Ludwig Binswanger (existential analysis), and others.

Frankl (1946/1986) developed logotherapy as a psychotherapeutic school with its own perspective on the human being and its constitutive elements based on the main postulate that "*being human means being conscious and being responsible*" (p. 5). According to this anthropological model, a human being is an irreducible whole of three dimensions, namely *somatic*, *psychic*, and *noëtic*, each of them having unique characteristics. The somatic or bodily dimension stands for biological and chemical processes of the body; the psychic or mental dimension represents emotional and cognitive processes of human experience; and the noëtic, spiritual dimension outlines the moral and ethical processes of the human experience (DuBois, 2004, pp. xiii–xiv; Lukas, 2000, p. 9).

The three dimensions are inter-related insofar as a change in one dimension influences the other two in a particular manner. In *Der Wille zum Sinn,* Frankl termed the dynamics between somatic and psychic dimensions "psychophysical parallelism" (Frankl, 2004, p. 63). This can be understood in terms of contemporary medical psychosomatic understanding that the changes in biochemical processes of the body affect psychological content of the human experience, and that the modification of psychological content of the human experience brings about the change in the biological processes occurring in the body. Frankl explored this dynamic, particularly in the context of mental disorders, where he distinguishes between the given human experience based on its etiology (somatogenic, psychogenic, noögenic) and symptomology (pheno-somatic, pheno-psychological) (2004, pp. 44–49).

Frankl termed the dynamics between the noëtic and psychosomatic dimensions of the human being as "psychonoëtic antagonism" (Frankl, 2004, p. 63). This is distinct from the psychophysical parallelism insofar as the changes in psychosomatic dimensions don't constitutively affect and change the noëtic dimension (in terms of potentiality of freedom to will, will to meaning, meaning to life, conscience, responsibility, etc.) but rather it only limits the potential expression and influence of noëtic constituents onto the rest of experiential constituents of human being.

Frankl (2000) also integrated into this three-dimensional anthropological model the psychoanalytical structure of the mind. From a psychoanalytical perspective, the structure of a human mind can be outlined in three layers, namely (1) the *unconscious* mind, representing those aspects of one's experience that are usually not easily accessible to awareness (such as primitive, instinctual desires and impulses); (2) the *preconscious* mind, outlining those aspects of one's experience that are not in a foreground of one's experience but can nevertheless be accessed by awareness when approached with sufficient amount of attention; and (3) the *conscious* mind, standing for the immediate aspect of one's experience deriving from sensory inputs and mental processing (Luborsky et al., 2011, p. 24). This threefold categorization of the human experience interacting with the three dimensions of human being sheds additional light on the variety of processes manifesting in each of the three dimensions. Particularly interesting is the outlining of the noëtic dimension in terms of these three layers of human experience, since according to Frankl (2000), the unconscious layer of human experience is not only constituted out of biological impulses but also of noëtic qualities or potentials, such as conscience, a nonreflected state of being, etc. (pp. 31, 36). Since the brief summary of these three dimensions has already been explored elsewhere (Srakar & Virtbauer, 2015, pp. 17–20), this chapter focuses particularly on outlining the active constituents of these dimensions relevant for further discussion.

The concept of dimensional anthropology can be approached from two theoretical angles, firstly from the third-person perspective and secondly from the first-person perspective. The third-person perspective can be observed in Frankl's formulation of the three dimensions and their constituents as static categorical units, while the first-person perspective can be observed in his formulation of the interdimensional dynamics, where dimensional constituents become the bearers of processes occurring between the three dimensions. The process-oriented aspect of his theoretical model is an important theoretical opening highly relevant for further discussion. As such, an attempt is made in the following few paragraphs to briefly present and situate Frankl's constituents of three dimensions as various processes rather than static theoretical units.

Although a human being's experience is a unique, indivisible whole of *being* (Frankl, 1946/1986, p. xvi), concepts of the psychophysical parallelism and psychonoëtic antagonism outline a constant process of interdimensional changing in the context of three conditions, namely "(1) the instincts; (2) inherited disposition; and (3) environment" (p. xxiv). As such, somatic, bodily processes influence the experience of psychological processes (and vice versa), and the experience of noögenic processes conditions the overall outcome of the experience of somatic and psychological processes in terms of potential suffering arising from the moral sensibility regarding the effects of one's reaction to the previous experiential moment. From a process-oriented perspective, the experiential bearers of this interdimensional dynamic can be summarized as follows: (a) the somatic dimension comprising of biochemical processes within the body and various sensory-motor processes related to them; (b) the psychological dimension comprising of processes of cognition, emotion, perception, attention, memory etc., which are manifesting as "emotional states, its moods, sensation of drives, instincts, desires and passions… [as well as] intellectual talents, acquired behavior patterns and social impressions" (Lukas 2000, p. 9); and (c) the noëtic dimension comprised of processes of "independent decisions of will ('intentionality'),[6] material and artistic interests, creative design [(creativity)], religious and ethical sensitivity ('conscience'), understanding of values, and love" (Lukas 2000, pp. 9–10). Among various interdimensional processes, two of them hold key therapeutic positions: *self-detachment* and *self-transcendence*. Self-detachment is the process of shifting the attention or embracing a less-identified attitude (for example through humor) towards the experiential content of suffering (deriving either from the environment or from within); self-transcendence is the process of shifting attention from motivation for action based on egoistic wishes and desires to motivation for action based on ethical understanding and fulfillment of meaning through creative, experiential, and attitudinal existential values (Frankl 1946/1986, pp. 290–294; 1969/1988, pp. 70–74).

> With the deriving of human beings [sic] capacity to distance themselves out of the noö-psychic [psychonoëtic] antagonism, the concept of "dealing with oneself" is initiated. This concept describes the high pedagogic-therapeutic goal of logotherapy, a goal that is appraised higher than self-awareness. Sufficient awareness in and of itself can never remain its ultimate purpose; rather it is much more a transitional stage that ought to lead beyond the self. Logotherapy's requirement for such "aiming-beyond-the-self" turns itself into a life-training course that breaks open the confining sphere of psychotherapy and leads into a "training towards accountability." (Lukas 2000, p. 54)

In the context of ethical processes manifesting in the noëtic dimension, one of the key concepts relevant for later discussion is also the concept of conscience, which represents a particular process of ethical perceiving, valuing, deciding, and responding. According to Frankl (1969/1988), the meaning to be fulfilled in any particular moment of existence manifests as an intuitive discovery of one's conscience rather than a cognitive construction of one's inference etc., since conscience "has the power to discover unique meanings that contradict accepted values" (p. 63). As such, the content of this ethical process (termed as conscience) is not a prescription of set of values and rules of certain tradition, but rather a set of values characterized by ontologization, existentialization and phenomenologization of morality.

[6] *Intentionality* should be understood in its narrower meaning in the context of logotherapy and its motivational theory. In this sense, it does not refer to "intentionality" as a technical term used within phenomenological discourses (as an experience of being conscious of something); rather, it contains a slight notion of action or orientation towards activity, which is absent in the traditional definition.

According to Frankl (2000), this process experientially culminates as a "pre-reflective ontological self-understanding" (p. 122), described as "the premoral understanding of meaning [...] rooted in the prelogical understanding of being" (p. 127). Frankl expanded this idea:

> By virtue of what I call the *pre-reflective ontological self-understanding*, or what is also called "the wisdom of the heart," [the man in the street] knows that being human means being responsible for fulfilling the meaning potential inherent in a given situation. What is even more important, [he] knows that meaning may be found not only in creating a work and doing a deed, not only in encountering someone and experiencing something, but also, if need be, in the way in which he stands up to suffering. (p. 122)

*The Five Aggregates (**pañcakkhanda**)*

The anthropological model of Theravāda Buddhism was orally outlined by a wandering ascetic (*samaṇa*) Siddhattha Gotama also known as the Buddha or "Awakened One" somewhere between 500 and 400 BCE in eastern India. It was written down in a textual form of Pāli Canon around first century CE (Gethin, 1998, p. 42; 2008, pp. xv–xvii). This model has emerged as a response to contemporary theories and explorations on the topic of unchangeable, permanent nature of self (*attā*), developed within Jain and brahmanical (Upaniṣadic) traditions, as well as in later periods within the traditions of *Sāṃkhya* and *Yoga* (Gethin, 1998, p. 134). The Buddhist thought explored the human experience from a different perspective than other Indian schools, as it critically examined the above-mentioned postulate in terms of "descriptive analysis of the nature of experience, or, to put it simply, of just what it is that seems to be going on all the time" (Gethin, 1998, p. 135). As such, the Buddha formulated the concept of five aggregates (*pañcakkhanda*) "as a scheme of categories for analysing human identity and for explicating the structure of experience [as-such]" (Bodhi, 2000a, p. 840). According to this model, a human experience can be outlined in terms of five experiential categories, namely, materiality (*rūpa*), feeling (*vedanā*), perception (*saññā*), volitional formations (*saṅkhāras*), and consciousness (*viññāṇa*) (*Saṃyutta Nikāya*, trans. 2000, pp. 886–887, *SN III 47*), which are perpetually held together by their mutual causal connectedness.

The Buddha described in detail the process of mutual interconnectedness of constituents of human experience with the concept of dependent origination (*paṭiccasamuppāda*), which elaborates (through outlining 12 mutually interconnected links with numerous persistent feedback loops) a complex nonlinear causality present in the underlying patterns of one's everyday experience (*Saṃyutta Nikāya*, trans. 2000, pp. 533–534, *SN II 1*). Although a complete survey of this concept is beyond the scope of this work, it should be perceived as highly relevant for tackling the dynamics between the various manifestations of the five aggregates (*pañcakkhanda*). One of the key points put forth by the concept of dependent origination (*paṭiccasamuppāda*) is namely the experiential insight, that what binds the five constituents of human experience (*pañcakkhanda*) is not the experiential self (*attā*), but the causality as such. As Gethin (1998) pointed out, "the fact that experiences are causally connected is not to be explained by reference to an unchanging self that underlies experience, but by examining the nature of causality" (p. 139). As such, from the first-person perspective, each one of these five categories contains "a multiplicity of phenomena that share the same defining characteristic" (Bodhi, 2000a, p. 840), and are according to the Buddha's analysis perceived as impermanent (*aniccā*), painful (*dukkha*), and non-self (*anattā*) (*Saṃyutta Nikāya*, trans. 2000, pp. 868–870, *SN III 21–23*). Any identity that a human being assumes, or a self that one presupposes to exist, is regarded as a wrong view of self (*sakkāyadiṭṭhi*), which experientially manifests due to human being's habitual clinging (*upādāna*) to one's bodily sensations, emotions, thoughts, etc. As long as clinging (*upādāna*) persists as the main perpetual manifesting force of human experience, the five aggregates (*pañcakkhanda*) are addressed as the five aggregates subject to clinging (*pañcupādānakkhandha*) (*Saṃyutta Nikāya*, trans. 2000, pp. 863–864, *SN III 14*), sometimes also translated as "the five 'bundles of grasping-fuel'" (Harvey, 2013a, p. 32). As such, this early Theravāda Buddhist anthropological model perceives a human being as an interconnectedness of five categorically different experiential functions (*pañcakkhanda*), which are distinctively lacking any unchanging experiential substance that might be referred to as the self (*attā*) of the human being (Bodhi, 2000a, p. 841).

The aggregate of materiality (*rūpakkhanda*) is classified into two subgroups (Ñāṇamoli, 1999, p. 898, Table 1). Firstly, there is the so-called primary materiality (*mahābhūta*) constituted out of four elements (*dhātu*), namely, earth (*pathavi*), fire (*tejo*), water (*āpo*), and air (*vayo*), manifesting as constituents of the biology of human body as well as the experiential qualities of hardness, fluidity, warmth, and motion (Buddhaghosa, trans. 1999, pp. 343–347, *Vism 348–351*; see also Anālayo, 2003, p. 164). Out of these four primary elements, the second subgroup manifests as the so-called derived materiality (*upādā-rūpa*), which represents 24 forms manifested as a result of clinging (*upādāya*). The 24 derived forms stand for: five sense organs [eye (*cakkhāyatana*), ear (*sotāyatana*), nose (*ghānāyatana*), tongue (*jivhāyatana*), body (*kāyāyatana*)]; four objects of sensing [visible datum (*rūpāyātana*), sound (*saddāyatana*), odor (*ghandāyatana*), flavor (*rasāyatana*)];[7] three faculties [femininity faculty (*itthindriya*), masculinity faculty (*purisindriya*), life faculty (*rūpajīvitindriya*)]; heart-basis (*hadaya-vatu*); two modes of expression [bodily intimation (*kāyaviññatti*), verbal intimation (*vacīviññatti*)]; space element (*ākāsadhātu*); three characteristics of materiality [lightness of matter (*lahutā*), malleability of matter (*mudutā*), and wieldiness of matter (*kammaññatā*)]; four phases of materiality [growth of matter (*upacaya*), continuity of matter (*santati*), ageing of matter (*jaratā*), and impermanence of matter (*aniccatā*)]; and physical nutriment (*āhāra*) (*Saṃyutta Nikāya*, trans. 2000, p. 895, *SN III 59*; Buddhaghosa, trans. 1999, pp. 358–359, 442–444, *Vism 364, 443–444*; see also Boisvert, 1995; Ñāṇamoli, 1999).

[7] Touch is regarded as a component of the three primary elements (earth (*pathavi*), fire (*tejo*), and air (*vayo*)) and is as such excluded from this list (Ñāṇamoli, 1999, p. 805).

The aggregate of feeling (*vedanākkhanda*) stands for "bare affective quality of an experience" (Dhamma & Bodhi, 2000b, p. 80) and is usually outlined in three types, namely, pleasant (*sukha*), unpleasant (*dukkha*), and neutral (*adukkhama-sukha*) (*Saṃyutta Nikāya*, trans. 2000, pp. 914–916, *SN III 86–87*; Buddhaghosa, trans. 1999, pp. 462–463, *Vism 460*; see also Anālayo, 2003). It arises together with the contact (*phassa*) between the consciousness (*viññāṇa*) and the bodily or mental object received through one of the six senses (*indriya*), namely the five sense organs [eye (*cakkhāyatana*), ear (*sotāyatana*), nose (*ghānāyatana*), tongue (*jivhāyatana*), body (*kāyāyatana*)] and the mind (*mano*) (*Saṃyutta Nikāya*, trans. 2000, pp. 895–896, *SN III 59–60*; see also Boisvert, 1995; Hamilton, 1996). The aggregate of perception (*saññākkhandha*) stands for the cognitive function of apperceiving the distinct features of encountered object and it arises similarly as the aggregate of feeling (*vedanākkhanda*), namely based on the contact (*phassa*) of consciousness (*viññāṇa*) either with the five senses and their objects or with the mental objects manifested in the mind. As such, it can be understood as a process of organization of received sensory and mental experiential inputs into the recognizable, knowable qualities of encountered object (*Saṃyutta Nikāya*, trans. 2000, pp. 915–916, *SN III 87*; Buddhaghosa, trans. 1999, pp. 464–465, *Vism 462*; see also Dhamma & Bodhi, 2000b; Hamilton, 1996; Harvey, 2013a).[8] The aggregate of volitional formations (*saṅkhārakkhanda*), conditioned in the same manner as the previous two aggregates, stands for all of the remaining aspects of human experience,[9] such as intentionality, emotions, reasoning, intellectual and creative processes, described as various combinations of 50 distinct components that together form or construct a stable connection between the rest of aggregates, thus putting forth a multilayered but coherent experience. These 50 distinct components are further organized into three groups based on their ethical characteristics as (a) meritorious, beautiful, or profitable (*kusala*); (b) demeritorious, unwholesome, or unprofitable (*akusala*); and (c) neutral or indeterminate (*avyākata*) mental activity (*Saṃyutta Nikāya*, trans. 2000, pp. 895–896, 915–916, *SN III 60, 87*; Buddhaghosa, trans. 1999, pp. 464–478, *Vism 462–472*; see also Boisvert, 1995; Harvey, 2013a; Ñāṇamoli, 1999). The aggregate of consciousness (*viññāṇakkhanda*) stands for the cognitive function of being aware of or being conscious of the present experiential content arising from the biological or psychological sources and it is conditioned by name-and-form (*nāmarūpa*),[10] described as the five senses and the mind (*Saṃyutta Nikāya*, trans. 2000, pp. 896–897, 915–916, *SN III 61, 87*). The condition of name-and-form

[8] The latter two aggregates, although represented as a distinct, standalone aggregates, are nevertheless regarded by later Abhidhammic categorization as subcategories of the aggregate of volitional formations (*saṅkhārakkhanda*) reformulated as mental factors (*cetasika*) (Anuruddha, trans. 1993, pp. 77–78, *Abhidh-s II 2*).

[9] Excluding the function of knowing or cognizing, which is assigned to the aggregate of consciousness (*viññāṇakkhanda*).

[10] The term is sometimes translated also as mind-and-body. This translation might be more appropriate in the current discussion, but for the sake of uniformity with Ñāṇamoli's translation of *Visuddhimagga* (Buddhaghosa, 1999), the translation "name-and-form" is used.

(*nāmarūpa*) represents the key principle of the uniqueness of each individual human being and can be understood as the "conceptual and formational individuality" (Hamilton, 1996, p. 135) derived from the dynamics between the rest of aggregates (Harvey, 2013a, p. 33; Ñāṇamoli, 1999, pp. 900–901, Table 3; Olendzki, 2013, p. 57).

An important developmental step in expression and organization of the Buddha's teachings in the Theravāda tradition took place with a formulation of the third part of the Pāli Canon[11] also known as *The Basket of Higher or Further Dhamma* (*Abhidhamma Piṭaka*). It is constituted out of seven books, namely, *The Enumeration of Phenomena* (*Dhammasaṅgaṇī*), *The Book of Analysis* (*Vibhanga*), *The Discourse on Elements* (*Dhātukathā*), *The Concepts of Individuals* (*Puggalapaññatti*), *The Points of Controversy* (*Kathāvatthu*), *The Book of Pairs* (*Yamaka*), and *The Book of Conditional Relations* (*Paṭṭhāna*), which elaborately tackle various doctrinal aspects of the Buddha's teaching and systemize them into a complete psychological and ethical presentation of the full-fledged soteriological system of early Buddhist thought (Dhamma & Bodhi, 2000a, pp. 11–13; Gethin, 1998, pp. 46–48). In these texts an important shift occurs in the presentation of anthropological model, since the concept of the five aggregates (*pañcakkhanda*) is replaced and reinterpreted by the concept of four ultimate realities (*dhamma*s), which outlines four irreducible components of existence (*dhamma*s) namely, materiality (*rūpa*), mental factors (*cetasika*s), consciousness (*citta*), and *nibbāna*. This model of human experience reshapes and elaborates the aggregate of materiality (*rūpakkhanda*) into 28 types of materiality (*rūpa*), the aggregates of feeling (*vedanākkhanda*) and perception (*saññākkhandha*) into 2 mental factors (*cetasika*s), volitional formations (*saṅkhārakkhanda*) into remaining 50 mental factors (*cetasika*s), and the aggregate of consciousness (*viññāṇakkhanda*) into 89 and 121 types of consciousness (*citta*). From the first-person perspective, materiality (*rūpa*) stands for a cognizable object, mental factors (*cetasika*s) stand for various cognitive procedural elements occurring simultaneously with the cognition of the object, and consciousness (*citta*) stands for the cognition-as-such. An ordinary, conditioned human experience is a combination of various components of the first three ultimate realities (*dhamma*s), while *nibbāna* stands for the unconditioned aspect of reality, outside of the triadic experiential framework of cognizable object, cognitive procedural elements and cognition-as-such (Dhamma & Bodhi, 2000b, pp. 26–27, 76).

> A… distinguishing feature of the *Abhidhamma* is the dissection of the apparently continuous stream of consciousness into a succession of discrete evanescent cognitive events called *citta*s, each a complex unity involving consciousness itself, as the basic awareness of an object, and a constellation of mental factors (*cetasika*) exercising more specialized tasks in the act of cognition. Such a view of consciousness, at least in outline, can readily be derived from the Sutta Piṭaka's analysis of experience into the five aggregates, among which the four mental aggregates are always inseparably conjoined, but the conception remains there merely suggestive. In the Abhidhamma Piṭaka the suggestion is not simply picked up, but is expanded into an extraordinarily detailed and coherent picture of the functioning of consciousness both in its microscopic immediacy and in its extended continuity from life to life. (Dhamma & Bodhi, 2000a, pp. 8–9)

[11] The first two parts of Pāli Canon are namely *The Basket of Discourses* (*Sutta Piṭaka*) and *The Basket of Monastic Discipline* (*Vinaya Piṭaka*).

Mindfulness (*sati*) and Its Cultivation

According to the analysis put forth in the Abhidhammic textual sources, mindfulness (*sati*) is understood as a universal beautiful mental factor (*sobhanasādhāraṇa*), situated in a group of mental factors (*cetasika*s) that are ethically wholesome or beautiful (*sobhanacetasika*) (Anuruddha, trans. 1993, p. 85, *Abhidh-s II 5*). "Ethically wholesome" in this context refers to a mental moment infused with non-greed (*alobha*), non-hatred (*adosa*), and non-delusion (*amoha*), which is conducive for arising of future ethically wholesome mental moments that altogether stimulate the progress towards cessation of one's experiential suffering (Dhamma & Bodhi, 2000b, pp. 85–86). According to Gethin (2013), mindfulness (*sati*) is outlined in the early Abhidhammic texts as a "recollection (*anussati*), recall (*paṭissati*), remembrance (*saraṇatā*), keeping in mind (*dhāraṇatā*), absence of floating (*apilāpanatā*), [and] absence of forgetfulness (*asammussanatā*)" (p. 270).

> As a mental quality, *sati* represents the deliberate cultivation and a qualitative improvement of the receptive awareness that characterizes the initial stages of the perceptual process. Important aspects of *sati* are bare and equanimous receptivity, combined with an alert, broad, and open state of mind. One of the central tasks of *sati* is the de-automatization of habitual reactions and perceptual evaluations. *Sati* thereby leads to a progressive restructuring of perceptual appraisal, and culminates in an undistorted vision of reality "as it is". The element of non-reactive watchful receptivity in *sati* forms the foundation for *satipaṭṭhāna* [or presence of mindfulness (Anālayo, 2003, p. 43)] as an ingenious middle path which neither suppresses the contents of experience nor compulsively reacts to them. (Anālayo, 2003, p. 266)

According to the Theravāda Buddhist tradition, cultivation (*bhāvanā*) of mindfulness (*sati*) represents a key element on the eight-fold noble path (*ariya-aṭṭhaṅgikamagga*), since it leads towards the development of one of its factors (*aṅga*), namely, the right mindfulness (*sammā-sati*) (Harvey, 2013b, p. 83). Right mindfulness (*sammā-sati*) is described as having four characteristics, namely, diligence (*ātāpī*), mindfulness (*sati*), freedom from desire and aversion (*vinneya abhijjhādomanassa*), and clear comprehension (*sampajāna*). *The Discourse on the Establishment of Mindfulness* (*Satipaṭṭhāna Sutta*) (Anālayo, 2003; *Dīgha Nikāya*, trans. 1995, *II 290–315*; *Majjhima Nikāya*, trans. 1995, *I 55–63*), one of the key early instructional texts on cultivation of mindfulness (*sati*), outlines four objects of contemplation that lead to cultivation of right mindfulness (*sammā-sati*), namely the body (*kāya*), feelings (*vedanā*), states of consciousness (*citta*), and the mental objects (*dhammas*) (*Dīgha Nikāya*, 1995, pp. 335–350, *DN II 290–315*; *Majjhima Nikāya*, trans. 1995, pp. 145–155, *MN I 55–63*; see also Anālayo, 2003; Dhamma & Bodhi, 2000b).

The cultivation of mindfulness (*sati*) is in Buddhist tradition a component of two types of meditation practices, namely the meditation for calm (*samatha*) and for insight (*vipassanā*). The two types differ from each other, in that *samatha* leads to concentration absorptions whereas *vipassanā* develops insight into the three characteristics of existence, i.e., impermanence (*anicca*), non-satisfactoriness (*dukkha*) and non-self (*anattā*). In the practices for calm (*samatha*) one develops and holds attention (*manasikāra*) on the chosen object for a prolonged period of time with the aim to naturally calm the mental and physical reactions to the present experience. According to Virtbauer (2016), "the point of this practice is to concentrate entirely on an embodied process that is concretely and directly connected to one's life in the present moment" (p. 74). The calming of mental and physical reactions cultivates the arising of beautiful mental factors (*sobhanasādhāraṇa*) that are conducive for early developmental aspects of the mental factor of wisdom (*paññā*) to arise and, together with attention (*manasikāra*), form the so-called wise attention (*yoniso manasikāra*). The cultivation of wise attention (*yoniso manasikāra*) further provides a stable foundation for arising of mindfulness (*sati*) and clear comprehension (*sampajāna*). Such intense concentration can lead to highly peaceful and joyful experiential states known as full absorptions (*jhāna*). But these states are still not the ultimate goal of the practices (Anālayo, 2003, p. 60; Dhamma & Bodhi, 2000b, pp. 79, 90; Gethin, 2004, p. 213). In the practices for insight (*vipassanā*) one observes, with the help of both mindfulness (*sati*) and clear comprehension (*sampajāna*), not any particular object but rather the process-oriented nature of reality itself or experience-as-such, with the aim of cultivating wisdom (*paññā*), which can be defined as a clear insight into the three characteristics of every single phenomenon, namely, impermanence (*anicca*), painfulness (*dukkha*), and non-selfness (*anattā*), ultimately leading to *nibbāna* (Gethin, 2004, p. 215).

Theoretical Introduction of Mindfulness (*sati*) into Frankl's Dimensional Anthropology

As mentioned, logotherapy and Theravāda Buddhism derive from distinct cultural backgrounds and consequently their descriptions of the human being and its ontological characteristics differ in many ways. As such, the first part of this section explores the possibility of introducing the five aggregates (*pañcakkhanda*) into dimensional anthropology, while the second part attempts to outline mindfulness (*sati*) and its cultivation as an ethical embodied process that could potentially be situated in a noetic dimension of human being.

Potential Accommodation of Two Anthropological Models

According to Walsh and Shapiro (2006), the reconciliation of such culturally different anthropologies, as in the case of a dimensional anthropology and the five aggregates (*pañcakkhanda*), can theoretically be approached through the process of so-called *accommodation*, which stands for "expanding and enriching conceptual categories" (p. 228) of one system with the ideas of another, in this case of dimensional anthropology with those of five aggregates (*pañcakkhanda*). A dimensional anthropology offers a broad theoretical framework to approach the model of the five aggregates (*pañcakkhanda*), since it aims as a model to describe a human being as holistically as possible within the given limitations of its linguistic and cultural context. On the other hand, the model of five aggregates (*pañcakkhanda*) outlines the human being not so much as a whole but rather as various interconnected processes. In this context, it is worth mentioning Gendlin's (1999, p. 233) observations that both reductionistic and holistic anthropological models shed light onto the human being in a particular manner but nevertheless can be complemented with a process-oriented approach. As such, the following attempt at accommodation of the two models can be perceived as a potential enrichment of Frankl's (1969/1988, pp. 22–30) anthropological combination of reductionistic (three ontologically different dimensions of human being) and holistic (interconnectivity of the three dimensions of human being forming an anthropological unity) model with the process-oriented model of Theravāda Buddhism.

In this case, the somatic dimension—the biological and chemical processes of the physical body (as outlined through the findings in the field of natural and medical sciences)—can be accommodated with the aggregate of materiality (*rūpakkhanda*), particularly with a part of the aggregate describing the physical parts of body. The psychological dimension can be accommodated with various aspects of aggregates of materiality (*rūpakkhanda*), feeling (*vedanākkhanda*), perception (*saññākkhanda*), and volitional formations (*saṅkhārakkhanda*). First, it can include psychological aspects of the aggregate of materiality (*rūpakkhanda*), which relates to the experiential aspects derived through the body, such as the experience of hardness, fluidity, warmth, and motion (Buddhaghosa, trans. 1999, pp. 343–347, *Vism 348–351*). Second, it can situate the aggregate of feeling (*vedanākkhanda*), which can be located on the border between the somatic and psychological dimensions of the human being, since it can arise together with cognition either through the five "body" doors (objects put forth by five sense organs) or the "mind" door (mental objects put forth by memory) (Buddhaghosa, trans. 1999, pp. 463–464, *Vism 461*). Third, it can accommodate the aggregate of perception (*saññākkhanda*) in its totality, and fourth, it can also include those 11 volitional formations (*saṅkhārakkhanda*), that are ethically neutral (*avyākata*), five of which are present in every single moment of experience regardless of the presence of the rest of experiential ingredients (ethically beautiful (*kusala*) or unwholesome (*akusala*)), while the remaining six are appearing only occasionally. In this context, it is worth mentioning that the aggregate of feeling (*vedanākkhanda*) shouldn't be understood as a synonym for emotions. According to Kuan (2008), "emotion can be [understood as] the transition from the original feeling [(*vedanā*)] to *saṅkhāra* (volitional formation)" (p. 28), and thus is a mixture of many different elements besides the affective tone accompanying them.

The noëtic dimension can be accommodated with the remaining 39 constituents of volitional formations (*saṅkhārakkhanda*), since the noëtic is a dimension of ethical sensitivity (Lukas, 2000, p. 10). As such, it can embrace 25 beautiful or ethically wholesome (*kusala*) formations as well as 14 ethically unwholesome (*akusala*) ones (Ñāṇamoli, 1999, p. 899, Table 2). In this context, it is worth mentioning Frankl's (2000, p. 126) exploration of the concept of conscience, which is described in terms of ontologization, existentialization and phenomenologization of morality. Such a description of the characteristics of ethical processes can be argued to resemble the embodied ethics of Theravāda Buddhist thought and can be correlated to the constituents of the volitional formations (*saṅkhārakkhanda*) and their division into beautiful or ethically wholesome (*kusala*), unprofitable or ethically unwholesome (*akusala*), and neutral or indeterminate (*avyākata*) mental factors (*cetasika*). Furthermore, it is worth mentioning Crumbaugh's (cited in Frankl, 2000) interpretation of the logotherapeutic concept of will to meaning as a form of perceptual organization:

> Man not only strives to perceive his environment as a meaningful totality, but he strives to find an interpretation which will reveal him as an individual with a purpose to fulfil in order to complete this total Gestalt—he strives to find an *apologia pro vita sua*, a justification for his existence. The Gestalt laws of organization, subsumed under the law of *Prägnanz*, or filledness, represent an unlearned striving to construct meaningful, unified Gestalten from all elements of experience. Frankl's will to meaning can be considered another way of looking at the same concept, though there is an advantage in his thinking, for it is a particularly human idea, pointing up man's distinctive ability to perceive or find meaning not merely in what is, but in what can be. This is the ability which Max Scheler has called the capacity for free contemplation of the possible, and which he considers the factor that separates man from the lower animals....
>
> The will to meaning is primarily a perceptual phenomenon. It follows that if innate tendencies toward perceptual organization exist, it may be claimed that they manifest a striving toward organization of experience into ontologically significant patterns. (p. 114)

As such, striving toward organization of experience into ontologically significant patterns could perhaps be related to the processes outlined by volitional formations (*saṅkhārakkhanda*), since it points towards a crucial aspect of one's existence, namely that the manner in which one perceives the current experience and interprets it ("how" one experiences) clearly conditions one's reaction to that experience. According to the model of dependent origination (*paṭiccasamuppāda*) (*Saṃyutta Nikāya*, trans. 2000, pp. 533–534, *SN II 1*), the five aggregates (*pañcakkhanda*) represent various elements of the 12 links, which point toward the fact that all five aggregates (*pañcakkhanda*) always arise together and condition each other nonlinearly. Hence, in every single moment the volitional formations (*saṅkhārakkhanda*) condition consciousness or cognition (*viññāṇa*), which in turn conditions the cognized name-and-form (*nāmarūpa*) or newly assembled perception of the aggregates. The response to the experiential outcome of these conditions is also a combination of particular types of volitional formations (*saṅkhārakkhanda*), consciousness (*viññāṇa*), etc., which again condition the cognized name-and-form (*nāmarūpa*) of the "response." In this manner, the flux of experience is continuously being reshaped by its active elements. In this context, one can observe that both logotherapy and Theravāda Buddhism aim to cultivate—through the process of organizing experiential content into ontologically significant and ethically informed patterns—the human being's capability of meaningfully responding to life. Of course, the complete survey of the proposed compatibility between will to meaning and components of volitional formations (*saṅkhārakkhanda*) is beyond the scope of this chapter. Nevertheless, further research in this area might be relevant, since the discussed models of organization of experience can perhaps be related to the logotherapeutic techniques as well as to the contemplative practices of Theravāda Buddhism.

In the context of interdimensional dynamics between the three dimensions as described by Frankl, one can further observe some similarities with Theravāda Buddhism. Firstly, both systems of thought understand a human being as being conditioned by somatic and mental influences and that the exchange between the somatic and psychological dimension occurs through mutual conditionality, explained by Frankl through the concept of "psychophysical parallelism" (Frankl, 2004, p. 63), and by the Buddha through the concept of dependent origination (*paṭiccasamuppāda*) (*Saṃyutta Nikāya*, trans. 2000, pp. 533–534, *SN II 1*). Furthermore, both systems of thought understand that human beings are capable of changing their attitudes towards their experience (be it benevolent or painful). Frankl put forth this idea through the concept of "psychonoëtic antagonism" (Frankl, 2004, p. 63), while the Buddha expressed it through its outline of transcendental dependent origination (*lokuttara-paṭiccasamuppāda*) (*Saṃyutta Nikāya*, trans. 2000, pp. 555–556, *SN II 31–32*; Ṭhānissaro, 2008, pp. 72–74). According to Bodhi (2000b, p. 1045), one can find instances in the textual sources of Theravāda Buddhism, where it is clearly expressed that even the Awakened ones (*arahant*s), those who have reached the peak of insight into the nature of human being, still experience the pain deriving from the body, but despite that pain, their minds remain free from mental suffering. Such attitude closely resembles Frankl's approach towards the unchangeable suffering deriving from the somatic and psychological dimensions in which he outlined the human capacity to rise above the pain and live a meaningful life despite the chronic bodily pain.

As shown in Fig. 1, the aggregate of consciousness (*viññāṇakkhanda*) hasn't been situated in any particular dimension, since with its triadic correlation with the contact (*phassa*) and the experienced object (*nāmarūpa*), it cannot be located in any of the particular dimensions, but can best be perceived as a joint connecting them and arising in every moment together with several components from all of the three dimensions. Despite being present in every single dimension, it is explained exclusively only as the process of cognizing and hence shouldn't be misunderstood as any sort of self, since according to Theravāda Buddhism, "[t]he self as an independently existing, stable, and substantive agent that exerts downward control over mental activity is seen as a by-product of ignorance, a misguided reification of disparate mental processes" (Kudesia & Nyima, 2015, p. 912).

> The *Nikāyas* tell us that every cognitive event depends not upon a duality between subject and object, but upon a trinity of sense organ, sense object and consciousness. The coming together of these three constitutes contact (*phassa/sparśa*), the starting point of any episode of knowing.... The events cognized by cognition are the collisions between inner and outer world, the interaction of stimuli such as light and sound waves (etc.) upon the sensitive matter of retina and inner ear (etc.) that translate these modulations into the neuronal activity we call consciousness. The knowing of an object by means of an organ is not the same as the subject-object relation. Consciousness is not a subject, but an activity, a process, an event occurring moment after moment. It is a relationship between organs of sensation and thought on one hand, and objects of sensation and thought on the other. It is a natural inter-

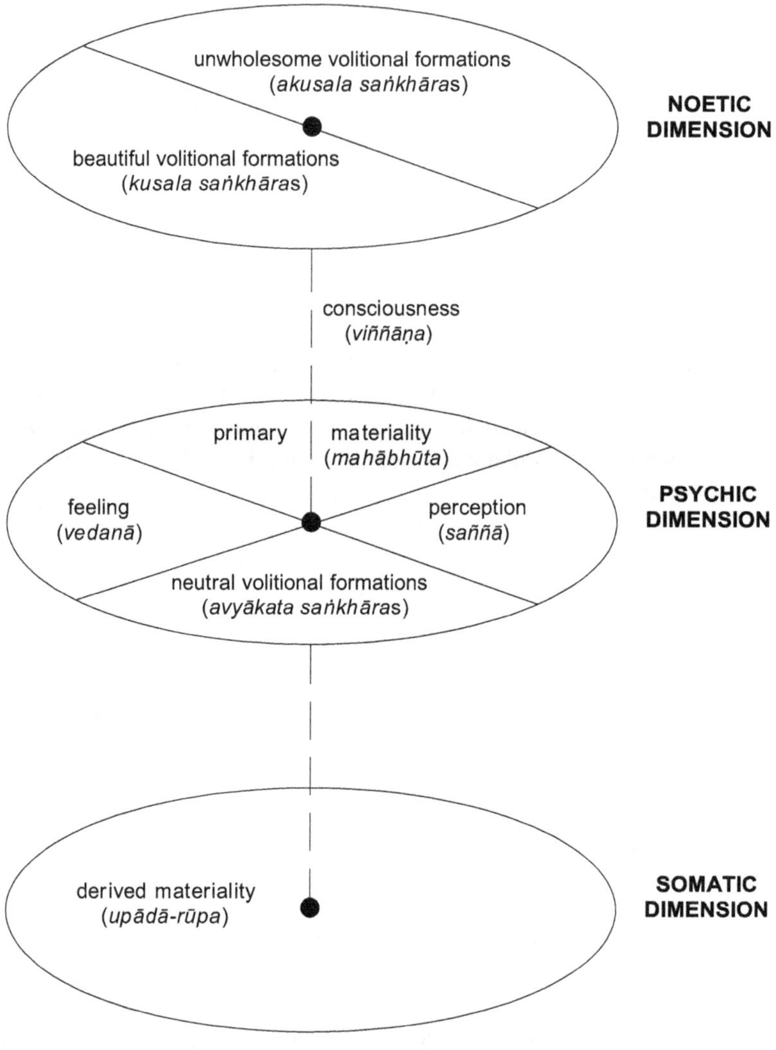

Fig. 1 Accommodation of constituents of the five aggregates (*pañcakkhanda*) into three dimensions of Frankl's anthropology (Although Fig. 1 outlines dimensional anthropology and the five aggregates (*pañcakkhanda*) in terms of various static components they should nevertheless be understood in terms of interrelated processes. According to the logotherapeutic concepts of psychophysical parallelism and noëtic antagonism as well as Theravāda Buddhism (dependent origination (*paṭiccasamuppāda*)) all statically represented components are actually dynamically interrelated in every single moment of one's experience.)

face between the sensitive matter of the body's sense receptors (which would include the brain) and the data contained in the surrounding (and internal) environment that is mediated by mental states of knowing. This mentality is likely an emergent property of materiality, but the virtual world constructed of this mental activity presents as a robust phenomenology of experience. (Olendzki, 2013, pp. 67–68)

This points towards one of the most obvious distinctions and potential incompatibility between the two systems, since logotherapists explain the human being at the core of its noëtic dimension as an existential self (person), capable of rising above the given situation and choosing a meaningful attitude towards one's experience. On the other hand, Theravāda Buddhist practitioners point to the human being at the core of its conditionality as a non-self (*anattā*). The questions of whether a human being is a self or non-self and in what way can a lived experience of these notions be theoretically conceptualized have already been approached within contemporary scientific dialogue. These attempts opened up many new dilemmas and showed that the concepts of self and non-self due to their highly complex and multilayered nature cannot be easily outlined in a uniformed theoretical presentation, and that further interdisciplinary investigation is still needed (Gallagher, 2011, pp. 27–28; Olendzki, 2006, p. 250). Nevertheless, if one takes into consideration this basic anthropological difference between logotherapy and Theravāda Buddhism, a few interesting questions arise within the context of theoretical accommodation and its potential practical applications. Can logotherapy exist as a therapeutic system without the fundamental premises of a permanent self? What are the implications for logotherapeutic practice if there is no permanent self? In what ways would logotherapeutic techniques change if the fundamental premises of permanent self are altered? Do they change at all? Does their therapeutic effect change? Does the change occur perhaps only at the level of the language through which the technique is mediated and contextualized during logotherapeutic sessions and as such, does not impact the desired effects? The following brief reflection should be regarded only as a preliminary attempt at tackling some of the above-mentioned questions. These issues require an in-depth exploration and comparison of both discourses, something which is beyond the scope of this work. As such, further research in this area is recommended.

One could argue that, despite the differences in formulation of the anthropological models, they could perhaps point towards the same thing, albeit in a different terminology, expression, and scope. This can be observed in instances in which Frankl (2000) described the self in a quite similar way to the Theravāda Buddhist understanding of conditionality of the human being. For example: "The self does not yield to total self-reflection. In this sense, human existence is basically unreflectable, and so is the self in itself. Human existence exists in action rather than reflection" (p. 36). Similar approaches to human experience can be perceived in the Buddha's description of 62 wrong views of self (*sakkāyadiṭṭhi*) (*Dīgha Nikāya*, trans. 1995, pp. 73–90, *DN I 13–46*) highlighting various forms of discursive cognitive reflection on the notion of self, all of which are being perceived as unconducive for overcoming suffering (*dukkha*) and should be abandoned by direct experiential insight into the nature of human existence (Gethin, 1998, p. 162). As already mentioned, the concept of non-self (*anattā*) aims at dissolving the process of habitual clinging (*upādāna*) and identification to phenomena, which is perpetuated through the manifold expressions of the idea of "inherent subject" to whom phenomena manifest. In this context, it is worth mentioning an attempt made to explain in

Western philosophical terminology the issue of habitual clinging (*upādāna*) (addressed by the concept of non-self (*anattā*)) as the so-called *ontological addiction*, which

> is defined as "the unwillingness to relinquish an erroneous and deep-routed belief in an inherently existing 'self' or 'I' as well as the 'impaired functionality' that arises from such a belief."... The ontological addiction formulation is a means of operationalizing within Western clinical domains the Buddhist view that suffering, including the entire spectrum of distressing emotions and psychopathologic states, results from adhering to a false view of self and reality. Therefore, within Buddhism, wisdom refers to the gradual development of insight that allows and facilitates an individual to undergo recovery from ontological addiction by reconstructing their view of self and reality. (Shonin et al., 2014, p. 125)

In this context, ontological addiction could perhaps be related to the neurotic mindset characterized by excessive occupation with one's own self (in a form of discursive thinking) also known in logotherapeutic literature as *hyperreflection.* As shown in the above paragraph, the concept of non-self (*anattā*) has a clear soteriological function in the system of Theravāda Buddhism and thus it could be in some of its aspects (particularly in its aim to change the experiential framework of currently experienced content) related to Frankl's approach outlined in his theory of meaning and values, in which he explained the means to bypass or overcome the hyperreflective tendencies of the neurotic mindset particularly through the usage of two logotherapeutic methods, namely dereflection[12] and paradoxical intention,[13] in order to lower the level of so-called "anticipatory anxiety" and "compulsive self-observation" (DuBois, 2004, p. xxxiii; Fabry, 1975, pp. 274–275; Frankl, 1946/1986, pp. xix–xx). The similarity between logotherapeutic techniques and aspects of Theravāda Buddhist contemplative practices is an interesting and important topic for further investigation, since it might shed additional light on the differences and commonalities between their understanding and application of the concepts of existential self and non-self (*anattā*).

[12] Dereflection deals with excessive attention to one's own self, and it helps the patient "to ignore the symptoms" (Frankl, 2004, p. 207) by addressing ones "capacity for self-transcendence" (DuBois, 2004, p. xxxiii), thus shifting the patient's focus from the symptom to something other than the self. As a consequence of the shifted focus, the natural processes, which before were inhibited by the attention itself, slowly begin again to unwind effortlessly at their natural pace.

[13] Paradoxical intention deals with excessive attention to one's perseverance against an undesired situation or object. It directs the patient's focus on the very thing, situation, or action he or she is afraid of. "Encouraging the patient to do, or wish to happen, the very things he fears engenders an inversion of intention" (Frankl, 1969/1988, p. 103). By doing this, "the human capacity of 'self-distancing'" (DuBois, 2004, p. xxxiii) is mobilized, and the patient's habit of fighting against or fleeing from the feared situation, deed or thing, is slowly supplemented by a playful attitude towards the fear, which is often filled with and enhanced by the humor of the patient.

Cultivation of Mindfulness (sati) *as a Noëtic Process*

Since both systems of thought developed their anthropological models based on ethical qualities of human existence, the main solid point for the dialogue and potential enrichment of the practice of logotherapy with Theravāda Buddhist teachings and contemplative practices for establishment of mindfulness (*sati*) lies in their common understanding of the human as being conscious and responsible. The teachings of early Buddhism outlined its soteriological approach through the eightfold noble path (*ariya-aṭṭhaṅgikamagga*), traditionally summarized or grouped into three interconnected categories, namely morality (*sīla*), concentration (*samādhi*), and wisdom (*paññā*) (Harvey, 2013b, p. 83). Likewise, Frankl outlined a logotherapeutic approach towards relieving human suffering through an orientation to meaning and values, formulating a dynamic map of three existential forms, namely creative, experiential, and attitudinal values, through which one can discover a meaning to fulfill in every single situation (Frankl, 1969/1988, pp. 70–74; 1946/1986, pp. xix–xx). Although their general goals to some extent perhaps differ (logotherapists aiming towards a meaningful existence in the mundane world (*samsara*), while Theravāda Buddhists aiming experientially beyond the mundane existence (*samsara*)), they both nevertheless understand the human being as being capable of conscious ethically infused change or transformation, and are thus bringing forth a similar necessity to cultivate one's responsibility towards life.

According to Virtbauer (2016), the Theravāda Buddhist approach to suffering should be regarded as "a kind of pragmatic spiritual psychology and ethics.... [These are expressed through] an applied first-person psychology of analysing and understanding the mind-and-body through an embodied meditation practice" (p. 72). The practice of logotherapy is theoretically similar to the contemplative practices of Theravāda Buddhist (and vice versa), particularly in the context of so-called attitudinal values, where one is called upon to change oneself when facing unchangeable suffering such as pain (incurable diseases), guilt, and death. "It is prerogative of being human, and a constituent of human existence, to be capable of shaping and reshaping oneself" (Frankl, 1969/1988, p. 73). According to Frankl, the human being's action and realization of potentiality of one's existence is directed forth in every single moment by one's will to meaning, which puts a human being into a clear position of decision-making and ethical evaluation of one's potential response to the present experience of his existence. These types of attitudinal change manifest in the noëtic dimension of the human being through one's ability of self-detachment and self-transcendence. Although the intensity of application of these two abilities (self-detachment and self-transcendence) might differ between the two systems due to their cultural and historical contexts of usage, one can nevertheless observe similar principles (perhaps expressed differently) at the very core of Theravāda Buddhist contemplative practices, where "the most obvious 'health-psychological' and therapeutic benefit of mindfulness practice refers to the ability to train oneself in greater psychological flexibility [deriving from] the mental capacity to concentrate willingly" (Virtbauer, 2016, p. 76). For example, one can observe such principal commonalities in the contemplative practices that aim at cultivation of four immeasurables or divine abidings (*brahma-vihāras*), namely, loving-kindness (*mettā*), compassion (*karuṇā*), empathetic joy (*muditā*), and equanimity (*upekkhā*) (Buddhaghosa, trans. 1999, pp. 288–319, *Vism 295–325*), where one uses a mental image of other living beings as a meditation object and actively cultivates an attitude of non-greed (*alobha*) and non-hatred (*adosa*) towards them. These four qualities are described by some authors also as "conduct-related terms" (Shonin et al., 2014, p. 131), since they are not only highly relevant for the meditative process as such, but rather have strong implications for the everyday ethical behavior of an individual. As such, mental ethical focusing of one's attention on someone other than oneself could perhaps be related to the process of self-distancing, while the cultivation of specific benevolent ethical attitudes that accompanies it might be pointing towards the process of self-transcendence.

> Part of meditation training has to do with learning to focus the mind on a particular object or on a series of emerging objects, but most of the training has more to do with cultivating particular qualities of mind by means of which the object is regarded. The technology of awareness is a matter of how the aggregate of consciousness (*viññāṇa*) interacts with the aggregate of material form (*rūpa*) as it manifests in the sense organs of the body and the sense objects of the environment; but the development of mindfulness and insight is rather a matter of how the aggregate of formations (*saṅkhāra*) co-arises with the other aggregates. (Olendzki, 2013, p. 57)

According to the above-presented potential accommodation of the five aggregates (*pañcakkhanda*) into dimensional anthropology (Fig. 1), one can observe that the aggregate of volitional formations (*saṅkhārakkhanda*) is situated both in psychic and noëtic dimensions of human existence and hence is highlighting the implicit position of mindfulness (*sati*) within the proposed theoretical accommodation. Since mindfulness (*sati*) is categorized as a universal beautiful mental factor (*sobhanasādhāraṇa*), which is traditionally positioned in terms of aggregates under the beautiful volitional formations (*kusala saṅkhāra*), one could argue that mindfulness (*sati*) can be potentially situated in the noëtic dimension. Furthermore, one could closely relate mindfulness (*sati*) and its various aspects also to the aggregate of perception (*saññākkhanda*), which as already mentioned, is in the later Abhidhammic thought regarded as one of the universal (neutral) volitional formations (*saṅkhārakkhanda*) or mental factors (*cetasika*). According to Kuan (2008, pp. 41–56), there are four aspects and functions of mindfulness (*sati*): (a) simple awareness functioning as perceiving of the currently manifesting sensory objects, (b) protective awareness functioning as conscious regulation of mind's reaction to sensory data by sense restraining and moral evaluation, (c) introspective awareness functioning as monitoring of the regulation of mind's reaction to sensory data, and (d) deliberately forming conceptions functioning as bringing to mind the experientially invoked remembering of experiences conducive to the development of concentration (*samādhi*) and wisdom (*paññā*). Kuan also noted:

> The practice of mindfulness consists in conducting the wholesome functioning of *saññā* (apperception/conception), one of the five components of personality [(five aggregates (*pañcakkhanda*))] according to Buddhism. It also shows that *saññā* is linked with cognition and also emotion, which includes the secondary feeling (*vedanā*) as a subjective reaction to the mere reception and registration of sensation. Avoiding cognitive problems, mindfulness prevents *saññā* from going astray to conceptual proliferation (*papañca*), which is obstructive to the insight that leads one to liberation. On the other hand, mindfulness prevents feelings from developing into emotional disturbances; through transformation of *saññā* it conduces to the surmounting of emotional agitation and hence the attainment of… equanimity (*upekkhā*). This practice helps to achieve an optimal cognitive capability and emotional state, and thereby enables one to attain the ultimate religious goal. (p. 10)

In this sense, could mindfulness (*sati*) relate to what Frankl (2000) termed the prereflective ontological self-understanding, described as "the premoral understanding of meaning… rooted in the prelogical understanding of being" (p. 127)? In the context of contemporary Western psychological idiom various interpretations of the term mindfulness (*sati*) are being developed, but for the purpose of this discussion the following attempt at description might be appropriate: "*Mindfulness is a state of heightened meta-awareness in which discursive cognition is diminished and attention is solely focused on and receptive to goal-relevant aspects of the present moment*" (Kudesia & Nyima, 2015, p. 923). To some degree, mindfulness (*sati*) could be perceived as prelogical understanding of being, since it stands for the process of immediate experiential "perceiving" of the human being in form of various sensations, thoughts, emotions, etc. (rather than thinking about these aspects of human experience). At the same time, it could be described as premoral understanding of meaning, since according to practitioners of Theravāda Buddhism, with such immediate experiential "perceiving" of the human being, a specific knowing (*sampajāna*) accompanies it, which is incompatible with ethically unwholesome states of being or responses to one's experience (ethically characterized by greed (*dosa*), hatred (*lobha*), and delusion (*moha*)). To some extent, this also overlaps with Frankl's (1969/1988) formulation of the human being's main motivational source as the will to meaning, which was contrasted in his writings to Freud's will to pleasure and Adler's will to power.[14] Additionally, an important aspect of cultivating mindfulness (*sati*) that shouldn't be neglected is that the goal is not the development of attention (*manasikāra*) or any other particular psychological ability, but rather wisdom (*paññā*), since "ancient Buddhist texts understand the presence of mindfulness as in effect reminding us of who we are and what our values are" (Gethin, 2013, p. 270). This makes additional theoretical opening in terms of proximity of ethical understanding of human being between logotherapy and Theravāda Buddhism, since mindfulness (*sati*) doesn't represent only a psychological function

[14] In this context, will to pleasure might be interpreted as action derived from greed (*lobha*), while will to power might be interpreted as action derived from partly greed (*lobha*) and partly hatred (*dosa*), since comparison with the other has to contain in itself a simultaneous non-acceptance of the self and other.

or trait, but stands as "*an embodied ethical act, process, and practice*" (Grossman, 2015, p. 17), a characteristic very similar to Frankl's (2000) pointing towards the present moment of actualization of ethics (p. 29).

Future Perspectives

There are various points that would require further investigation of potentially enriching dialogue between proponents of logotherapy and Theravāda Buddhism. Although description of dimensional anthropology in this work attempts at clear and summarized presentation, additional research needs to be conducted about its existential and phenomenological philosophical roots, in order to fully grasp the theoretical width and depth of Frankl's anthropological model and its various applied forms in psychotherapeutic contexts (Correia et al., 2016, p. 16). Similarly, a much more detailed inquiry into Theravāda Buddhism and analysis of its approach to human experience needs to be conducted in order to truly grasp the depth and complexity of its refined teachings.[15]

From the perspective of accommodation, one of the most critical points to be addressed in future dialogue is to first establish a precise translation of logotherapeutic concepts into the vocabulary of Theravāda Buddhism and vice versa in order to find the points at which these concepts collide, differ, or are unique in themselves. As Shonin, Van Gordon, and Griffiths (2014) observed, "there currently is no unified and structured system for the effective interpretation, classification, and operationalization of Buddhist terms, principles, and practices within [psychological and psychotherapeutic] clinical settings" (p. 124), which brings a huge challenge to the future explorations in these fields.

Through the investigation of these topics, a few directions might be valuable for future research. First, one can observe an interesting parallel between Frankl's concept of meaning (and its related expressions) and the Theravāda Buddhist concept of mental factors (*cetasika*). In this context, it is worth mentioning the mental factor (*cetasika*) of desire (*chanda*), which could, in combination with wholesome (*kusala*) mental factors (*cetasika*), perhaps enrich and more precisely define Frankl's terminology, such as will to meaning and freedom to will (Dhamma & Bodhi, 2000b, pp. 82–83). Second, the concept of conscience (Frankl, 2000, p. 119) could be explored in more depth through the lenses of both the theoretical and practical aspects of Theravāda Buddhism—theoretical in terms of Abhidhammic analysis of human experience, and practical in terms of contemplative methods for calm (*samatha*) and insight (*vipassanā*). Finally, it might be fruitful to compare the Theravāda Buddhist contemplative methods with logotherapeutic techniques, since

[15] Additionally, practical application of these two approaches to life should also be cultivated in order to get a first-person experience of the two systems and their similarities as well as differences.

the mechanisms of achieving the ethically desired change in the experience of human beings seem to be (at least from the perspective of current preliminary research) quite similar in terms of directing and applying attention towards a meaningful object (be it a deed, a human being, or a particular attitude towards experience) in order to alleviate human suffering.

Conclusion

Research of mindfulness (*sati*), as currently approached within psychological and psychotherapeutic scientific circles, emphasizes particularly its cognitive and behavioral aspects, which often situate Buddhist-derived interventions into a limited paradigm of contemporary psychoanalytic and cognitive-behavioral therapeutic approaches. The dialogue between proponents of logotherapy and Theravāda Buddhism can be perceived as an attempt made within existential-humanistic tradition of psychotherapy to introduce Buddhist-derived interventions, particularly those which foster the cultivation of mindfulness (*sati*), into their current approach towards relieving human suffering. As noted, the practice of logotherapy can be enriched by the Theravāda Buddhist concept of five aggregates (*pañcakkhanda*) to such a degree that it could theoretically incorporate in its anthropological model the concept of mindfulness (*sati*) without neglecting its ethical foundation. The introduction of mindfulness (*sati*) into a therapeutic tradition, which is highly characterized by tackling ethical aspects of human living as a means to relieve human suffering, can potentially have strong implications for contemporary developments in the research field of Buddhist-derived interventions. It can offer a fruitful theoretical framework from which Western psychotherapeutic and psychological discourses can approach mindfulness (*sati*) with the inclusion of its ethical aspects as emphasized within the traditional teachings of Theravāda Buddhism. As such, this work attempts to contribute to the currently almost-nonexistent or rather highly preliminary dialogue between logotherapy and mindfulness (*sati*) by providing an initial anthropological framework that could serve as a solid theoretical foundation for further research in the area of applying the methods for cultivation of mindfulness (*sati*) into the logotherapeutic clinical setting. Furthermore, within a broader context, it aims to contribute to the enrichment of the dialogue between practitioners of existential-humanistic psychotherapeutic paradigms, Theravāda Buddhism, and Buddhist-derived interventions (Fabry, 1975, pp. 274–275; Littman-Ovadia & Niemiec, 2016, p. 388; Nilsson, 2014, p. 168; Virtbauer, 2016, p. 72).

Acknowledgments The author expresses deep gratitude to Dr. Tamara Ditrich, Dr. Royce Wiles, and Dr. Borut Škodlar for proofreading earlier versions of the text, Tim Somerset for linguistic polishing, and Charles Wang and Nan Tien Institute for financial support that made this research possible.

References

Anālayo. (2003). *Satipaṭṭhāna: The direct path to realization*. Windhorse.

Anuruddha, A. (trans. 1993). Abhidhammattha Sangaha: A comprehensive manual of Abhidhamma (M. Narada & B. Bodhi, Trans.). In B. Bodhi (Ed.), *A comprehensive manual of Abhidhamma: The Abhidhammattha Sangaha of Acariya Anuruddha* (pp. 23–366). Buddhist Publication Society Pariyatti Editions.

Berry, J. W., Poortinga, Y. H., Breugelmans, S. M., Chasiotis, A., & Sam, A. (2011). *Cross-cultural psychology: Research and applications* (3rd ed.). Cambridge University Press.

Bodhi, B. (2000a). Introduction [to The Book of Aggregates (Khandhavagga)]. In B. Bodhi (Ed.), *The connected discourses of the Buddha: A new translation of the Saṃyutta Nikāya* (pp. 839–852). Wisdom Publications.

Bodhi, B. (2000b). Notes. In *The connected discourses of the Buddha: A new translation of the Saṃyutta Nikāya* (pp. 1043–1105). Wisdom Publications.

Boisvert, M. (1995). *The five aggregates: Understanding Theravāda psychology and soteriology*. Wilfred Laurier University Press.

Brown, C. G. (2017). Ethics, transparency, and diversity in mindfulness programs. In L. M. Monteiro, J. F. Compson, & F. Musten (Eds.), *Practitioner's guide to ethics and mindfulness-based interventions* (pp. 45–85). Springer International Publishing.

Buddhaghosa, B. (1999). *The path of purification: Visuddhimagga* (B. Ñāṇamoli, Trans.). Buddhist Publication Society; Pariyatti Editions.

Chakkarath, P. (2012). The role of indigenous psychologies in the building of basic cultural psychology. In J. Valsiner (Ed.), *The Oxford handbook of culture and psychology* (pp. 71–95). Oxford University Press.

Cooper, M. (2003). *Existential therapies*. Sage Publications Ltd.

Correia, E., Cooper, M., & Berdondini, L. (2016). Worldwide list of existential psychotherapy institutions. In S. Schulenberg (Ed.), *Clarifying and furthering existential psychotherapy: Theories, methods, and practices* (pp. 83–131). Springer International Publishing.

Dhamma, U. R., & Bodhi, B. (2000a). Introduction (M. Narada & B. Bodhi, Trans.). In B. Bodhi (Ed.), *A comprehensive manual of Abhidhamma: The Abhidhammattha Sangaha of Acariya Anuruddha* (pp. 1–20). Buddhist Publication Society Pariyatti Editions.

Dhamma, U. R., & Bodhi, B. (2000b). Explanatory guide. In B. Bodhi (Ed.), *A comprehensive manual of Abhidhamma: The Abhidhammattha Sangaha of Acariya Anuruddha* (pp. 23–366). Buddhist Publication Society Pariyatti Editions.

Dīgha Nikāya. (trans. 1995). (M. Walshe, Trans.): Wisdom Publications.

Ditrich, T. (2013). The concept of smṛti in the Yogasūtra: Memory or mindfulness? *Asian Studies, 1*(1), 45–62. https://doi.org/10.4312/as.2013.1.1.45-62

DuBois, J. M. (2004). Understanding Viktor Frankl's *Theory and Therapy of Mental Disorders* [Editor's Introduction] (J. DuBois, Trans.). In *On the theory and therapy of mental disorders: An introduction to logotherapy and existential analysis* (pp. ix–xliii). Brunner–Routledge.

Fabry, J. B. (1975). Logotherapy and eastern religions. *Journal of Religion and Health, 14*(4), 271–276.

Frankl, V. E. (1946/1986). *The doctor and the soul (Original work published 1946 as Ärztliche Seelsorge; Vienna: Franz Deuticke.)* (R. Winston & C. Winston, Trans.). Alfred A. Knopf.

Frankl, V. E. (1969/1988). *The will to meaning: Foundations and applications of logotherapy*. Meridian. (Original work published 1969)

Frankl, V. E. (2000). *Man's search for ultimate meaning*. Perseus. (Original work published *Der Unbewusste Gott*, 1948 and English translation, *The Unconscious God*, 1975)

Frankl, V. E. (2004). *On the theory and therapy of mental disorders: An introduction to logotherapy and existential analysis* (J. DuBois, Trans.). Brunner–Routledge. (Original work published *Theorie und Therapie der Neurosen Einfuhrung in die Logotherapie und Existenzanalys*)

Frankl, V. E. (2010). *The feeling of meaninglessness: A challenge to psychotherapy and philosophy*. (A. Batthyany & A. Tallon Eds.). Marquette University Press.

Gallagher, S. (2011). Introduction: A diversity of selves. In S. Gallagher (Ed.), *The Oxford handbook of the self* (pp. 1–29). Oxford University Press.
Gendlin, E. T. (1999). A new model. In J. Shear & F. J. Varela (Eds.), *The view from within: First-person approaches to the study of consciousness*. Imprint Academic.
Gethin, R. (1998). *The foundations of Buddhism*. Oxford University Press.
Gethin, R. (2004). Lecture transcript: "On the practice of Buddhist meditation according to the Pali Nikāyas and exegetical sources." In *Buddhism in Past and Present* (Vol. 9, pp. 201–221). University of Hamburg, Asia-Africa-Institute, Department for Indian and Tibetan Studies [Continuing Academic Education]. https://www.buddhismuskunde.uni-hamburg.de/pdf/4-publikationen/buddhismus-in-geschichte-und-gegenwart/bd9-k12gethin.pdf
Gethin, R. (2008). *Sayings of the Buddha: A selection of suttas from the Pali Nikāyas*. Oxford University Press.
Gethin, R. (2013). On some definitions of mindfulness. In J. M. G. Williams & J. Kabat-Zinn (Eds.), *Mindfulness: Diverse perspectives on its meaning, origins and application* (pp. 263–279). Routledge.
Grossman, P. (2015). Mindfulness: Awareness informed by an embodied ethic. *Mindfulness, 6*(1), 17–22. https://doi.org/10.1007/s12671-014-0372-5
Hamilton, S. (1996). *Identity and experience: The constitution of the human being according to early Buddhism*. Luzac Oriental.
Harvey, P. (2013a). Dukkha, non-self, and the teaching on the four "noble truths". In S. M. Emmanuel (Ed.), *A companion to Buddhist philosophy* (pp. 26–45). Wiley Blackwell.
Harvey, P. (2013b). *An introduction to Buddhism: Teaching, history and practices* (2nd ed.). Cambridge University Press.
Kristeller, J. L., & Rikhye, K. (2008). Meditative traditions and contemporary psychology. In K. R. Rao, A. C. Paranjpe, & A. K. Dalal (Eds.), *Handbook of Indian Psychology* (pp. 506–538). Foundation Books.
Kuan, T.-F. (2008). *Mindfulness in early Buddhism: New approaches through psychology and textual analysis of Pali, Chinese and Sanskrit sources*. Routledge.
Kudesia, R. S., & Nyima, V. T. (2015). Mindfulness contextualized: An integration of Buddhist and neuropsychological approaches to cognition. *Mindfulness, 6*(4), 910–925. https://doi.org/10.1007/s12671-014-0337-8
Lavelle, B. D. (2016). Against one method: Contemplation in context. In R. E. Purser, D. Forbes, & A. Burke (Eds.), *Handbook of mindfulness: Culture, context, and social engagement* (pp. 233–242). Springer International Publishing.
Littman-Ovadia, H., & Niemiec, R. M. (2016). Character strengths and mindfulness as core pathways to meaning in life. In P. Russo-Netzer, S. E. Schulenberg, & A. Batthyany (Eds.), *Clinical perspectives on meaning: Positive and existential psychotherapy* (pp. 383–405). Springer International Publishing. https://doi.org/10.1007/978-3-319-41397-6_19
Luborsky, E. B., O'Reilly-Landry, M., & Arlow, J. A. (2011). Psychoanalysis. In D. Wedding & R. J. Corsini (Eds.), *Current psychotherapies* (9th ed.). Brooks/Cole.
Lukas, E. (2000). *Logotherapy textbook: Meaning-centered psychotherapy* (T. Brugger, Trans.). Liberty Press. (Original work published *Lehrbuch der Logotherapie*)
McCown, D. (2013). *The ethical space of mindfulness in clinical practice: An exploratory essay. Jessica Kingsley Publications.*
Majjhima Nikāya. (trans. 1995). (B. Ñāṇamoli, Trans., B. Bodhi Ed.). Buddhist Publication Society.
Manickam, L. (2008). Research on Indian concepts of psychology: Major challenges and perspectives for future action. In K. R. Rao, A. C. Paranjpe, & A. Dalal (Eds.), *Handbook of Indian psychology*. Foundation Books.
Monteiro, L. M., Musten, R. F., & Compson, J. (2015). Traditional and contemporary mindfulness: Finding the middle path in the tangle of concerns. *Mindfulness, 6*(1), 1–13. https://doi.org/10.1007/s12671-014-0301-7

Ñāṇamoli, B. (1999). Index, glossary, tables. In *The path of purification: Visuddhimagga* (B. Ñāṇamoli, Trans.) (pp. 857–904). Buddhist Publication Society; Pariyatti Editions.
Nilsson, H. (2014). A four-dimensional model of mindfulness and its implications for health. *Psychology of Religion and Spirituality, 6*(2), 162–174. https://doi.org/10.1037/a0036067
Olendzki, A. (2006). The transformative impact of non-self. In D. K. Nauriyal, M. S. Drummond, & Y. B. Lal (Eds.), *Buddhist thought and applied psychological research* (pp. 286–297). Routledge.
Olendzki, A. (2013). The construction of mindfulness. In J. M. G. Williams & J. Kabat-Zinn (Eds.), *Mindfulness* (pp. 55–70). Routledge.
Rhys Davids, T. W., & Stede, W. (Eds.). (1921–1925). *Pāli-English Dictionary*. Pāli Text Society. https://dsal.uchicago.edu/dictionaries/pali/.
Saṃyutta Nikāya. (trans. 2000). (B. Bodhi, Trans.). Wisdom Publications.
Shonin, E., Van Gordon, W., & Griffiths, M. D. (2014). The emerging role of Buddhism in clinical psychology: Toward effective integration. *Psychology of Religion and Spirituality, 6*(2), 123. https://doi.org/10.1037/a0035859
Srakar, D., & Virtbauer, G. (2015). Logotherapy and Advaita Vedānta: Steps towards an integration. *SFU Forschungsbulletin, 3*(1), 11–27. https://doi.org/10.15135/15.3.1.11-27
Ṭhānissaro, B. (2008). *The shape of suffering: A study of dependent co-arising*. Metta Forest Monastery.
Trenckner, V., Andersen, B., Smith, H., Hendriksen, H., von Hinüber, O., Holten Pind, O., & others (Eds.). (1924–1992). *A Critical Pāli Dictionary* (Vols. 1–3). The Royal Danish Academy of Sciences and Letters. https://cpd.uni-koeln.de/intro/
Virtbauer, G. (2012). The Western reception of Buddhism as a psychological and ethical system: Developments, dialogues, and perspectives. *Mental Health, Religion & Culture, 15*(3), 251–263. https://doi.org/10.1080/13674676.2011.569928
Virtbauer, G. (2016). Presencing process: Embodiment and healing in the Buddhist practice of mindfulness of breathing. *Mental Health, Religion & Culture, 19*(1), 68–81. https://doi.org/10.1080/13674676.2015.1115474
Walsh, R., & Shapiro, S. L. (2006). The meeting of meditative disciplines and western psychology: A mutually enriching dialogue. *American Psychologist, 61*, 227–239. https://doi.org/10.1037/0003-066X.61.3.227

David Srakar (1989) graduated in Psychotherapy Science (BA. pth.) from Sigmund Freud University Vienna (2014) and postgraduated in Applied Buddhist Studies (MA) at Nan Tien Institute (2016). He also holds a Certificate of Training in Logotherapy and Existential Analysis (2015) and a European Certificate of Psychotherapy (2023). Currently, he works in a private practice in Ljubljana (Slovenia), providing individual and couples psychotherapy, as well as facilitating trainings in contemplative skills. His areas of interest include existential psychotherapy, cross-cultural psychotherapy, Indian indigenous psychology, and the dialogue between psychotherapy and Indian contemplative traditions.

Nature, Nurture, and the Noëtic: Addressing Flawed Assumptions of Galton's Paradigm

Charles L. McLafferty, Jr.

The idea of nature vs. nurture is a foundation of psychological theory. Sir Francis Galton (1869/1892) was not necessarily the first to propose the idea, but became so interested in the idea that genius was inherited that he developed a statistical method that was the forerunner of modern-day correlation; he termed it "the law of deviation from the average" (p. vi). Nature–nurture was featured prominently in the March and April, 2004 issues of the *Monitor on Psychology* and infused throughout the January, 2005 issue of *American Psychologist*. Sternberg, Grigorinko, and Kidd (2005) offered insights into the study of intelligence and race, requiring us to discern between science and folk tales. We need to use an equal level of discernment to examine the assumptions behind the studies of nature vs. nurture, which are based on the premise that Galton's idea is foundational to our understanding of the person.

Admittedly, it is an oversimplification to reduce all studies of the nature–nurture paradigm to the concerns noted herein, and the more recent contributions of large-scale genotyping to the research (Friedman, Banich, & Keller, 2021) must be acknowledged. And at least one researcher has concluded—twice—that "the nature–nurture debate is over" (Turkheimer, 2000, 2022).

Though the twin studies applied to this paradigm have long been presented as the "gold standard" of psychological research, three assumptions have never been questioned, and they must be considered and validated in order to confirm Galton's theory. If any one of these assumptions can be proven wrong, the theory of

With kind reprint permission; adapted and updated from *The International Forum for Logotherapy* (originally published in Vol. 46, No. 2).

C. L. McLafferty, Jr. (✉)
Purpose Research, Charlottesville, Virginia, USA

Viktor Frankl Institute of Logotherapy (USA), Stamford, TX, USA
e-mail: charles@purposeresearch.com

C. L. McLafferty, Jr., J. I. Levinson (eds.), *Logotherapy and Existential Analysis*, Logotherapy and Existential Analysis: Proceedings of the Viktor Frankl Institute Vienna 2, https://doi.org/10.1007/978-3-031-48922-8_27

nature–nurture must be reconsidered. These assumptions are so rudimentary that perhaps we should be asking why nature vs. nurture has been universally accepted for so long.

Assumption 1: Unitivity

The first assumption, termed *unitivity*, is based on the idea that "heritability and environmentality add to unity" (Sternberg et al., 2005, p. 53); in other words, they add to one.

$$\text{Hereditability}(\text{nature}) + \text{environmentality}(\text{nurture}) = 1$$

Thus, variability from any other source must be incorporated into heritability, environmentality, and/or their interaction, and therefore precluded from consideration outside of the paradigm. From this assumption, consideration of alternative factors is precluded, as the very design of studies begins with the purpose of teasing apart the variability of nature vs. that of nurture. Therefore, the assumption of unitivity means that *only* nature and nurture make us who we are.

For example, one type of twin study used in the study of nature vs. nurture has involved comparing identical twins adopted at birth to two different families; because they are genetically identical, the assumption of unitivity allows for all differences between the twin pairs to be attributed to environmentality. Once the influence of environment (nurture) has been determined, it is possible to derive the genetic component by subtracting the influence of nurture from 1 to determine hereditability.

$$1 - \text{Environmentality} = \text{Hereditability}$$

To be sure, in recent decades twins are no longer separated when adopted for ethical and social reasons, so this specific experimental design is no longer available.

Another type of twin study determines the influence of hereditability by comparing identical twins (genetically identical) with fraternal twins (as genetically similar as any nontwin siblings), both types of twin pairs raised in the same household. By determining the difference between these two sets of pairs, researchers can determine the hereditability of given traits. With this design (and the assumption of unitivity), environmentality is derived from the formula:

$$1 - \text{Hereditability} = \text{Environmentality}$$

More recently, researchers have begun to point out that the environmental component is not so uniform for twins, arguing that this factor must be divided into the *shared* environment for the twin pair and the unique, *unshared*, environment for each member. This is an important insight: Though it maintains the idea of unitivity, it makes it more difficult (if not impossible) for researchers to determine hereditability (and environmentality) in such a clear manner.

As an aside, I would postulate that it is likely that identical twins spend more time together than fraternal twins, resulting in more shared environmental influences. In my experience, it is not uncommon for identical twins to report having a tight bond, and reports in the literature note instances of a twin knowing when the others are injured or in danger [see, for example, anecdotal reports from The Stanford Twin Registry (Stanford Medicine, 2023)]. This difference further confounds the determination of hereditability when comparing identical to fraternal twins.

Overall, the intent and design of twin studies has been to determine the relative influences of nature and nurture. The assumption of unitivity is required for these studies to be valid, as the existence of any other influence on human development must be "folded" into the nature or the nurture component. In fact, if there is any other factor, it is precluded from consideration by this assumption.

Assumption 2: Unidimensionality

The second assumption is related to the first. In order for the variability of nature and nurture to show unitivity, to add to one, they must be measured in similar units or be complementary parts of a whole; we cannot add together apples and oranges. As Sternberg et al. (2005) noted, "heritability has a complementary concept, that of environmentality" (p. 53). *Unidimensionality* refers to the assumption that nature and nurture are complementary, constituting a linear dichotomy. Under this concept, genetic and environmental influences constitute extremes of a continuum, a theoretical line that represents influences and interactions of both factors. This assumption requires that the human being lives only in the singular dimension of nature and nurture and their intersection.

Assumption 3: Universality

The third assumption is implicit in the range of its application in research and theory. *Universality* requires that the nature–nurture paradigm is automatically valid, regardless of the trait studied, such as giftedness, substance use, intelligence, language acquisition, as well as psychological disorders such as anxiety, depression, and schizophrenia. This reinforces the idea that nature and nurture are *the only two influences on human development, intelligence, and behavior in every circumstance and experience of human life*.

Under this assumption, for example, if the researcher is studying use of substances, it is only necessary to examine the factors of nature and nurture, because there are no other causative agents possible. If a researcher wanted to study intelligence or mental health, every variable would have to be a part of hereditability, environmentality, or a combination of the two.

Examining the Assumptions

Phenylketonuria (PKU), the inability to metabolize phenylalanine, is regularly cited as an example of nature–nurture interaction (e.g., Sternberg et al., 2005). Decades ago, PKU caused severe mental deficiencies. In 1934, Asbjørn Følling examined two siblings with severe intellectual and developmental impairments; their parents had noticed a strong smell in their urine; it was so pronounced that the father "found it difficult to tolerate" (Christ, 2003, p. 46). Følling detected something wrong with ketones in their urine, but it took him several months to determine that the problem was caused by phenylpyruvic acid, which resulted from an inability by the body to break down phenylalanine. He prescribed a palliative diet deficient in phenylalanine, revealing an environmental component. As will be demonstrated, this discovery also illustrates violations of all three assumptions.

Galton's (1869/1892) postulates can be addressed through the use of a dimensional ontology, which allows a more parsimonious understanding of human development. Viktor Frankl (1967) proposed three interpenetrating dimensions of the human being: *soma* (the physical body), *psyche* (the emotions and intellect), and the *noëtic* (the soul). The noëtic dimension includes self-transcendence, choice, free will (required for choice to exist), responsibility (which naturally emerges from having choice), spirituality, and the unique meaning capacity of *Homo sapiens*. While animals and humans both have the dimensions of soma and psyche, Frankl noted that the noëtic dimension differentiates human beings from animals.

In this ontology, genetic expression and hereditability are by definition somatic in origin—genes synthesize amino acids, full stop. Given that most people today have adequate physiological support for normal genetic function (PKU being a notable exception), nurture has greatest variability in the psyche. Given this perspective, it is more accurate to consider nature and nurture as *dimensionally distinct* rather than unidimensional and complementary.

This relates to the example of PKU, as science (a uniquely human function, which unquestionably involves some measure of the noëtic dimension) has given the person the *choice* of whether to follow the diet and thus ameliorate the symptoms. The human ability to choose is unique to the noëtic dimension. The existence of another factor means that nature and nurture are not unitive. The discovery of PKU's cause has virtually eliminated heritability, but the variability that has increased as a result has been choice, not environmentality. Choice creates a multivariate relationship between nature, nurture, and *the person who chooses*. In this respect, nature and nurture are no longer additive and unidimensional.

Note, however, why PKU is considered to be exemplary of the idea of nature vs. nurture: PKU has a genetic origin, but the symptoms result from the influence of environmental factors on this defective genotype. It is easy to see that altering the environment corrects the genetic deficiency, resulting in a cure. The influence of the noëtic factor, choice, is taken for granted by "folding" it into the environmental portion of the equation.

This single exception also invalidates the universality assumption; once we understand the existence of a third factor related to PKU, then we can no longer assume that the nature–nurture paradigm is universal.

By extension, *on that theoretical day when the human genome is completely understood, Galton's (1892) theory will be refuted: Scientists will have maximized human choice while minimizing adverse aspects of heritability and environmentality* (McLafferty, 2006). In short, the influences of nature and nurture will no longer be seen as "adding to one" or "complementary," as Sternberg et al. (2005) noted, nor can these influences be seen as universal.

The Danger of Reductionism

At the moment the human genome is completely understood, scientists may declare that all behavior is hereditary. Ironically, they will be making this conclusion under the assumption that the discovery of the genetic basis of all behavior also required that the discovery itself was caused by genetic factors—and the now-maximized choice to control the expression of the human genome is also the result of genetic expression. I have termed this the assumption of *supergenetic determinism.* Frankl (1969/2014) addressed this tendency toward reductionism more than half a century ago:

> I once came across a quotation defining man as "nothing but a complex biochemical mechanism powered by a combustion system which energizes computers with prodigious storage facilities for retaining encoded information." Now, as a neurologist, I stand for the justification of using the computer as a model, say, for the activity of the central nervous system. It is perfectly legitimate to use such an analogy. Thus, in a certain sense the statement is valid: man is a computer. However, at the same time he also is infinitely more than a computer. The statement is erroneous only insofar as man is defined as "nothing but" a computer. (p. 8)

In the same way, defining the human being as "nothing but" the expression of DNA is to leave out any sense of agency, personhood, free will, responsibility, and choice. Though researchers may eventually be able to point to a genetic basis of any *possible* behavior that can be observed, thus "proving" that 100% of behavior is genetically based, they will be unable to show specific mechanisms by which the expression of our genes explains every individual behavior; after all, correlation does not imply causation.

Thus, even with the eventual arrival of a complete understanding of the human genome, we must return to Anne Anastasi's (1958) insight: We must not only understand *how much* genetics and environment affect the person, we must also understand *how*—the process by which the individual becomes a human being. And to that we must add: We may come to understand how environment and genetics result in human behavior, but we must also understand the *why* of human existence. Frankl

(2006) was fond of paraphrasing Nietzsche: “He who has a *why* to live for can bear almost any *how*” (p. 104).

Theorists have proposed factors that operate in conjunction with genetics and environment, such as symbol systems (language, science, math, musical notation) (Gardner, Hatch, & Torff, 1997) and human agency (Biddell & Fischer, 1997; Frankl, 1967). Assuming that animals do not have language, science, and math symbol systems, nor the existence of some arena of choice and free will (Frankl, 1967) needed for agency, these distinctly human variables are noëtic. How do they affect nature–nurture research?

Inclusion of the Noëtic Dimension

As noted, the noëtic dimension is that which defines the human being as distinct from the animal. Studies of twins regarding language development and IQ invariably involve the measure of noëtic symbol systems, using the manipulation of language and/or representations of math or logic. Research regarding substance use (or abuse) involving twins ignores the noëtic dimension. For example, the most successful treatment involves 12-step programs that invoke a “Higher Power” to strengthen the ability to choose; both the “Higher Power” (however defined by the individual) and choice are functions of the noëtic dimension. Twin studies of career selection assume nature and nurture alone determine choice, precluding the Jungian sense of “finding one’s calling”; again, choice and “calling” are noëtic concepts. For each of these fields of study, the noëtic dimension is a confounding variable, its variability subsumed into genetic and/or environmental components.

As noted earlier, researchers have begun to look at environmentality differently, by recognizing that part of a twin pair’s experience is their *shared environmental experience*, but that each has an independent, nonshared component. Though researchers are still referring to this as *nonshared environmentality* (folding it into the nurture component), it is also an implicit recognition that each twin has choice and free will, revealing the inherent flaws in these three assumptions of the nature–nurture idea. This represents a further theoretical fracture of the “gold standard” of twin studies.

From a clinician’s standpoint, the tiny arena of choice that each of us possesses is likely the most powerful fulcrum available for change. The healer’s role is arguably to help the client discover and develop a sense of agency capable of harnessing and transcending nature and nurture. With choice comes responsibility and the realization of freedom, which cannot occur without meaningful and purposeful options. Indeed, it is through exercising our ability to choose that we become fully human (Frankl, 1967). *Galton’s* (1892) *paradigm ultimately assumed that the person has no true freedom.* Perhaps it would be more appropriate to rephrase Frankl (1967): Nature and nurture represent our fate, while the noëtic represents our capacity to take a stand toward that fate (see also Lukas, 2015, “From fate to freedom,” pp. 205–230).

For over a century, Galton's (1892) nature–nurture paradigm has anchored psychological research and theory. Though renowned, his idea and its derivations were never scientifically validated. Examination of the assumptions of unitivity, unidimensionality, and universality indicate that Galton's idea, and all studies based on it, bear reconsideration. Inclusion of the noëtic dimension and its interaction with genetics and environment allows the researcher to consider the whole person—the human as a multidimensional being—in studies of human development.

It is time for a new paradigm: Nature, nurture, and the noëtic.

References

Anastasi, A. (1958). Heredity, environment, and the question "How?". *Psychological Review, 65*, 197–208. https://doi.org/10.1037/h0044895

Biddell, T. R., & Fischer, K. W. (1997). Between nature and nurture: The role of human agency in the epigenesis of intelligence. In R. J. Sternberg & E. Grigorinko (Eds.), *Intelligence, heredity, and environment* (pp. 193–242). Cambridge University Press.

Christ, S. E. (2003). Asbjørn Følling and the discovery of phenylketonuria. *Journal of the History of the Neurosciences, 12*(1), 44–54. https://doi.org/10.1076/jhin.12.1.44.13788

Frankl, V. E. (1967). *Psychotherapy and existentialism*. Washington Square Press.

Frankl, V. E. (2006). *Man's search for meaning*. Beacon Press. (Original work published 1946)

Friedman, N. P., Banich, M. T., & Keller, M. C. (2021). Twin studies to GWAS: There and back again. *Trends in Cognitive Sciences, 25*(10), 855–869.

Galton, F. (1892). *Hereditary genius: An inquiry into its laws and consequences* (2nd ed.). MacMillan and Co. (Original work published 1869). http://www.mugu.com/galton/books/hereditary-genius/index.html

Gardner, H., Hatch, T., & Torff, B. (1997). A third perspective: The symbol systems approach. In R. J. Sternberg & E. Grigorinko (Eds.), *Intelligence, heredity, and environment* (pp. 243–268). Cambridge University Press.

Lukas, E. (2015). *The therapist and the soul: From fate to freedom*. Purpose Research.

McLafferty, C. L., Jr. (2006). Examining unproven assumptions of Galton's nature-nurture paradigm. *American Psychologist, 61*, 177–178. https://doi.org/10.1037/0003-066X.61.2.177

Stanford Medicine. (2023). *The Stanford Twin Registry: Twin stories*. Retrieved from https://med.stanford.edu/twin-registry/photo-story/stories.html

Sternberg, R. J., Grigorinko, E., & Kidd, K. K. (2005). Intelligence, race, and genetics. *American Psychologist, 60*(1), 46–59.

Turkheimer, E. (2000). Three laws of behavior genetics and what they mean. *Current Directions in Psychological Science, 9*(5), 160–164.

Turkheimer, E. (2022). This time I mean it: The nature–nurture debate is over. *Behavioral and Brain Sciences, 45*. https://doi.org/10.1017/S0140525X21001771

Charles L. McLafferty, Jr., PhD, has served on the faculties of the University of Virginia and the University of Alabama at Birmingham. He is the founder and president of Purpose Research, which seeks to incorporate meaning and purpose into the research, theory, and practice of the helping professions. McLafferty has edited and/or published more than a dozen books on logotherapy by authors such as Joseph Fabry, Elisabeth Lukas, Paul Wong, and Ann Graber. He has earned an educational diplomate from the Viktor Frankl Institute of Logotherapy (US). As a National Certified Counselor (US), he volunteered for five years at a regional crisis center as part of the National Suicide Prevention Lifeline network and for which he developed a logotherapeutic in-service training module.

From Meaning to Purpose: Finding the Heart of a Living Logotherapy

Charles L. McLafferty, Jr.

The compass was indispensable for long distance travel for much of our history. Most people don't know that the compass, when it was originally invented about 2500 years ago, was used for divination. It was used for Feng Shui, for orienting and finding the best location for buildings by the Chinese. They invented the compass by tying a thread of silk to a piece of lodestone, or magnetite, which would orient itself in space.

The compass as we know it is obsolete, but for the last millennium it revolutionized shipping because until then sailors could only use the stars or landmarks for navigation. But with a compass, they could navigate even in cloudy or stormy weather; they could veer further and further from the shore. And it became possible to make shipping runs twice a year instead of once a year. Though the compass as we know it is obsolete, in this new millennium we need a new compass. Viktor Frankl has shown us what that will be.

It was 40 years ago, plus or minus a week or two, that I met my spiritual mentor. In that meeting she introduced me to many different schools of thought, including the logotherapy of Viktor Frankl. I would not be here today if it were not for her.

Little did I know that, 20 years later and 20 years ago, I would be completing my dissertation on three of those very theories to which she introduced me, each of which originates in a completely discrete school of thought, each one supporting

With kind reprint permission; adapted and updated from *The International Forum for Logotherapy* (originally published in Vol. 46, No. 1). This was originally presented as a plenary address at the World Congress of Logotherapy, June, 2017.

C. L. McLafferty, Jr. (✉)
Purpose Research, Charlottesville, VA, USA

Viktor Frankl Institute of Logotherapy (USA), Stamford, TX, USA
e-mail: charles@purposeresearch.com

C. L. McLafferty, Jr., J. I. Levinson (eds.), *Logotherapy and Existential Analysis*, Logotherapy and Existential Analysis: Proceedings of the Viktor Frankl Institute Vienna 2, https://doi.org/10.1007/978-3-031-48922-8_28

and expanding the others. In fact, for the past few decades I have conducted research and presented in several areas related to logotherapy—nature vs. nurture vs. noös (McLafferty, 2006), applying the dimensional ontology to research methods (McLafferty, et al., 2010), stages of meaning development (McLafferty, 2014), ethics of long-term medical care in persistent vegetative states (McLafferty, 2016a), and training of crisis center counselors with logotherapeutic principles (McLafferty, 2012). But the work I keep returning to is the work that began with my dissertation.

Humanity's Historic Transition: From the World of Knowledge to the World of Meaning

I will pick up where I left off in 2015 here in Dallas, when I spoke about meaning as a bridge from the past of authoritarianism to a future of freedom and responsibility (see McLafferty, 2016b). As a brief review:

I used the metaphor of the Edmund Pettus Bridge in Selma, Alabama, where I lived during the turbulent 1960s, in the times of the famous march from Selma to Montgomery. I noted that we are in a time of transition unlike any that we have seen in human history. Perhaps there has never been a period of time in which humanity had the choice of whether to cause its own extinction—whether by nuclear annihilation, wasting of our resources, or poisoning our planet—or to ensure that humanity not only survives, but thrives in finding what Frankl (2010) called "unity in spite of diversity" (p. 158). Even the United States, where I am speaking, has aspirations that resonate with Frankl's idea of unity in diversity: E pluribus unum means "out of the many, one."

The emphasis of "self"—the pedestal of "me first" has as a potential counterweight the logotherapeutic idea of self-transcendence. Make no mistake—the stage of identity development, of forming a coherent self—is important, if not critical, in development (whether for an individual, a family, or a nation). Though there are exceptions, self-transcendence is only possible to the extent that there is a self to be transcended. Thus, the application of logotherapy becomes possible at the point that the self emerges.

There are "helps" along the path of development. Rules and authority help us to acknowledge social rules that guide us to live harmoniously. But some courageous souls are not content to be what Frankl (1985, p. 26 ff) called *peacemakers* (i.e., settling for comfort at any cost) but are rather *pacemakers* (setting a new path for the next generation based on their conscience). Joseph Fabry (2013) noted that pacemakers initiated the civil rights movement in the 1950s and 1960s.

This is related to that transition through which humanity is passing—collectively, we are leaving a past of external authority and entering the bridge to a new freedom, a freedom with a terrifying responsibility not just for ourselves, but for each other, for the entire human race. Pictures of the horrors of humanity, movies of unspeakable acts, recordings of conversations between government officials—all virtually impossible a century ago—are now omnipresent. The power of the printing press—and the corporations who controlled it—have been supplanted by the Internet, social media, and desktop publishing. Today, an individual with an idea can publish it and have it distributed to the entire world in hours or even minutes. We are in a time of revolution. Truly, humanity is mastering the *world of knowledge*.

The bridge on which we are entering as humanity is the *world of meaning*. Viktor Frankl correctly foresaw the human need for meaning more than 80 years ago, and his work remains as relevant and needed today as it was when he was helping unemployed workers during the Great Depression (Batthyány, 2010). But where does the bridge lead? What's on the other side of the bridge of meaning? And that is where I continue today.

Finding Direction in the World of Meaning

Anthony de Mello (1982/1984) told the story of "The Explorer":

> The explorer returned to his people, who were eager to know about the Amazon. But how could he ever put into words the feelings that flooded his heart when he saw exotic flowers and heard the night-sounds of the forests; when he sensed the danger of wild beasts or paddled his canoe over treacherous rapids?
>
> He said, "Go and find out for yourselves." To guide them, he drew a map of the river.
>
> They pounced upon the map. They framed it in their Town Hall. They made copies of it for themselves. And all who had a copy considered themselves experts on the river, for did they not know its every turn and bend, how broad it was, how deep, where the rapids were and where the falls? (pp. 32–33)

This is one of the paradoxes of logotherapy. Frankl has drawn a map. He has described the exotic flowers and treacherous rapids of meaning that we face. It is too easy to frame the copies and hang them on the wall and point to them as proof that we, too, have found meaning.

But as logotherapists we have a different approach: We seek to live logotherapy, to center ourselves on meaning so that we can help others do the same. We need, at the least, a compass to orient us to our new landscape. The search for authenticity, for a living logotherapy, involves a series of questions:

- Is there a "heart" of logotherapy, central concepts without which it cannot exist?
- How can these concepts be useful in our lives and work?
- What is the meaning of meaning, and how does that relate to the power of purpose?

In order to proceed, it is necessary to establish a common foundation for discussion by defining some key words and concepts:

- *Spirituality* is that which is distinctly human and superhuman. The word does not necessarily refer to religion (Frankl, 2014, p. 5).

- *God*: "the partner of your most intimate soliloquies" (Frankl, 1978, p. 63). That's a definition Frankl came up with when he was 16 years old, according to Don Klingberg (2001) in his biography of Frankl. It's probably not coincidental that it was at about this time that Frankl went through a nihilistic period—he understood the perils of going through deep doubt and came out of it with a definition of God, one that he said no atheist ever objected to.
- *Religion*: This is important, because Frankl was not talking about Presbyterian or Baptist or Jew or Hindu or Muslim. As just noted, he was referring to the relationship of the person with God. Each person has their own religion; in his words, "an expression of 'man's search for ultimate meaning'" (Frankl, 1986, p. xii).
- *Responsibility*: the ability to respond, to be "response-able" (Fabry, 2013, p. 16).
- Finally, we have *conscience*: the imperfect meaning-organ, found in the noëtic dimension.

Research of Theories Incorporating Spirituality

As noted, 20 years ago, my dissertation project involved evaluating three theories of psychology that included a spiritual dimension. Each of these theories derives from very different sources, and each has central assumptions, parts of the theory that form a core. In qualitative research and naturalistic inquiry, comparison of different sources is known as *triangulation* (Lincoln & Guba, 1985; Patton, 2002). Perhaps "unity in spite of diversity" (Frankl, 2010, p. 158) applies to this approach. Today, as I look across theories, with a couple minor adjustments, it is possible to reconcile logotherapy with other theories and works that have been part of my exploration.

The research involved the preparation of three case studies. The three theories were: (a) the logotherapy of Viktor Frankl and Elisabeth Lukas, based on existential philosophy and therapy; (b) *Psychosynthesis*, a book written by Roberto Assagioli (1965) with Robert Gerard, who sat with Assagioli in a room for several weeks with a tape recorder running—together they laid out Assagioli's theory; and (c) the spiritual psychology of Meredith Sprunger, a psychologist and minister who was a student of *The Urantia Book* (1955; cf. an abridged version, Sprunger, 2012) and wrote *Spiritual Psychology* (Sprunger, 2009) as a primer on the applications of spiritual principles to psychology.

The idea behind this study was that, if a spiritual psychology is possible, then it should be based on universal principles. I looked for ideas that were congruent across the theories in order to demonstrate their universality.

These theories have completely different sources as their foundations. Thus, it was an exploration to see how they connected. Frankl, I believe, had very carefully defined a spiritual psychology. Frankl's (1969/1988) dimensional ontology was a perfect framework for mapping the theoretical stances onto each other. The dimensions of soma, psyche, and noös provided an easy match.

Each cell in the human body has at its core the DNA needed to create it. The curious thing about DNA is that these complex strands of protein have all of the blueprints needed to recreate *every other cell in every organ* in the human body. My search has led me to look for prototypes, for exemplars, in logotherapy. Aside from looking for connections between these three theories, I looked for what was essential to logotherapy. What examples lead to the DNA—the heart—of Frankl's thinking?

The Scales of Existentialism: A Thought Experiment (Fig. 1)

The *scales of existentialism* are a good place to begin. In 1993, when I came to my first World Congress in Toronto, Rosemary Henrion and Tom McKillop began the introductory course on logotherapy with the scales of existentialism. Two years later, Elisabeth Lukas (2020) focused on the scales of existence in her keynote address to the Tenth World Congress of Logotherapy in Dallas.

On the one side is a mechanical, materialistic existence, depicted as a rock in the figure. This is the stance of what is traditionally thought of as existentialism or nihilism. From this perspective, we are merely random combinations of DNA, a fluke of the cosmos. A life has emerged from molecules which happen to coexist, and then is gone forever. In this viewpoint, we are floating on a rock hurtling through space, the result of random events. The universe is hostile and uncaring. It does not matter if we are poor or rich, educated or illiterate, sick or whole; it doesn't matter if we heal the sick, it doesn't matter if we educate the illiterate, because, in a million years it won't even matter that we existed. Looking at it this way, our choices and decisions are meaningless. There is no good or evil, just relativity. If we are willing to face that terror, then are we confronted with the necessity to create meaning. But if we are truly honest with ourselves in this philosophical stance, we can only conclude that such a self-created meaning is a delusion (cf. Lukas, 2020). So that is one side of the scales.

On the other hand, there is the teleological side. On this side, the universe was created with purpose. Indeed, each of us is created with purpose. The universe is supportive, beyond our ability to see and know. Even our genetic inheritance, our DNA, has purpose. Our choices and decisions are important. Each choice toward

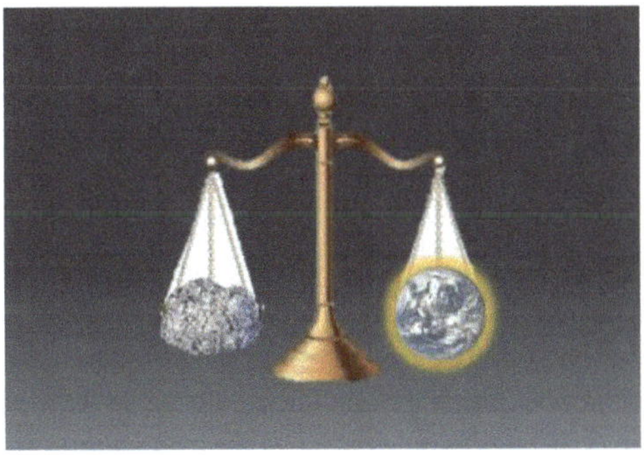

Fig. 1 The scales of existence

truth, beauty, and goodness is important, and becomes a monument in eternity. Nothing of goodness is ever lost in time. Each of us has a unique meaning and purpose to give to the world.

The scales of existence are the first example of one of the core statements of logotherapy; it is possible to think of these scales when discerning our choices and when we help others to do the same. Frankl pointed to this existential question, as cited in Lukas (2020):

> The question is: "Is existence nothing but a mass of nonsense, or is it a mass of ultimate meaning?" This question cannot be answered by the natural sciences alone. It cannot be answered at all; it is a completely unsolvable problem—rather, it must be decided. All being is ambiguous: Both interpretations—both the interpretation "nonsense" and the interpretation "ultimate meaning"—are possible. Both are thinkable: that being is total nonsense, and that it is total ultimate meaning; but these are indeed only two "thinkables," two thought possibilities, and not thought necessities. With respect to the decision we are called upon to make, there is no logical coercion; in no way are we logically forced, logically obligated to decide for one or the other. Both interpretations are logically of equal status. Logically there is as much which speaks for the one interpretation as for the other. The equal status of the two answers: the answer "absolute nonsense" and the answer "absolute ultimate meaning"—results in the responsibility of the respondent. He is not only faced with a question—No: He is faced with a decision, and, in fact, an existential decision, but not an intellectual decision. What he must perform is not the "intelligere," not a factual realization—but rather a personal commitment. (pp. 22–23)

Frankl's Dimensional Ontology

In order to better understand this idea, we need to move into what is commonly taught as Frankl's (2014) *three-dimensional ontology*. I have used a symbolic diagram to portray these dimensions. The first dimension is the *soma*, the physical dimension; the *psyche*, the emotions and the intellect; we share both soma and the psyche with the animal kingdom. The third dimension is the truly human, the *noëtic*, the dimension of choice, responsibility—Frankl calls it the soul, the human spirit, the uniquely human dimension (Fig. 2).

Conscience is the organ of meaning (DuBois, 2004); it is a uniquely noëtic function (Frankl, 2000). Out of the constellation of choices, there is one choice that is the best (Lukas, 2015). Viktor Frankl (2000) tells us that there is one choice among many that is the best one. But conscience is not perfect:

> Conscience is a definitely human phenomenon. But we must add that it is also "just" a human phenomenon. It is subject to the human condition in that it is stamped by the finiteness of man. For he is not only guided by conscience in his search for meaning, he is sometimes misled by it as well. Unless he is a perfectionist, he also will accept this fallibility of conscience. (Frankl, 2014, p. 45)

The noëtic is uniquely human. Free will and responsibility are part of the noëtic dimension. The noëtic requires choice in action. Choices can be wrong or right, evil or good, false or true. They can lean toward impartiality or wholeness, separativeness or inclusiveness. The human being in the noëtic dimension is potentially

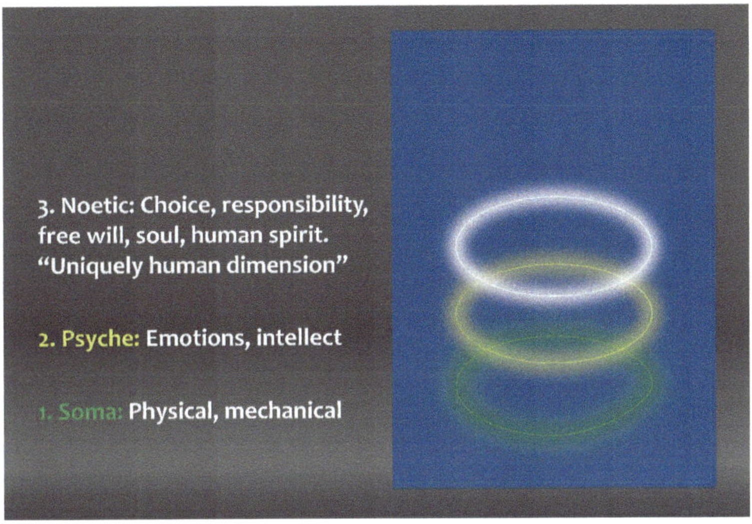

Fig. 2 Frankl's three-dimensional ontology

perfectible. If that is true, the noëtic must also be potentially corruptible. This is the soul, the *human* spirit.

The noëtic dimension contains *within it* the treasure chest of healing. Frankl has said there are no neuroses possible in the dimension of the spirit because the spirit cannot get sick.[1] In my dissertation (McLafferty, 1997) I had some difficulties in resolving this point with the other two theories. One anecdote in Frankl's writing opened a window into my understanding.

"How Can I Know?"

The second example is contained in an apocryphal anecdote told by Frankl: After a lecture, a student approached Frankl and asked "But how can I know that there really is a God?" And Frankl answered, "The fact that you have asked the question is proof that you know the answer already." This exchange raised questions for me. How was Frankl able to reply with such certainty to that student? How could he *know* that this was true for that person? From what point of view of existentialism—or logotherapy—was he able to respond this way?

Interestingly, the other two theories I examined for my dissertation agreed with Frankl's response. Sprunger (personal communication, 1996) noted that "the

[1] However, Frankl (2000) also stated: "Mental illness may be psychogenic (neurosis) or somatogenic (psychosis) in nature and origin. But noögenic and (psych-) iatrogenic (pseudo-) neuroses also exist" (p. 134).

existence of the question of God is proof that God has already found the individual." Assagioli (1965) began with the spiritual dimension as a statement of fact.

Anthony de Mello (1982/1984) told the story of *The Question*:

> Said the monk: All those mountains and rivers, and the earth and stars, where do they come from?
>
> And the master answered: Where does your question come from? (p. 28)

Frankl's answer to the student may be consistent with several schools of thought, but how does the philosophy of logotherapy explain the answer if the scales were equally balanced and the answer was unknowable? Frankl's answer stimulated thought for years, as I wondered if it might hold a key to logotherapy. I asked many logotherapists about it, but my questions weren't resolved. The key took years to find, a puzzle I had already been wrestling with in my dissertation: Frankl's dimensional ontology.

Frankl's Fourth Dimension

I suspected there had to be a fourth dimension in logotherapy as I worked on my dissertation project, but didn't have a clear definition for it. However, I was able to use Frankl's three dimensions as a backbone for the three theories. For the theory of logotherapy I didn't have, per se, a discrete delineation between the uniquely human dimension, the noëtic, or "the *human* spirit" and what is termed "the *divine* spirit," which was part of the other two theories.

To gain some clarity, I corresponded with Elisabeth Lukas, who was very open in her training classes regarding the presence of the divine. In correspondence, Lukas did allude to it by saying, "meaning is the voice of the divine spirit to be heard through conscience" (personal communication, 1996).

It was years later that I began to find this fourth dimension was already in Frankl's books; it was "hiding in plain sight." The first realization happened as I was rereading *Man's Search for Ultimate Meaning* (Frankl, 2000) and was well into the first chapter when I had the sense that I had missed something on the previous page. It was an "aha" moment. I circled back, and there it was:

> A higher dimension, by definition, is a more inclusive one. The lower dimension is included in the higher one; it is subsumed in it and encompassed by it. Thus biology is overarched by psychology, psychology by noölogy, and *noölogy by theology* [emphasis added]. (p. 16)

In this passage Frankl defined *four* dimensions. But note that he is not talking about "theology" as we know it—the use of that word may have been a translational artifact. "Theology" is derived from "theos" and "logos," and we need to consider that he may not have been referring to "theology" as the academic study of religion but rather as the individual's relationship with "the partner of one's most intimate soliloquies."

Over the following months and years, I found other indications of a fourth dimension. This quote was also from *Man's Search for Ultimate Meaning*: "In my book

The Will to Meaning I have expressed my conviction that there is a dimensional barrier between the human world and the divine world…" (Frankl, 2000, p. 156). A "dimensional barrier" indicates that there is a human dimension and a divine one.

And in a footnote in *Psychotherapy and Existentialism:* "In German there is a distinction between *geistig* and *geistlich*, the former indicating the human dimension and the latter indicating the religious one…" (Frankl, 1985, p. 65).

More recently, on rereading *The Will to Meaning* (Frankl, 2014), I realized that an entire chapter, titled "Dimensions of Meaning," has a number of differentiations between the human and divine dimensions. These distinct dimensions further define the theory of logotherapy as a four-dimensional theory.

Frankl, therefore, included four dimensions in logotherapy: (a) the somatic, the biophysical, the genetic expression, which has to do with our appearance in the world; (b) the psychic, the emotions and the intellect; (c) the noëtic, the human spirit or the soul; and (d) a fourth dimension, as referred to by Frankl. The best I can define it, and I can only approximate it in words: the eternal and infinite, beyond language, "Source," perfection, the Life that calls to us through conscience.

To return to the symbolic line drawings, the fourth dimension (depicted in Fig. 3 as a glowing sphere) is a source of illumination, of hope, of healing for the entire person. It goes by many different names across the literature. These are not necessarily the names that Frankl gave to it, though a few of these you will recognize: Ultimate Meaning, the "partner of our most intimate conversations," Spirit, Life (as in "Life calls to us"), Transcendence; our true compass [more correctly, the True North to which our inner compass points] Without Name or Number; the great I AM; a fragment of Infinity; the Divine Indweller; Cosmic Consciousness… there

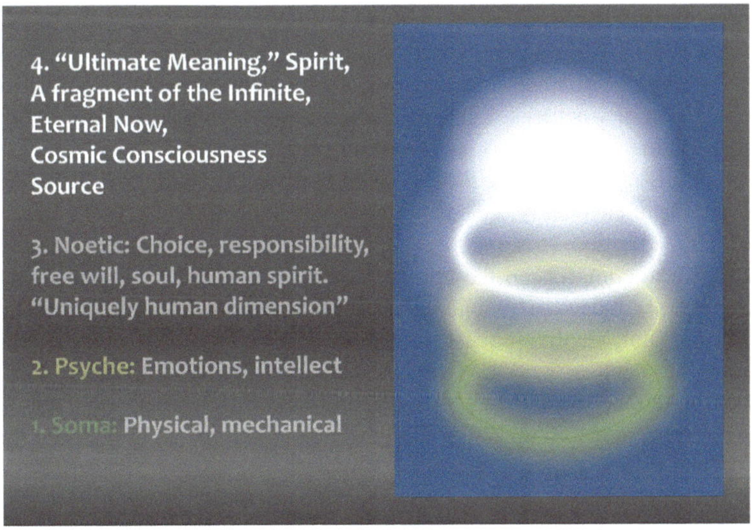

Fig. 3 Frankl's fourth dimension

are many different names, “key words” that are used in many of these schools of thought to refer to and differentiate between the human and divine dimensions.

All of these refer to the same thing; it is a dimension beyond the human, beyond the noëtic. There’s nothing… there’s no word, no phrase, no single prescription that can be given, because this dimension is beyond human understanding. Frankl (2000) noted this idea in *Man’s Search for Ultimate Meaning*. And this is one of the keys: By pointing out this dimension, there’s no single approach or method, no system for discovery that is possible. If each of us is responsible—uniquely—to find meaning, then this fourth dimension is even more uniquely discovered by each one of us. We acknowledge this when we use the phrase “The One About Whom Naught May Be Said.” In some faith traditions, the holy name cannot be written or spoken. The most that can be done is to indicate a direction, because each of us must take the responsibility to look for it, to find it, to define it, and to develop our understanding and relationship with it. Each one of us must determine the name(s) by which we know “the partner of our most intimate soliloquies.”

Coupling Being and Meaning

To return to the student who asked “How can I know that there really is a God?” I finally concluded that Frankl knew that the student was experiencing a fourth dimension. If we look at the converse, if we flip it around to say that there could be no God, the student would not be asking the question. The pull from the spark of the Infinite that indwells us, the pilot light of eternity… by whatever name we know it, brings forth the question.

But doesn’t this also relate to those existential scales? The fact that Frankl asked us the question about the scales meant that he already knew the answer. But Frankl didn’t give us the answer; simply by asking us the question *he makes us responsible for determining our existential stance toward Life*. Each of us must answer to Life for the question of whether life has meaning and in so doing place the “weight of our being” on the side of the scales that we choose.

It should also be noted that Frankl stated that we cannot answer *logically*, we cannot answer intellectually. This is because the intellect, by itself, is incapable of answering the question. It is only by opening the door to the noëtic dimension that we can begin to comprehend the immensity of Life, the facticity of meaning, the pull of purpose. Indeed, I maintain that the “Scales of Existentialism Thought Experiment” catalyzes that process *if the person is ready to open that door*. And if they are not, it plants a “seed thought” that perhaps will grow over time.

But consider this: If life were only mechanical, then each of us would not be asking the question of meaning. We would have no *being* to place on the side that we choose! Thus meaning would be arbitrary and self-created. As Lukas (2020) noted in her keynote address:

> The "primal therapeutic act" therefore consists of coupling being and meaning. And there is no treatment and no support of a suffering person which can do without it. For where being is not coupled with meaning, human health, happiness, bravery, etc. have no meaning; therapy would, in fact, be pointless. All values would then be merely human evaluations and could be cancelled again by human evaluations. Even the value "patient" would be only a fiction pertaining to a meaningless heap of matter. And the value "recovery of the patient" would also amount to an equally arbitrary subjective judgement. It would then be, in objective terms, a matter of indifference, whether the world exists or not, whether people, animals, plants, cultural achievements, continue to exist—their being would not be any better than their non-being, their preservation not better than their destruction. (p. 24)

Computers and machines, in my experience, do not have insight, conscience, or intuition, and they never ask questions like this. (In fact, computers don't ask questions.) Computers don't have a noëtic dimension. Computers are unable to ask the questions of meaning. Recently, I "conversed" with two of the new Artificial Intelligence programs, ChatGPT (https://chat.openai.com) and BardAI (https://bard.google.com), and the only way they could answer questions of meaning is to regurgitate what they have harvested on the web—or what their programmers have coded as responses. [Both AI programs, when asked the meaning of life, were coded to note that (to anthropomorphize) "they" were not capable of answering the question.] It is only because we have the presence of a living Spirit that the question of meaning or of the existence of God arises deep within us.

To extend this insight, this is why Frankl was able to state that the presence of an existential vacuum is a sign of growth, not of regression. The questions of existence are evidence (if not proof) that the individual is experiencing an emergence, a growth, of the human spirit, of the noëtic dimension.

Living in the Dual World: We Are Mediators

Returning to the scales of existence: It is possible to turn them on the side in order to see them from a different perspective. We can translate these two viewpoints, mechanical and teleological, into *matter* and *spirit*. We have the essence of these symbolized in the earth as a rock vs. a living planet. Helena Blavatsky (1888, p. 633) stated that matter is spirit at its lowest point of manifestation and spirit is matter at its highest. To her, it was a question of vibration (Fig. 4).

We don't have to rely on metaphysics; we can look to the greatest physicist of all time for his answer: Einstein stated that $E = mc^2$. What he said in a simple, scientific formula was "matter and energy (light) are interchangeable." He gave us a mathematical formula to interrelate the highest and the lowest.

Between spirit and matter is the human being. We are the mediators between spirit and matter, and between matter and spirit. It is by acting on this dimensional tension that we are able to manifest the soul, the noëtic. Every religion throughout time has had some form of mediator between spirit and matter, a bridge between the highest and the lowest that we can know. What Viktor Frankl did was to show us *meaning* as a mediator between the highest and the lowest in our nature. So we can

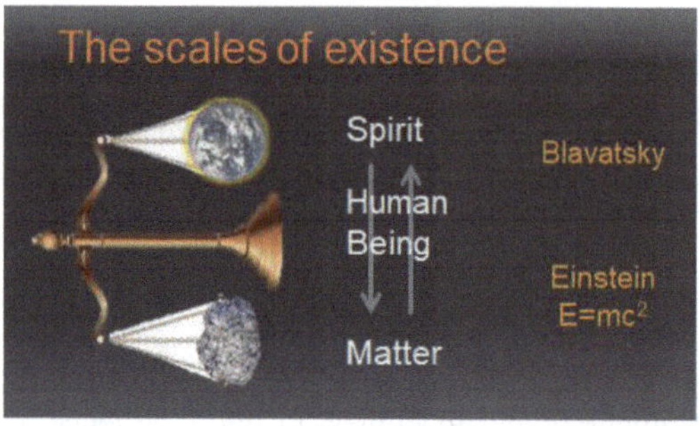

Fig. 4 The duality of matter and spirit

think of spirit and matter as we make decisions. And as we act on them, we create—we *co-create* the soul, the noëtic dimension. We develop it through our choices and decisions—and how we act on them—like a muscle that's being strengthened.

We can see that meaning changes dimensionally as we are developing. The meaning of words, for example, gives us a bridge between our inner world and the environment in which we live. The word "chair" is a mediator between the object upon which we sit and a representation that we hold in the mind that allows us to communicate with each other about it.

In the soma we find the outer world of action; in the psyche, the world of emotion and knowledge. As we move into awareness and recognition of the world of meaning—the noëtic dimension—we begin to discover a meaning that is greater than ourselves, an entire world of meaning. As we listen to the still voice of the conscience, we discover the source of conscience, the echo of an infinite silence. We discover the fact that we are connected in ways that we cannot image. And that is the Ultimate Meaning of Viktor Frankl (2000). Just as we move from the world of knowledge to the world of meaning, now we open to the *world of purpose and of ideas*. In this regard, Carl Jung (1989) noted: "The decisive question for man is: Is he related to something infinite or not?" (p. 325).

However, I propose that, from this perspective, having to make a choice between the two sides of the scales of existence is an illusion. It's like the old Buddhist koan that forces a choice between a false dichotomy: What is the sound of one hand clapping? We are *both* matter and spirit, we're not one or the other; we must navigate both at once if we are to fully live our lives. If we choose one or the other, we are still incomplete. If we choose only mechanistic logic, we become crystallized in our own worn-out intellectual grooves, like a digital loop of sampled house music. If we choose only teleology, pure spirit, we can easily get distracted in contemplating our navels or become lost in space. Or, worse yet, we can demand that everyone has exactly the same relationship with Life that we do. We must find "the path between the opposites" or what is commonly known as "The Great Middle Way" of Buddhism in order to grow noëtically.

All too often our society, our culture, our media, our theories, our research methods, our television ads begin with a zero-sum game. We have a great deal of mechanistic programming built into our minds. What happens if we start in the other direction? What would happen if education began with the purpose for which a Kindergartner was created instead of "we have a lot of facts to cover today, so let's get started"? If we begin with meaning and purpose, there will be a different stance toward education, counseling, ministry, business, and medicine—indeed, our entire society will be transformed.

Just imagine, when one day we are able to demonstrate the fact of the noëtic dimension—the soul—then we will know, as a fact, when human life actually "begins" on a spiritual basis. More importantly, we will know at the end of life, when a soul begins to separate from its physical mechanism and to withdraw its energy and attention, the point at which we can allow the natural process of life and death to ensue… we can "let go" instead of spending so much of our life energy and healthcare resources frantically keeping alive a person who—in essence—is ready to move on (cf. Graber, 2009, McLafferty, 2016a). We will know this as a scientific fact, and we will accept it as part of the flow and continuity of Life.

Our Imperfect World

Viktor Frankl (1985) made a statement about our imperfect world that may be surprising:

> I prefer to live in a world in which man has the right to make choices, even if they are wrong choices, rather than a world in which no choice at all is left to him. In other words, I prefer a world in which, on the one hand, a phenomenon such as Adolf Hitler can occur, and on the other hand, phenomena such as the many saints who have lived can occur also. I prefer this world to a world of total, or totalitarian, conformism and collectivism in which man is debased and degraded to a mere functionary of a party or the state. (p. 28)

When we look at purpose more deeply, then we find that there are certain inevitabilities, as Meredith Sprunger (2012) stated. If our universe is created with purpose, if we are created with purpose (and with the free will to follow it), then there are implications of this idea. In line with Frankl's thinking about our imperfect world, "The Inevitabilities" is a passage that Sprunger quoted from *The Urantia Book* (1955):

> The uncertainties of life and the vicissitudes of existence do not in any manner contradict the concept of the universal sovereignty of God. All evolutionary creature life is beset by certain inevitabilities.
>
> Consider the following…

1. Is courage—strength of character—desirable? Then must man be reared in an environment which necessitates grappling with hardships and reacting to disappointments.…
5. Is the love of truth and the willingness to go wherever it leads, desirable? Then must man grow up in a world where error is present and falsehood always possible.…
8. Is unselfishness—the spirit of self-forgetfulness—desirable? Then must mortal man live face to face with the incessant clamoring of an inescapable self for recognition and honor. Man could not dynamically choose the divine life if there were no self-life to forsake. Man could never lay saving hold on righteousness if there were no potential evil to exalt and differentiate the good by contrast. (p. 51)

In a similar vein, Robert Gerard (personal communication, 1996) stated that our troubles can be seen as the gymnastic bars on which we exercise our mental and emotional bodies to strengthen them against the blows of fate (cited in McLafferty, 1997).

The point here is that all too often we know our role on the scales of existence but we forget. We forget that we are here on this planet with meaning and purpose and that through the entirety of existence we are supported. In that regard, our trials and tribulations are inevitabilities.

Our Imperfect Selves

Each of us is unique. Each of us is important. Each of us is needed for a specific purpose, though none of us can see it readily. Frankl (1986) noted that if we were perfect, we would be interchangeable, replaceable. But we know all too well that we are not perfect. And we are unique—there will never be others exactly like us in all of eternity:

> If all men were perfect, then every individual would be replaceable by anyone else. From the very imperfection of men follows the indispensability and inexchangeability of each individual; for each is imperfect in his own fashion. No man is universally gifted; but the bias of the individual makes for his uniqueness. (p. 69)

In reflecting on Frankl's ideas, some insights have emerged: If we are created with purpose, then even our imperfection is purposeful. Perhaps this imperfection contains a clue to the very purpose at the core of our being: Isn't it interesting that we spend our entire lives trying to stamp out this imperfection? The tension between our imperfect outer selves and the faint sense that we have a source of perfection and purpose is needed and necessary. If we are the bridge between spirit and matter, then perhaps it is built of this very tension between our own imperfection and an inner core that is incapable of illness or imperfection. That tension becomes the path itself, the bridge. If we focus on our imperfections, we destroy ourselves; if we focus on the perfect, we become paralyzed, unable to act. But if we allow both our imperfection and what Fabry (2013) called "the medicine chest" found in the noëtic dimension to coexist, then we can use that tension for the work of meaning and purpose. Isn't this what Frankl (1985) was referring to when he spoke of the *noödynamic tension* between who we are and who we can be?

Importantly, often there is a gift that corresponds with the seeming weakness. For example: ADHD—someone with the symptoms of attention deficits and hyperactivity pays attention to everything; they have the gift of attention: It's not focused, but these individuals often notice a lot more than most people. For those who exhibit perfectionism—intense, one-pointed thought. For procrastinators—perhaps some of them are good contemplators.

We have both perfection and imperfection, coexisting, at once—and by moving to a simultaneous inclusion of both, we become more than can we can imagine. Frankl (1986) was fond of paraphrasing Goethe: "If we take people as they are, we make them worse. If we treat them as if they were what they ought to be, we help them to become what they are capable of becoming" (p. 8). We can do that for others, and we can do that for ourselves.

My thinking led to a conclusion that was initially surprising: *In our imperfection lies hid the secret of our indispensability*. If we were perfect, there could be no tension between the imperfection of our present and the hope and possibilities of the future. Is it possible that our imperfection is the outward manifestation of Purpose itself?

How Do These Ideas Fit with Logotherapy?

Viktor Frankl (1986) defined logotherapy as "ultimately education toward responsibility" (p. xxii)—the *ability* to *respond*. It involves an active participation in life, dynamic interaction with life. Living logotherapy requires the ability to respond.

Frankl (1985, p. 43) also said that logotherapy leads to the door of religion, but can go no further. He added that "logotherapy does not cross the boundary between psychotherapy and religion. But it leaves the door to religion open and it leaves it to the patient whether or not to pass the door" (Frankl, 2014, pp. 109–110). Is this not what Viktor Frankl did? He pointed us in a direction, then left us responsible for the rest. He does not give us the name that cannot be said—we must find that for ourselves.

Why did he say that logotherapy couldn't go any further? Because once we move to that door, we are on our own. We are responsible. Frankl (2014) added: "It is the patient who has to decide whether he interprets responsibleness in terms of being responsible to humanity, society, conscience, or God. It is up to him to decide to what, to whom, and for what he is responsible" (p. 110). Every choice, every decision has the potential to bring us closer to this threshold. Once we move to that door, there is nothing else that the study or practice of logotherapy can reveal to us. That is the true choice, the reason for our greatest gift of free will.

Perhaps this is why only three dimensions are formally stated in Frankl's logotherapy, and this is an important point: It is not necessary to include a fourth dimension to practice logotherapy, on ourselves or others. The pursuit of Ultimate Meaning (the fourth dimension) is only possible once we become aware of and committed to free will, conscience, and responsibility, and as each of us becomes responsible for recognizing and responding to "the partner of our most intimate conversations."

The Source of Existential Terror

To the nihilist who says there is no meaning and we are terrified to face the futility of our existence, I would answer that perhaps the truth is that we are afraid to encounter something that is greater than we can imagine. Could it be that William

James (1985) described this phenomenon a century ago in *The Varieties of Religious Experience*? He recorded various accounts of encounters with a Source of infinity and eternity, with a light that is brighter than the sun, with a pure love whose presence is so powerful that those who experienced it were certain that their very being would be dissolved. This is the power of purpose, from which all meaning is derived.

Finding the Meaning of Meaning

Meaning always points to something outside of itself. Meaning is not self-referential. As mentioned, even the definition of a chair points to something other than the word. Using the *Complete Oxford Dictionary*, one of the words of "mean" is a bridge between two sides. One of the different origins of the word (moan) means "sex between a man and a woman," a definition from centuries ago. The word "mean" is used to indicate the average between two or more numbers. The most recent definition of "mean" derives from a root word which means "mind." It is only in the last century, according to Oxford, that the word *meaning* has come to be associated with *purpose*. The evolution of the word has a parallel in the development of humanity.

More importantly, meaning always has a basis in something greater than itself. The meaning of meaning is that it is always a bridge, a connector; it always points to or connects with something else.

Finally, Frankl stated that meaning is available in every situation. How could meaning be available in every situation? How could Frankl say that? If our universe is created with purpose, (the teleological side of the scales of existence) then meaning is available in every situation. As we align with purpose, with the dimension of transcendence, meaning is no longer needed… because it is *everywhere*.

The Heart of Logotherapy

This brings us back to the compass as a metaphor for the conscience. As mentioned, the first use of the compass was for Feng Shui—the correct placement of objects in the physical dimension. The compass worked without understanding its mechanism. And its second usage was for navigation and shipping, as a tool in the psyche.

The compass is imperfect, error-prone: If we look at the compass from the side, we cannot see the direction correctly; this is called parallax error. You have to look at it head on. If there's metal nearby, it throws it off. And the compass requires a source, a field in which it works. The earth's magnetic field is the arena in which it works.

The future compass of conscience has many of those things in common. Our reading of conscience is imperfect; it is inconstant. It's affected by objects nearby such as the other influences in our lives, or by a kind of parallax error: We can look at it and see something different than the conscience is telling us. At first, the compass of conscience works without us knowing how.

And conscience requires a source, a field in which it operates. Without that source, it would not show us a direction. At first, we seek to read the compass, to know our conscience. With practice over time, we become the compass itself, the conscience; like iron filings near a magnet, we align with the source of meaning. This is what is meant by living logotherapy—we are magnetized by meaning.

In living in the heart of logotherapy there is a core of Being, a pure Spirit that we are called to and somehow have a relationship with. It is that part of ourselves—Spirit—that cannot get sick. Our choices and decisions and actions develop the noëtic; they strengthen it—or corrupt it. They make Spirit more apparent to us, so that we can move into the source of it. Our perception of conscience may be imperfect, but we are working toward perfection, the Source of conscience. Frankl's Ultimate Meaning points us to meaning, to responsibility, to our greatest gift: free will. Frankl emphasized that it is in our choices and decisions—and in activating them—that we grow noëtically. We create the bridge to Ultimate Meaning, our potential perfection.

When we can stand in the tension between an overwhelming perfection that we sense, and the awful imperfection of who we are—knowing that we are not only spirit *and* matter, we are also the *bridge between* the highest and the lowest that we can know—then we can discover the heart of logotherapy. We can know the meaning of meaning. We can increasingly live in the power of purpose.

Here we depart from the metaphor of the compass. When we become the compass, we are not content to simply give direction to others as much as we help others to discover—and to become—the compass themselves. In the old way of doing it, we became gurus that gave others direction but, in so doing, created dependency; in the new way, we can help each person become his and her own guru, to discover meaning and align with its source. This is what Frankl (2014) wanted. We become the compass itself, and help others to do the same.

And that, in my opinion, is the heart of logotherapy. This is the true compass to which Viktor Frankl pointed the future of humanity.

References

Assagioli, R. (1965). *Psychosynthesis*. Penguin Books.

Batthyány, A. (2010). Viktor E. Frankl and the development of logotherapy & existential analysis [Introduction]. In *The feeling of meaninglessness* (pp. 7–39). Marquette University Press.

Blavatsky, H. P. (1888). *The secret doctrine, Volume I: Cosmogenesis* (Vol. 1, 3rd ed.). Theosophical Publishing Society.

de Mello, A. (1982/1984). *The song of the bird*. Image Books.

DuBois, J. M. (2004). Understanding Viktor Frankl's *Theory and Therapy of Mental Disorders* [Editor's Introduction] (J. DuBois, Trans.). In *On the theory and therapy of mental disorders: An introduction to logotherapy and existential analysis* (pp. ix–xliii). Brunner-Routledge.

Fabry, J. B. (2013). *The pursuit of meaning: Viktor Frankl, logotherapy, and life*. Purpose Research. (Original work published 1968)

Frankl, V. E. (2014). *The will to meaning: Foundations and applications of logotherapy* (Expanded ed.). Plume. (Original work published 1969)

Frankl, V. E. (1978). *The unheard cry for meaning: Psychotherapy and humanism*. Simon and Schuster.

Frankl, V. E. (1985). *Psychotherapy and existentialism*. Washington Square Press. (Original work published 1967)
Frankl, V. E. (1986). *The doctor and the soul (Original work published 1946 as Ärztliche Seelsorge;* Vienna: Franz Deuticke.) (R. Winston & C. Winston, Trans.). Alfred A. Knopf.
Frankl, V. E. (2000). *Man's search for ultimate meaning*. Perseus. (Original work published *Der Unbewusste Gott*, 1948 and English translation, *The unconscious God*, 1975)
Frankl, V. E. (2010). In A. Batthyany & A. Tallon (Eds.), *The feeling of meaninglessness: A challenge to psychotherapy and philosophy*. Marquette University Press.
Graber, A. V. (2009). *The journey home: Preparing for life's ultimate adventure*. Purpose Research.
James, W. (1985). *The varieties of religious experience*. Penguin. (Original work published 1902)
Jung, C. G. (1989). *Memories, dreams, reflections* (R. Winston & C. Winston, Trans., Rev. ed.). Vintage.
Klingberg, H. (2001). *When life calls out to us: The love and lifework of Viktor and Elly Frankl*. Doubleday Books.
Lincoln, Y. S., & Guba, E. G. (1985). *Naturalistic inquiry*. Sage.
Lukas, E. (2015). *The therapist and the soul: From fate to freedom*. Purpose Research.
Lukas, E. (2020). *Understanding* Man's Search for Meaning*: Reflections on Viktor Frankl's logotherapy* (J. B. Fabry, H. T. Smith, B. Z. Hirsch, & J. O'Meara, Trans. C. L. McLafferty, Jr. Ed.). Purpose Research.
McLafferty, C. L., Jr. (1997). Spirituality in three theories of psychology: A qualitative study. *Dissertation Abstracts International, 58*(03b), 1567.
McLafferty, C. L., Jr. (2006). Examining unproven assumptions of Galton's nature-nurture paradigm. *American Psychologist, 61*, 177–178. https://doi.org/10.1037/0003-066X.61.2.177
McLafferty, C. L., Jr. (2012). *Training lay counselors in logotherapy at the Birmingham Suicide Help Line/Crisis Center*. Paper presented at the First Future of Logotherapy Congress, Vienna, Austria.
McLafferty, C. L., Jr. (2014). *Stages of meaning development: Unconsciousness, consciousness, mastery*. Paper presented at the Future of Logotherapy II, Vienna, Austria.
McLafferty, C. L., Jr. (2016a). Meaning "until the last breath": Practical applications of logotherapy in the ethical consideration of coma, brain death, and persistent vegetative states. In A. Batthyány (Ed.), *Logotherapy and existential analysis: Proceedings of the Viktor Frankl Institute Vienna* (Vol. 1, pp. 365–376). Springer. https://doi.org/10.1007/978-3-319-29424-7_31
McLafferty, C. L., Jr. (2016b). Meaning as the bridge from crumbling traditions of the past to a future of freedom: Frankl's contribution to peace and purpose. *The International Forum for Logotherapy, 39*, 15–21.
McLafferty, C. L., Jr., Slate, J. R., & Onwuegbuzie, A. J. (2010). Transcending the quantitative-qualitative divide with mixed methods research: A multidimensional framework for understanding congruence and completeness in the study of values. *Counseling and Values, 55*(1), 46–62.
Patton, M. Q. (2002). *Qualitative research and evaluation methods* (3rd ed.). Sage.
Sprunger, M. (2009). *Spiritual psychology: A primer*. Purpose Research. (Original work published 1988)
Sprunger, M. (2012). *The abridged Urantia papers*. Square Circles Publishing.
The Urantia book. (1955). The Urantia Foundation.

Charles L. McLafferty, Jr., PhD, has served on the faculties of the University of Virginia and the University of Alabama at Birmingham. He is the founder and president of Purpose Research, which seeks to incorporate meaning and purpose into the research, theory, and practice of the helping professions. McLafferty has edited and/or published more than a dozen books on logotherapy by authors such as Joseph Fabry, Elisabeth Lukas, Paul Wong, and Ann Graber. He has earned an educational diplomate from the Viktor Frankl Institute of Logotherapy (US). As a National Certified Counselor (US), he volunteered for five years at a regional crisis center as part of the National Suicide Prevention Lifeline network and for which he developed a logotherapeutic in-service training module.

How Values Motivate Actions

Daniel von Wachter

The Belief-Desire Theory of Action

What motivates human actions? According to a widespread view, all actions are motivated by *desires*. And "desires" here means drives, or impulses, or urges. So all human actions are motivated by impulses. The person uses his beliefs in order to decide what he should do in order to satisfy his desires. If you are hungry, you satisfy that desire by consulting your belief that there are apples in the cellar and then going to the cellar in order to eat an apple. This is the "belief-desire theory" of human action, propagated by David Hume (McNaughton, 1988). In the Old Testament (2 Sam 11, King James Version), King David desired his neighbor's wife Bathsheba. He satisfied that desire by sending her husband Uriah to the front lines of battle so that he was killed. In this, David used his beliefs cleverly in order to have his desire satisfied.

The belief-desire theory presents a mechanistic view of action. Desires are seen to be similar to physical forces, such as the force that a stone exercises on the table on which it is lying. This may have some plausibility for actions that are motivated by drives. But in ordinary discourse it seems that some of our actions are against our desires, motivated by a conviction. So some of our actions seem to be motivated by beliefs. Sometimes we resist our desires or drives. In such cases, we call the desires "temptations." In ordinary discourse, we would say, for example, that I stayed at home in order to care for my old father instead of going skiing with my friends because I believed that I had a duty to do so. I acted on that conviction, although I had a strong desire to go skiing. According to the common-sense view, sometimes we do something out of a conviction against our desires and drives.

D. von Wachter (✉)
Ludwig-Maximilians-Universität München, Munich, Germany
e-mail: epost@von-wachter.de

C. L. McLafferty, Jr., J. I. Levinson (eds.), *Logotherapy and Existential Analysis*,
Logotherapy and Existential Analysis: Proceedings of the Viktor Frankl Institute
Vienna 2, https://doi.org/10.1007/978-3-031-48922-8_29

Humeans reject this view because, they say, beliefs are something passive. Beliefs present something as it is. About people who are self-sacrificing in their help to others, Humeans say that they have a desire to help other people. The impression that they are motivated by beliefs is a deception.

On the Humean view, there are no beliefs about what is good or bad or about somebody having a certain duty. What we ordinarily consider to be moral convictions and value beliefs are, according to the Humean, in fact *desires*. They say we need to distinguish been facts and values. There are no facts about values and duties. There are no true beliefs about values. There is no realm of values. Statements about values and duties are just expressions of desires or preferences. This is commonly known as the *fact-value distinction.*

This is of great importance to human beings and to logotherapists as well as their clients. If there are no truths about values and duties, then if I find in myself a certain desire, then there is no truth about whether that is a good desire, or whether that is a desire for something good. There is then no point in inquiring whether it is good to satisfy that desire. Except in the sense that I can inquire whether that desire is in conflict with another desire. For example, if I find in myself a desire for my neighbor's wife, then on the Humean view it is not *true* that it would be *wrong* to fulfill that desire. If I believe in the Humean view, I can only examine this desire by inquiring whether it conflicts with my other desires. In practice, in psychotherapy this view leads to the therapist asking the adulterous client just: "How do you feel about it?" This is a very different question from the question "Do you believe that your course of action is good?"

Some Actions Are Motivated by Beliefs

I want to dispute this Humean view by asserting that, while some actions are motivated by drives, others are motivated by *beliefs*. Sometimes I act against my desires because I believe that it is good to do so or that I have a duty to do so. This is the view that corresponds to the ordinary understanding. Before they are told otherwise at school, people believe that some actions are good and others are bad and that (of course) it is true that it is wrong to steal.

Let us examine moral beliefs and value beliefs. The moral beliefs that we need to consider first are not generalizations, such as "killing is wrong." The trouble with them is that that one can always construe unusual cases that are exceptions. Let us focus on *particular* moral beliefs, for example "King David's sending Uriah into war was reprehensible [that is, morally wrong]" or "It was very good of Miller to help Smith in that situation." These are beliefs about particular actions, actions at a certain time and place.

We can have beliefs about other people's duties. Of course, these beliefs cannot motivate actions. But beliefs about my duties can motivate my actions. Miller can be motivated to help Smith by the belief "I have a duty to help Smith." First person value beliefs can motivate actions. How can such a belief motivate? The Humean would say: A belief cannot motivate because it just presents things as being in a certain way.

My reply to this is that a belief can motivate if it presents a situation as requiring or requesting a certain action from the person. If I believe that I have a duty to pay back the money to Smith then, while I might have no desire to pay back the money, I believe that reality is calling me to act in a certain way. The situation and the things with their relationships toward each other are constituting a call to action. That is how things present themselves to the person. Later I shall discuss why we should accept that and why the Humean has no good reason for rejecting that. But first, in order to see the phenomenon more clearly, let us distinguish various kinds of such motivating beliefs.

1. Beliefs in duties: "I have a duty to do *x*." "I have a duty not to do *y*," that is, "It would be wrong to do *y*."
2. Beliefs about supererogatory actions: good actions that are beyond duty. "(It is beyond my duty but) it would be very good to do that." Analogously: actions that are bad but not wrong. We can call them "ugly actions."
3. "Value" in philosophy usually is not restricted to actions. Any state of affairs, any thing or situation, can be believed to be good or bad. The existence of a flower can be believed to be good. In Genesis it says that after each day of creation, God looked at what he had created, "and God saw that it was good" (Genesis 1; King James Version). Let us use the expression "value belief" in order to capture both, beliefs in duties as well as beliefs that something is good or bad.

Let me explain. Beliefs in duties say that a person has an obligation to do a certain action. More precisely, it entails that there is a certain range of possible actions within which the person has an obligation to action. If, for example, you have a duty to pay back the money before Friday, then you are free to do so today or tomorrow, but it must be before Friday. So duties leave open some range of allowed courses of action.

Duty is connected to guilt: If you do not fulfill a duty, you acquire guilt through this.

A correlate of duty beliefs are beliefs that say that a certain action is *forbidden*. In that case, reality is telling you that actions within a certain range are bad, so that if you do them, you acquire guilt.

Some good actions are beyond what one is obliged to do. They are *supererogatory* actions. Most people do not have a duty to go into the slums, build a relationship with people, and help them to get their lives in order. Which is what some Christians did in Britain in the nineteenth century. But it is very good to do so. It is supererogatory.

To a person who does a supererogatory action the situation presents itself as calling him to action. The person sees a need for action. The need or the calling comes from the situation, it "supervenes" on the situation, as we say today in philosophy. The person might in addition believe that God is asking or commanding them to act. But also then, the person has the belief that the situation is calling them.

Often there are people involved in the situations which call somebody to action. Then we say "My daughter needs me!" In my view, it is natural to limit the concept of "duty" to cases in which somebody has a duty towards somebody. But also situations in which there are no people suffering or lacking something can call us to action. They can give a purpose and meaning to life.

A person can believe that a certain thing would be good, and that can motivate him to create that thing. An artist can create a work of art with that motive. Belief in the value of research and knowledge can motivate scientists and philosophers. And God is motivated to create a universe, plants, animals, and many more things.

I conclude that some actions are motivated by beliefs. Sometimes we see that sometimes reality calls us to act.

Differences Between Value Beliefs and Desires

Often people say that "values are feelings." The meaning of this statement is a bit unclear. One might want to say that we "feel" values. When we think about the horrors of war, we feel the evil. This refers to the way we encounter values. But more often by the statement "values are feelings" people mean that there are no value beliefs and that evaluations are really are just expressions of desires or drives. Let us try to clarify the issue by listing differences between value beliefs and desires.

1. We can recognize whether something is a value belief or a desire. I can ask myself "Do I believe that this action is good?" And I can believe that the action is not good while I have a strong desire for it. Or I can believe that the action is good while that action for me is difficult and hard. I have an inclination against it. An inclination pushes me to act (or not to act) in a certain way. By contrast, a value belief is normative; it is like a compass, it gives me orientation. It judges the desires and tells me how I should deal with them and control them. In therapy I assume that you want to uncover both desires and value beliefs, but encourage the person to try to form true value beliefs and act on them rather than on the desires. The value beliefs lead to meaning.
2. Both, desires and value beliefs, reside in the subject, they are a property of the subject. But value beliefs present an object as being good (or bad) so that this does not depend on me. If the object is presented as calling me to action, then the object is calling even if I don't respond. A desire, by contrast, is a desire for some object, but it depends on me. The object is attractive to me because I have an appetite for that kind of thing.
3. A value response is not directed toward the satisfaction of my desires. It is not optimized for self-satisfaction, it is optimized for the object. Consider an act of helping: In an act of helping, you are concerned with what the other person needs and with his well-being. You might have a pleasant feeling after you have helped, but you cannot produce this feeling without being concerned for the other person's well-being. It is an important piece of advice to be really con-

cerned about the other person's well-being. By contrast, if you are motivated by a desire and thus act in order to satisfy the desire, you are guided by the desire; you ask: What do I need? How do I produce most pleasure for me?

Today in the West, certain currents encourage people to focus on their well-being. Feminism encourages women to "actualize themselves" and not stay at home in order to educate the children. In a slightly different way, men are being discouraged to take on the responsibility of a husband, father, and provider. But I suggest that the way to happiness is to focus not primarily on one's desires but to focus on how one can be of use to others. Paradoxically, the attempt to actualize oneself leads to dissatisfaction, while self-sacrificial attitudes lead to satisfaction and happiness. Christianity is teaching this. Thus, Jesus said: "For whosoever will save his life shall lose it: and whosoever will lose his life for my sake shall find it" (Matt 16:25, King James Version). Many other aspects of Christianity reflect this pattern as well.

Having spelled out these three differences between value beliefs and desires, let me turn to the question how value beliefs are justified and how we can know values and duties.

Value and Duties Are Visible

How do we acquire beliefs about values and duties? Subjectivists present the matter as if the more plausible view is that there are no truths about values and duties. They suggest that those who believe in such truths are positing something mysterious, something that boggles the mind, something that is against reason. But consider how obvious the existence of duties and values is.

Let's begin with ourselves. If I think about me, my character and my life, I easily think of ways how I could be better. If we think about what we could or should do, we are very quickly aware of what is good and what is bad. For practitioners of logotherapy this means that despite lethargy, if people ask themselves which actions would be good and worth doing, they can see something. The only way humans do not see that something is good or bad, is that they do not ask the question. Human beings are confronted with goodness and badness as a swimmer in the water is confronted with water. Or perhaps it is more like how humans are in contact with the air which they are breathing.

Evil imposes itself more aggressively than the good. We easily forget all the good things in our life and in the world, but the bad things we can hardly get out of our mind. If we have a good conversation or were helped, we can value that and have it enlighten our heart, but we can also easily forget it. By contrast, even if we just lose our wallet or have a car accident, it occupies our mind. If more catastrophic things happen, they press themselves upon our mind with irresistible force. If people have a hard life, they can learn to bear this with patience and avoid lamenting or bitterness. But they will hardly forget the evil. Evil is imposing itself upon our mind most impertinently. We can call this the obtrusiveness of evil and the discreetness of goodness.

(If intellectuals say that there are no truths about duties and values and that moral convictions are really only preferences or desire, what is the argument for that? Duties present themselves to us very much as facts; as something we discover. We have feelings—and they feel very different from an encounter with values or duties. We can be deceived about what is good or bad, and we can deceive ourselves about it. We can manipulate our moral beliefs to fit better with our desires. But we cannot avoid having beliefs about duties and values. And if we try to find true beliefs about duties and values, we see some moral facts very clearly. The sacrifices a mother makes in order to care for her children are very valuable. She gets up every three hours during the night in order to feed her child and in order to comfort the other child. That sacrifice is a good thing. Of course, she also has an instinct to care for her children. But when a human cares for his parents or for someone else, there is not this instinct. Therefore, it is clearer that the person is motivated by value beliefs. As I have explained, we see most clearly that beliefs can motivate actions if we consider cases in which somebody does something out of a moral conviction against his desires. But that does not mean that actions are only motivated by moral beliefs if they are done against the desires.)

The Principle of Phenomenal Conservatism

I have dwelled a little on how unavoidable beliefs about duties and values are because that is relevant to the justification of value beliefs. Why do the subjectivists say that there are no truths about values and duties? Why do they declare value beliefs to be feelings?

One argument is, as I have explained, that beliefs cannot motivate because they are passive. They present something as it is, therefore they cannot motivate an agent to act. For that they would need to point to some change or to some action. My response was that moral beliefs present things as calling the person to act in a certain way.

Another argument of those who deny that there are moral truths is that such facts would be "queer," as J. L. Mackie (1977) called them. If somebody tells you that he saw an animal with five legs and an iron tale, you might respond that this is unlikely because it is different from everything we know. But such an argument cannot be successful against truths about duties or values, because we are aware of values and duties all the time.

Until some time ago, in philosophy moral truths were usually defended just by refuting the various objections. More recently, a defense of moral truths was developed which is in my view more complete.

Consider sense perception. When you have a visual impression that there is a tree over there, then that perceptual experience justifies your belief that there is a tree. To this possibility means that it is rational to hold that belief; it is in accordance with all your other beliefs and with all our experiences.

But why does that perceptual experience justify the belief? Because in the perceptual experience the object presents itself as being there and being in a certain way. It seems to the person that the object presses itself on him. The object pushes the person to believe that it is there; it induces the belief. This quality of the experience is that in virtue of which the experience justifies the belief.

Some empiricists used to say that in perception we are actually only justified in believing that we are having the experience. You are justified not in believing that there is a tree, but only that there are certain phenomena in your visual field. This epistemology, fortunately, does not have many adherents any more. That is because in epistemology we are nowadays not requiring infallibility anymore, but we ask which beliefs are *justified* under which conditions, and we take justification to be a matter of degree. Thus, sense impressions justify the beliefs which they induce.

But if sense impressions justify beliefs because in them something presents itself to the subject, then there could be also other kinds of impressions which justify beliefs. And that takes us to beliefs about duties and values.

The principle of phenomenal conservatism was put forward which says: If it seems to S that P, then, in the absence of defeaters, S thereby has at least some justification for believing that P (Huemer, 2007, p. 30).

I prefer this formulation: If a person has a conscious impression of something, then, in the absence of reasons to believe that the impression is unreliable, he is justified in believing that the impression is true.

The implication for value beliefs is that they can be justified through value impression, or, as they are sometimes called, intuitions. There is no good reason for dismissing the fact that we are aware of duties and values most intensely. All our knowledge comes through impressions. All our knowledge is based on things appearing to us. This is how we obtain knowledge through sense perception, and our awareness of duties and of values is also an impression that justifies the beliefs induced. As it is irrational to dismiss perceptual experiences, it is irrational to dismiss our experience of values which we have when we ask ourselves what is good, and which we often have involuntarily, for example when our conscience is telling us that we have acted badly, or when evil hits us. It is highly irrational to say that there are no truths about values and duties, because someone who says this is clinging to some assumption and derives from it that there are no such truths and ignores the impressions, while a rational person is one who is receptive to the impressions.

This is an important new development in epistemology, and I believe that it is correct. A rational person is one who tries to see and who trusts the impressions thereby received. (To a degree that depends on the clarity of the impression and on the presence of reasons to believe that the impression is unreliable.) This applies to values as much as it applies to sense perception.

I conclude that we have value beliefs, that they can be justified, and that they are our guide to happiness.

References

Huemer, M. (2007). Compassionate phenomenal conservatism. *Philosophy and Phenomenological Research, 74*(1), 30–55.
Mackie, J. L. (1977). *Ethics: Inventing right and wrong*. Penguin.
McNaughton, D. A. (1988). *Moral vision: An introduction to ethics*. Blackwell.

Daniel von Wachter, a native German now living in the Principality of Liechtenstein, has a doctorate in philosophy from the University of Hamburg and a doctorate in theology from the University of Oxford. His area of specialization is free will, causation, ontology, and philosophy of religion. He is also interested in the Austrian School of economics, the Enlightenment, and Christian August Crusius. Most of his writings are available at www.von-wachter.de.

Part VII
Book Reviews

Book Review: *Viktor Frankl and the Book of Job: A Search for Meaning* by Marshall Lewis

Pninit Russo-Netzer

The fundamental question, "Why do righteous people suffer undeservedly?" reflects a challenge that has perplexed scholars and laypersons alike throughout the human history, in various forms and expressions. Frankl (1946/1986) wrote:

> We must perform a kind of Copernican Revolution, and give the question of the meaning of life an entirely new twist. To wit: It is life itself that asks questions of man… it is not up to man to question; rather, he should recognize that he is questioned, questioned by life; he has to respond by being responsible; and he can answer to life only by answering for his life. (p.62)

The potential metamorphosis implied in this attitudinal shift, suggested by Frankl, holds the precious gift this book offers to its readers.

Viktor Frankl and the Book of Job presents a rich and comprehensive exploration of Viktor Frankl's logotherapy as a foundation to a deep, experiential, and fascinating journey of meaning discovery in face of challenging suffering, doubt, and despair that are inevitably involved with human condition. Texts can touch us, they can open new horizons and call us to action, but most of all, as this book shows, they can also transform us and move us toward an attitudinal shift. Alongside the many existing theological readings and interpretations of the Book of Job, the personal, psychological, and existential reading offered here provides a refreshing and unique view of Job as one who personifies human confrontation with absurdity, turmoil, and the existential vacuum. As the journey unfolds, the reader is provided with keys to unlock the wisdom concealed in complex existential truths and delve into our own unique life story and meaning.

Suffering is an ever-present reality in our lives as humans. But it is not the existence of suffering that makes us miserable; rather, it is the lack of its meaning and purpose. We are capable, and willing, to bear suffering but not when it feels futile,

P. Russo-Netzer (✉)
Achva Academic college, Arugot, Israel

C. L. McLafferty, Jr., J. I. Levinson (eds.), *Logotherapy and Existential Analysis*, Logotherapy and Existential Analysis: Proceedings of the Viktor Frankl Institute Vienna 2, https://doi.org/10.1007/978-3-031-48922-8_30

incomprehensible, and senseless. Suffering shakes us and questions us. Unlike the more self-absorbed hedonism or prosperity, suffering always transcends itself. When we are enjoying ourselves, the question of "why" does not emerge or call for our attention and action. In this sense, the Book of Job, as presented by Marshall Lewis, can be seen as a call, a personal invitation to engage with life in a more profound way and to embark on a journey of uncertainty and discovery even when suffering is left unexplained.

As Frankl's (1946/1985) own experiences in the darkness of oppression and deprivation during the Holocaust and Job's experiences of unjust suffering teach us, even in unbearable conditions, one can still take a stand and choose their way to respond to life's questions and discern the meaning embedded in dire events. Even in the face of tragic life circumstances, we can still self-transcend and courageously rise above suffering and despair to take responsibility over our experience and eventually reconstitute life on renewed and more profound roots. In this sense, we are shaped by the choices we make. These fundamental choices imbue life with meaning as they are not externally given but gradually grow from one's direct confrontation with life's limitations and through existential self-analysis. As the idea of kintsugi ("golden rejoining" in Japanese) exquisitely suggests, if we have never been broken, fully involved, or touched by life, we can never be truly whole. The broken beauty not only survives but thrives. Rather than hiding the flaws, the cracks are highlighted in gold.

Taken together, this book's strength lies not only in its conceptual clarity and organization of core principles of logotherapy, but also in its capability to apply these ideas and demonstrate their tangible wisdom to unsettling human challenges, relevant to any individual from all walks of life. The delicate and careful attention given to sensitive issues that lie at the heart of the Book of Job from the viewpoint of logotherapy illustrates the beauty and gravity of human experience. The triumph of the human spirit emerges not from discarding our wounded parts but from embracing our imperfections and rejoining them as pieces of a unique masterpiece and a more complete whole.

References

Frankl, V. E. (1985). *Man's search for meaning* (3rd ed.). Washington Square Press/Pocket Books. (Original work published 1946)

Frankl, V. E. (1986). *The doctor and the soul* (R. Winston & C. Winston, Trans.). Alfred A. Knopf. (Original work published in 1946 as *Ärztliche Seelsorge*)

Pninit Russo-Netzer, PhD, is a senior lecturer and researcher and the head of both the Education Department and the Resilience and Optimal Development Lab at Achva Academic College. She is also the head of the Compass Institute for the Study and Application of Meaning and the founder and head of the Academic Training Program for Logotherapy at Tel-Aviv University. She has published numerous academic articles and chapters and is the coauthor of five books and coeditor of four books on the topics of meaning in life, positive psychology, existential psychology, as well as positive change and growth. Russo-Netzer serves as academic advisor and consultant to both academic and nonacademic institutions worldwide, including the World Trade Center (WTCHR). She is the recipient of the International Positive Psychology Association (IPPA) Spirituality and Meaning Researcher Award, recognizing exemplary professionals who have had—and continue to have—a substantially positive impact on research in spirituality/meaning.

Book Review: *Viktor E. Frankl's Logotherapy and Existential Analysis: Theory and Practice* by Maria Marshall and Edward Marshall

Andreas Schreiber

As I began this review, I wondered how a new logotherapy textbook could surpass the existing literature for trained and experienced logotherapists. The authors, Maria and Edward Marshall, had already published a comprehensive book on logotherapy 10 years ago. My questions were quickly put to rest: This book provides new and interesting perspectives on logotherapy, with structured and concise explanations of the theory. It includes some thoughts on the Covid pandemic from a logotherapeutic perspective, and connects logotherapy with a number of other psychotherapeutic theories.

In this book, the authors present a structured foundation of meaning-centered psychotherapy in order to give credit to Viktor Frankl, the founder of this existential and meaning-oriented psychology. The Marshalls wanted to foster understanding of the original principles, fundamentals, and clinical applications of logotherapy as a basis to anchor it with other psychotherapeutic schools that address meaning with much less rigor, often without reference to the ideas of Frankl. The authors succeeded in this task!

The first two chapters, "The Origins," and "Uniqueness," are introductory in nature, but the third chapter, "The Roots," gives a well-structured and thorough coverage of the biography of Viktor Frankl, including less-known events and background. Even the story of the incarceration in the Nazi concentration camps is not merely recounted, but structured in certain episodes and with regard to the application of logotherapy. The authors give a lively explanation as to how such basic concepts of logotherapy as attitudes, self-transcendence, self-distancing, gratitude, value orientation, choices—as well as art, prayers and contemplation—were applied by Frankl and others as survival strategies in the camps.

A. Schreiber (✉)
Private Practice, Freiburg, Germany
e-mail: schreiber@curavitae.eu

C. L. McLafferty, Jr., J. I. Levinson (eds.), *Logotherapy and Existential Analysis*, Logotherapy and Existential Analysis: Proceedings of the Viktor Frankl Institute Vienna 2, https://doi.org/10.1007/978-3-031-48922-8_31

The first three chapters convey quite a bit of background on logotheory and Frankl, particularly for those who are new to the concepts. The subsequent chapters dig deeper into the assumptions and practical applications of logotherapy. In the fourth chapter, "The Three Pillars," the three core tenets of logotherapy are presented: (1) the freedom of will, (2) the will to meaning, and (3) the meaning in life. Though the explanation of the third pillar is not expanded in this chapter, that topic reveals itself throughout this book.

Having set the basic foundations of logotherapy, the authors proceed in a concise and structured manner into the philosophical and anthropological depths of the background theory and assumptions. They explain the anthropological assumptions in the fifth chapter "Dimensional Ontology," which include the necessity of a noëtic tension (noö-dynamics) in the human being, which supersedes the homoeostasis principle that is predominant in the physical and mental/emotional dimensions as well as the importance of finding, having, and actualizing values in order to fulfill meaning. The Marshalls are careful to fill out the abstract philosophy and theory with explanatory quotes of other authors, mostly from Elisabeth Lukas or Joseph Fabry, but also many others, often with a broader perspective and relation to other common psychotherapeutic or psychological theories such as cognitive behavior therapy and positive psychology. Examples are used to illustrate the concepts, applications, and clinical implications of each topic.

The chapters "Suffering and Meaning" and "Existential Analysis" use the same approach to present psychological and therapeutic topics of finding meaning in spite of the presence of suffering, guilt, or death (the *tragic triad*), and where and how to find meaning once it seems to be lost. They detail the "three highways to meaning"—creativity, experience, and attitude—as well as six methods by which we can find meaning: self-discovery, uniqueness, choices, responsibility, self-transcendence, and self-distancing; each are illustrated with a thorough set of questions.

The next three chapters delineate the process and methods of logotherapy, illustrated with several lively examples including therapeutic work during the Covid pandemic. The explanation of logotherapeutic methods is thorough and illustrative and gives helpful insights in their usage and effectiveness.

What got me excited was the chapter "Other Methods," in which the authors give a comprehensive though concise summary of additional techniques and methods combined with new approaches to enhance the client's search for meaning. Their way of explanation and use of examples was enlightening; many of these approaches have remained obscure in other texts.

Having mentioned the effectiveness of logotherapy in the therapeutic process, the chapter "Evidence-Based Logotherapy" gives a broad insight into many of the assessment methods that help to assess the level of meaning at which an individual functions or—in the process of therapy—develops and increases. This gives a fairly good orientation of the current measures and their applications for the practitioner.

In "Logotherapy and Well-Being," interpretations and approaches to foster resilience are presented, followed by an emphasis on the role of finding meaning and having purpose, which may help to strengthen resilience.

The book closes with chapters that summarize and comment on two interviews given to the Austrian Radio (ORF): The first is of Alexander Batthyány and Elisabeth Lukas about the current status of logotherapy, with a compressed summary of the basic assumptions; the second is of Elisabeth Gruber, Director of the Viktor Frankl Museum, Vienna, about the lively exhibition of Frankl's work and life. The final chapter reminds us that "the work remains"; it is a call to live the message of logotherapy and to convey and spread its concepts into the world.

In summary, this new textbook provides some new insights into the wide realm of logotherapy and gives an organized presentation of the theory with illustrative examples. Further, it connects logotherapy to other theories of psychotherapy and psychology and thus helps to combine different approaches in the light of meaning-centered therapy. A big plus of this book are the extensive, detailed, and actual reference lists given at the end of each chapter.

Andreas Schreiber, PhD, is a philosophical counselor and psychotherapist according to the naturopathic law in Freiburg, Germany. He earned his PhD in philosophy from Albert-Ludwigs University in Freiburg, Germany. He is certified as a diplomate educator by the Viktor Frankl Institute of Logotherapy (US) and has been actively involved as a member of the Institute since 2007. He is author of several publications related to the theory and practice of logotherapy. He has been an instructor of logotherapy since 2007, and a faculty member of the Institute since 2012. His areas of interest are the theory of logotherapy (logophilosophy), finding meaning in periods of transition, personal development, burnout, adaptation, and anxiety disorder. He teaches for the associate credential and supervises diplomate students.

Index

C. L. McLafferty, Jr., J. Levinson (eds.), *Logotherapy and Existential Analysis*, Logotherapy and Existential Analysis: Proceedings of the Viktor Frankl Institute Vienna 2, https://doi.org/10.1007/978-3-031-48922-8